Stabilizing Empire

Stabilizing Empire

PSYCHOPHARMACY IN
THE US WAR ON TERROR

Jocelyn Lim Chua

UNIVERSITY OF CALIFORNIA PRESS

University of California Press
Oakland, California

Library of Congress Cataloging-in-Publication Data

Names: Chua, Jocelyn Lim author
Title: Stabilizing empire : psychopharmacy in the US war on terror / Jocelyn Lim Chua.
Description: Oakland, California : University of California Press, [2026] | Includes bibliographical references and index.
Identifiers: LCCN 2026026753 (print) | LCCN 2026026754 (ebook) | ISBN 9780520428638 cloth | ISBN 9780520428645 paperback | ISBN 9780520428669 epub
Subjects: LCSH: Military psychiatry—United States—History—21st century | Psychopharmacology—United States—History—21st century | Soldiers—Drug use—United States | Soldiers—Mental health services—United States
Classification: LCC UH629.3 .C48 2026 (print) | LCC UH629.3 (ebook) | DDC 355.3/45—dc23/eng/20260610
LC record available at https://lccn.loc.gov/2026026753
LC ebook record available at https://lccn.loc.gov/2026026754

GPSR Authorized Representative: Easy Access System Europe, Mustamäe tee 50, 10621 Tallinn, Estonia, gpsr.requests@easproject.com

35 34 33 32 31 30 29 28 27 26
10 9 8 7 6 5 4 3 2 1

For Jonas

Contents

Acknowledgments

Like many books, this one was a collective undertaking, despite its single authorship. It would not exist but for the generosity of those who shared their stories and others who helped and encouraged me throughout the years that it took to research and write it. First and foremost, I thank my interlocutors for their willingness not only to narrate their experiences but also to help me think through and theorize the place of medicine in war. For privacy reasons, I cannot name them individually, but I hope what I've written does justice to their accounts.

At the University of North Carolina at Chapel Hill, I am lucky to be part of supportive communities, including the Department of Anthropology and the Moral Economies of Medicine working group. Thanks to Isabel Abarca, Ben Arbuckle, Felicia Bajomo, Lydia Boyd, Rachel Briggs, Mara Buchbinder, Courtney Canter, Rudi Colloredo-Mansfeld, Emily Curtin, Sue Estroff, Qiuzi Gao, Sugandh Gupta, Ampson Hagan, Bevin Hardy, Anusha Hariharan, Morgan Hoke, Chu-Wen Hsieh, Arvid Kachurin, Martha King, Camille Kroll, Jeannie Loeb, Julia Mackessy, Elizabeth Manekin, Towns Middleton, Raúl Nechochea López, Chris Nelson, Rachel Niehuus, Charles Price, Dafna Rachok, Michele Rivkin-Fish, Parag Saikia, Mel Salm, Preethi Saravanan, Barry Saunders, Kumi Silva, Diane

Slocum, Sara Smith, Angela Stuesse, Ann Suk, Jane Thrailkill, Amanda Thompson, Silvia Tomášková, Julio Villa-Palomino, Ana Vinea, Rebecca Walker, and Margaret Wiener, for all the ways, large and small, that they create community. The world is dimmer for the loss of the fiercely funny and brilliant Jenny Tone Pah-Hote. Hillary Lithgow and Ashlyn Clark indulged a half-formed idea, and their dedicated efforts made possible the two-day conference that we cohosted on the theme of research with military communities at the UNC Institute for Arts and Humanities in December 2022. Irina Olenicheva, Megan Mccall, Katie Poor, and Melanie Wisnant deserve the sun and moon for their constant support and for keeping everything afloat. Jacqueline Solis at UNC Libraries made Freedom of Information Act (FOIA) requests an unexpectedly breezy process.

I am grateful to the adept research assistants who contributed to this project, each in their own meaningful way: Courtney Canter, Charles Howe, Lacy Jo Keller, Rob Meeker, Lauren Nareau, Veronica O'Kelly-Nickerson, Amanda Tucker, and Sarah Rae Weinstein. Ashlyn Clark was a tireless reader of thousands of pages of FOIA documents and a genius at color-coding excel spreadsheets. Matthew Troyer had a clear vision for the cover just as I was truly understanding what this book was about. Learn more about Matthew's work here: https://www.troyermatthew.com.

This project and its many forms have been nurtured over the years by conversations with and feedback from colleagues and friends. My thanks to Fernando Armstrong-Fumero, Orkideh Behrouzan, Ana Bezić, Amy Borovoy, Jason Cons, Jean Dennison, William Downey, Elizabeth Durham, Sherine Hamdy, Courtney Handman, David Kieran, Junko Kitanaka, Rijul Kochhar, Ting Hui Lau, Zhiying Ma, Kenneth MacLeish, Amber Mathwig, Galia Plotkin, Eugene Raikhel, Peter Redfield, Allen Tran, Matthew Wolf-Meyer, and Zoë Wool. Aalyia Sadruddin reminds me what it means to think and write with care. In their various paths through the research triangle, my writing-group mates—Dörte Bemme, Mara Buchbinder, Nadia El-Shaarawi, Harris Solomon, and Saiba Varma—have collectively read every word of this book, many of them multiple times. They've walked along with me through much of this project. Rachel Factor, Christina Ford, Grayson Hampson, and Shreya Nayak have kept me grounded with friendship, food, walks, and music. Long live mommy band.

Chapter 6 is based on an article previously published in *Ethos*. I have shared parts of this research at presentations and seminars including at Bucknell University, Harvard University, the University of Florida, the University of Virginia, the Veteran Studies Association, and the University of North Carolina, and am grateful to the discussants and audience members for helping me to refine ideas presented here. The seeds of this project were first planted at a seminar at the School for Advanced Research in Santa Fe organized by Elizabeth Davis and Li Zhang and at the Global Psyche workshop at Vanderbilt University organized by Dominique Béhague, Kenneth MacLeish, and Jonathan Metzl, where my co-workshop participants helped me give contour to amorphous beginnings. Early during the Covid pandemic and shutdown, when our meetings were confined to Zoom, my faculty cofellows at the UNC Institute for Arts and Humanities helped me articulate what is at stake in this project. The participants who joined us around the table at the IAH for a workshop on collaborative engagement with military communities provided inspiration and provocations that continue to guide me.

Thank you to Kate Marshall and Natalie Gomez at UC Press for their editorial labor and encouragement. Susan Weiner stepped in with a discerning eye in the final stages. This project was made possible with support from the National Science Foundation and the Wenner Gren Foundation. My gratitude and appreciation also go to the three anonymous reviewers for their generative comments and astute suggestions. Photographs reproduced in this book are from the Defense Visual Information Distribution Service (DVIDS) and use of them requires the following statement: "The appearance of US Department of Defense (DoW) visual information does not imply or constitute DoW endorsement."

My family keeps my feet on the ground. Thank you, mom and dad, for your encouragement, despite the foreignness of academia and anthropology. Achi, Anya, Evan, and Laura are steadfast in their love, care, and presence. My large family of in-laws is wonderful, and I wish we saw them much more than we do. It's been a gift watching my seven nieces and nephews grow into thoughtful, kind, and silly human beings.

My son Jonas grew up with this project. When, during the pandemic shutdown, he discovered that I was waking up at 5 a.m. to get a few hours of undisturbed work done before virtual kindergarten, he offered to keep me company by waking up early, too. He navigates this world with a profound empathy, open curiosity, and easy joy that give me hope. Luther, you are everything.

Abbreviations

AAA	American Anthropological Association
ACU	Army combat uniform
ADHD	Attention deficit hyperactivity disorder
AHLTA	Armed Forces Health Longitudinal Technology Application
AMEDD	Army Medical Department
APO	Army Post Office
ASR	Acute stress reaction
ASVAB	Armed Services Vocational Aptitude Battery
AVF	All-volunteer force
BCT	Brigade combat team
BHO	Behavioral Health Officer
BHT	Behavioral Health Technician
BICEPS	Brevity, immediacy, centrality, expectancy, proximity, simplicity
CI	Counterintelligence

COB	Contingency operating base
COIN	Counterinsurgency
COP	Combat outpost
COSC	Combat and operational stress control
COSR	Combat and operational stress reaction
CPT	Captain
CSH	Combat support hospital
CSR	Combat stress reaction
CQ	Charge quarters
DFAC	Dining facility
DHB	Defense Health Board
DMH	Division Mental Health
DoD	Department of Defense
DoDSER	*Department of Defense Suicide Event Report*
DOT	Directly observed therapy
DoW	Department of War
DSM	Diagnostic and Statistical Manual
DVIDS	Defense Visual Information Distribution Service
EMDR	Eye movement desensitization reprocessing
FDA	Food and Drug Administration
1LT	First lieutenant
FM	Field Manual
FSD	Full-spectrum dominance
FOB	Forward operating base
GWOT	Global war on terror
HUMINT	Human intelligence
HUMINTer	Human intelligence collector or analyst
HTS	Human Terrain System
ICD	International Classification of Diseases
IRF	Immediate reaction force

JDAM	Joint direct attack munition
LSCO	Large-scale combat operation
MARP	Medical Access Records Pilot
MDO	Multi-domain operation
MHAT	Mental Health Advisory Team
MHP	Mental health professional
MOS	Military occupational specialty
MP	Military police
MRE	Meal, ready to eat
NCO	Noncommissioned officer
NDAA	National Defense Authorization Act
NSAID	Nonsteroidal anti-inflammatory drug
ODA	Operational Detachment Alpha
OPTEMPO	Operational tempo
PA	Physician assistant
PERSTEMPO	Personnel tempo
PET	Prolonged exposure therapy
PFC	Private first class
PFC	Prolonged forward care
PIES	Proximity, immediacy, expectancy, simplicity
PNN	Private news network
POG	People other than grunt
PTs	Physical training uniforms
PTSD	Post-traumatic stress disorder
PX	Post exchange
QRF	Quick reaction force
R&R	Rest and relaxation
REMF	Rear echelon motherfucker
RoE	Rules of engagement
RRF	Rapid reaction force

RTD	Return to duty
SCIF	Sensitive compartmented information facility
SF	Special forces
SGB	Stellate ganglion block
SGT	Sergeant
SPC	Specialist
SSG	Staff sergeant
SSRI	Selective serotonin reuptake inhibitor
SRP	Soldier readiness processing
US	United States
USCENTCOM	US Central Command
VA	US Department of Veterans Affairs
VoIP	Voice over internet protocol
WRAIR	Walter Reed Army Institute of Research

Introduction

Where there is no doctor, there was Nate.[1] On his third deployment in seven years, the 29-year-old served as the medic and sole health care provider within miles for his eight-man team. In 2011, the team was stationed in northern Afghanistan, at a small combat outpost in a river valley that the US Army would describe as "remote." Nate's supervising physician assistant, the next echelon care provider, was at a large FOB, or Forward Operating Base, 30 miles away—a solid seven-to-nine-hour drive in an up-armored Humvee, depending on how the day was.[2] In that setting, Nate's team turned to him for anything and everything. "Honestly, those guys?" Nate said when we spoke years later. "They thought that I was a friggin' physician, right? They all thought that I was the damned surgeon general of the Army or something."

Surgeon general of the Army, maybe, but friend, certainly. To do his work well, Nate quickly learned that he had to be trusted. "The number one thing was that I wanted to know that every one of my guys trusted me 100 percent. Implicitly, right?" he recalled. "Like, they could tell me anything. And they did." Having never received formal training to address mental health, Nate said he ran mostly on intuition.[3] At their small outpost, where there was little else besides weapons, time, and each other's company, monitoring mental health meant "just spending time with my guys, talking to them every day about, you know, just the dumbest stuff." It also meant attuning to small details. A buddy hasn't received mail from his wife in nearly four weeks. Was that why he's been looking off? On edge?

"Most of the troubles that came up," reflected Nate, "was stuff back home spilling over into what we were doing there." Whatever the spill-over, it became Nate's problem. "Most of my friends were over there to kill bad guys. That's what they wanted to do," he told me earnestly. "But when we go out tomorrow, I don't want this guy making a decision that he normally wouldn't because he's pissed off, you know? I saw it many times, guys doing shit that I thought was inappropriate."

Like much of battlefield medicine, Nate's work as a medic was a continuous exercise in risk management. When a teammate was having a rough time, usually Nate could talk things out and "calm him down for the day." But there were a number of times when the unfolding situation was above his pay grade. In those instances, Nate got the guys through the night with what he had on hand: valium. "I can do the acute stuff," he would tell these soldiers frankly, "but with something bigger like this I'm going to have to kick you to a higher power in the morning." With help from the noncommissioned officer, or NCO, on their team, Nate would have the soldier's weapon confiscated and arrange for a helicopter to transport the soldier to the nearest FOB the next day.[4]

Days, or perhaps a week or two later, the soldier would return on new medication. Nate remembers having to read up on whatever had been prescribed and being instructed to keep an eye on the soldier. Such returns required magical thinking. "When they came back I kind of assumed that they'd been cleared and things had been handled," Nate explained. "I remember thinking, 'Okay, I think you've talked it through, gotten it off your chest, and now they've decided that you're going to take an antidepressant from now on.'" Where risk and gain are in perpetual counterbalance, Nate had to trust the decision of the docs and military command to return their guys back to the line. "If I kicked a soldier up to a higher level of care for mental health, the assumption when they got back was that they were good to go." He pauses, then adds, "I mean, I kind of had to, right? I didn't really have an option."

For the most part, Nate remembers returned soldiers fitting right back in. "I didn't see any real difference in the way that they acted from day to day. They all reintegrated right back into the group." Then, half joking but also deadly serious, he adds with a smirk, "They came back and still told the same filthy, horrible, awful, evil jokes about death, rape, pillaging, and plundering and all that." The pills, he concluded, were a good thing. "They probably did help take the edge off at the end of the day. My guys weren't getting so wrapped up with whatever it was that they were dealing with."

But there was also work to be done once new medications were in the mix. As the "eyes and ears" to the enlisted, medics like Nate must monitor soldiers when they are prescribed new psychopharmaceuticals—a job even more critical when the medic is the only provider. So, when a soldier would return on an antidepressant or antianxiety medication that he wasn't familiar with, Nate would read up on it the best he could using their spotty internet. Having soldiers on new psychotropic medications required "a solid understanding of how to handle them [the drugs] and what to watch out for." Increased risk for suicide and impacts on performance and behavior were top on the list. Once he knew "what to watch out for, how to manage it, how to handle it," Nate felt more confident. But he kept a nervous watch.

This book examines chemical efforts to sustain and stabilize the US military empire, and what these efforts reveal about the vigorous interventionist and expeditionary posture of contemporary American militarism.[5] During the war on terror, psychopharmaceuticals were granted a radical role, enabling soldiers to stay deployed and to deploy repeatedly, across multiple warfronts. As a strained all-volunteer force experienced historically unprecedented patterns of prolonged and repeat deployments in the longest overseas war in US history, antidepressants, antianxiety medications, and mood stabilizers emerged as a practical and modest means of keeping the empire running. Across the time-space of the war on terror, psychopharmaceuticals were tasked with stretching human capacities for indefinite, "everywhere war" and stabilizing those tasked with stabilizing nations.[6] As such, their use in global counterinsurgency offers a revealing view onto the volatile expanse of contemporary US hegemony.

FULL SPECTRUM

In 2006, for the first time, the US Department of Defense (DoD) developed official criteria governing the use of FDA-approved psychiatric medications "in theater"—that is, within the physical and tactical settings of military operations, including active combat. During the wars in Iraq and Afghanistan, psychiatric medications entered theater in bottles and bloodstreams alike: drug formularies grew to treat symptoms newly diagnosed in deployment and to supply ongoing medication needs, while soldiers with previous diagnoses were authorized to take 180-day bulk supplies with them. Incorporated as retention strategy, tactical resource, and would-be panacea, psychopharmaceuticals were given an untested role in keeping soldiers in place on the battlefield and returning them to war, often with psychiatric diagnoses. *Stabilizing Empire* examines this quiet revolution: the pharmaceuticalization of battlefield mental health care in the war on terror.

While focused on the US-led wars in Afghanistan and Iraq, *Stabilizing Empire* situates these conflicts within the context of a larger campaign for US military dominance, one which, at its inception, was conceived as a global campaign of unknown duration, waged under the ostensible banner of a "war on terror." The events of September 11, 2001—four coordinated terrorist suicide attacks carried out by Al-Qaeda against the United States—were the immediate catalyst for the US-led invasion of Afghanistan and would be later used to justify the invasion of Iraq in 2003.[7] But as Defense Secretary Donald Rumsfeld instructed commanders in a memo days after September 11, "The President has stressed that we are not defining our fight narrowly and are not focused only on those directly responsible for the September 11 attacks."[8] Within months, the Pentagon was ordering actions led primarily by special operations forces heading "nonconventional" missions in secondary theaters in sub-Saharan Africa, the Philippines, the ex-Soviet Republic of Georgia, and across the wider Caspian Sea region. As policymakers began to interpret Al-Qaeda-inspired terrorism as a transnational, networked phenomenon, the goal, as national policy documents made clear, was to evolve US military strategy toward what the Pentagon continues to call "full-spectrum dominance": dominance across the entire spectrum of warfare, from traditional state-based threats to networked nonstate actors. Full-spectrum dominance, proponents argued, would ensure US military preeminence in an era of globalization.[9]

The logic of full-spectrum dominance was mirrored in the use of psychopharmaceuticals in the war on terror. Capsules, tablets, and pills were portable and easy to administer in an ever-shifting battlespace. Tactically light and agile, psychopharmaceuticals could reach soldiers in operationally remote locations, like the small combat outpost where Nate was stationed with his team. They also traveled well in the crush-proof bottles and zip-top baggies soldiers kept on their bodies as they departed fortified bases on convoys and missions. With few mental and behavioral health care professionals deployed in the wars in Iraq and Afghanistan—generally one for every 1,000 troops—pills enabled treatment to move separately from provider, offering "treatment-in-place" and helping offset personnel shortages.[10] Compared with talk therapy, psychopharmaceuticals traveled with relative ease across the material, geographic, and tactical terrain of the global war on terror.

In this sense, psychopharmaceuticals in war epitomize what Peter Redfield has called the "vital mobility" of military and humanitarian medicine.[11] To evoke its own terminology and spatial imaginary, the objective of battlefield medicine is to push its reach and technical capacity as far "forward" to the frontlines as possible. Combat medicine is the paramount example. The very purpose of combat medicine—and the basis of its success in saving military lives in the wars in Iraq and Afghanistan—is to reach the wounded at the place and moment of injury, where and when stabilizing emergency measures can be critical to survival.[12] Psychotropic medications likewise seem to render definitive mental health treatment for soldiers vitally mobile, traversing the reach of the counterinsurgency battlespace to stabilize and ultimately sustain those who occupy and fight.

Psychopharmaceuticals would evolve yet a second role in the war on terror: enabling soldiers with psychiatric diagnoses to deploy, again and again. Compare this to how, during the Vietnam war, soldiers with severe psychological impairments requiring ongoing management were removed from military service and replaced.[13] The diagnosis of combat-related post-traumatic stress disorder (PTSD) arose as a postwar problem; it was understood to affect Vietnam veterans and treated by the Veterans Affairs (VA) medical system.[14] During the war on terror, protracted conflict on multiple fronts waged by an all-volunteer force, or AVF, meant that the same soldiers were returned to the same wars, some after receiving a PTSD or another psychiatric diagnosis, and many with the aid of medication. The normalization of psychopharmaceutical use coincided with the expansion of battlefield mental health care from the narrow focus on the expected and transient stresses of combat to a broad spectrum of conditions, ranging from what military clinicians refer to as "bread-and-butter" issues like marital problems and adjustment disorders to chronic psychiatric conditions. In its breadth and form, battlefield mental health care became something more akin to outpatient mental health care at home. In the wars in Iraq and Afghanistan, military providers became responsible for what they now called, in direct allusion to US military strategy, *full-spectrum mental and behavioral health care*.[15]

The US military's marked turn to psychopharmaceuticals underscores a basic reality. Despite the growing military investment in robotics and lethal autonomous weapons systems, both now and in the near future, the US goal to project military and political dominance across time and space still requires people: people to build and occupy bases, cook food, collect intelligence, conduct foot patrols, and fight.[16] It should come as little surprise, then, that US military medical planners embraced psychotropic medications as a response to empire's central problem of human endurance and volatility in the war on terror—a chemical bandage for the embodied dilemmas of chronic war and a full-spectrum policy stance.

Psychotropic medications join other technologies of psychology and psychiatry that have been increasingly mobilized by modern militaries to enable their personnel to withstand more for longer.[17] The use of these drugs by the US military in the war on terror must therefore be understood as key to what Nomi Stone has described as a "larger national project that normalizes war as a permanent and indefinite state."[18] The normalization of medicated military service can be connected to multiple world systems: among them, the global influence of pharmaceutical markets—but also the permanent war readiness of the US, the flow of military supply and commodity chains, and relations of imperial power.[19] Psychopharmacy as battlefield medicine is thus neither incidental nor marginal—nor is it an issue of only medical or ethical concern. It is vital to understanding US hegemony and militarism in the twenty-first century.

Pills enabled Nate's team to continue to hold and occupy territory and to fight until replacements came in: to endure more, and for longer. While antidepressants were hardly the solution to all the team's problems, they didn't have to be. The pills evened out the soldiers of concern—just enough and for just long enough. In this sense, the pills did precisely what they were intended to do: they kept Nate's team in that same river valley, conducting the same foot patrols; fighting the same skirmishes; and, as Nate put it, continuing to "go out looking for trouble whenever we thought we could justify it."

Yet, as I suggest throughout this book, the idea that psychopharmaceuticals can be a lifeline at the empire's edges is both a biomedical and imperialist fantasy. If, by Nate's account, antidepressants succeeded in drawing people, affects, and weapons into working alignments, they did so for a provisional time-being that was tenuous at best. In practice, their use required improvisation, risk management, continual surveillance, and magical thinking on Nate's part. And even then, antidepressants were hardly a magic bullet. Defying any easy definition of cure, antidepressants "took the edge off" male anger while still maintaining a level deemed necessary for war, all while displacing "whatever they were dealing with" to another time and place. They helped stabilize the soldiers in Nate's care, but they did so in settings of violence and violation, where ideas of stability—as the former medic's joking about raping, pillaging, and plundering made disquietingly clear—were contorted and vexed. Pills returned soldiers to teammates who needed them as a puzzle needs all its pieces but who quietly questioned their return. Drugs could muddle and compound risk, lashing together double binds upon double binds. Psychopharmaceuticals laid bare the nervous, vibrating state of US imperial war and occupation.

My central argument in this book builds on this disquiet. I contend that in the effort to sustain and stabilize those who fight and occupy, psychopharmacy on the battlefield reveals with exceptional clarity the fundamental volatility of the US military empire. Psychopharmaceuticals, I suggest, have both exposed and exacerbated the tenuous nature of US imperial overreach. The counterterror state, as the chemicals that course through its veins reveal, is one of profound *in*stability.

EMPIRE OF CHEMICALS

Empires have long sought to harness the power of chemicals. In the nineteenth century, substances like the antimalarial quinine facilitated the colonial control of sub-Saharan Africa, the American interiors, and beyond. British and US extraction of prized fertilizers like phosphorus and guano fueled the growth of human populations and the industrial conquest of the Pacific and the Caribbean. With the burgeoning of the field of chemistry would come the development and use of synthetic compounds, including pesticides and chemical weapons, which would blur lines between military, civilian, and genocidal applications.[20] Mined and stolen, synthesized and manufactured, chemicals are among the most vital materials that empires have pursued, weaponized, and exploited.[21]

Injected, ingested, and inhaled, empire's chemicals have also kept it emboldened, alert, numbed, and pulsing. Authorized and unauthorized substances have long been used to enhance performance and ease injury and boredom in war. Alcohol is one of the oldest and most versatile of these substances, having been used for centuries of warfare to raise courage, alleviate stress, and anesthetize the wounded before, during, and after battle.[22] While a more recent addition to the chemical profile of war, psychopharmaceuticals had their place on the battlefield well before the war on terror. For instance, since their widespread use by both Axis and Allied powers during World War II, natural and synthetic stimulants, including amphetamines, have featured prominently in the global military arms race to engineer soldiers who fight without fatigue.[23] The Vietnam War saw the unprecedented use of newly available psychotropic medications to calm soldiers in distress, and US military research today continues to actively seek pharmaceutical routes to armor the mind from combat injury and trauma.[24] In the meantime, conflict around the world has become progressively intertwined with the mass production and global spread of mind-altering substances.[25] Used to ramp up fighters for war, drugs also promise to bring them back into the fold after war's end. Recently, for example, the therapeutic potentials of psychedelics like psilocybin have attracted the attention of military and veteran clinical research communities. The relationship between chemicals and war runs so deep that the history of warfare could be written as the history of psychoactive substances. Indeed, such histories have been written.[26]

American life, too, is saturated with psychopharmaceuticals. The number of psycho- or neuroactive medications being prescribed in the US today is unprecedented, with their use garnering cataclysmic descriptions like "pharmageddon."[27] In 2020, more than 252 million prescriptions were written for psychiatric medication, with medications for attention deficit hyperactivity disorder (ADHD) constituting over a third of prescriptions that year.[28] Psychiatric polypharmacy—the ingesting of two or more psychiatric medications daily—"has become a social and medical fact for millions of patients."[29] US drug companies, meanwhile, continue to vie for footholds to expand the global psychotropic marketplace, transforming concepts of self and experiences of suffering in the process.[30]

Given the proliferation of drugs in contemporary life and the synergies between chemicals and empire, the turn to psychotropic medications in the war on terror may come as little surprise. Yet this development was neither a historical inevitability nor a mere extension of the routine and expanding use of these medications across American life. When viewed from the perspective of modern military psychiatry, the psychopharmaceutical solution to the suffering of soldiers on the battlefield is hardly an obvious one. Military psychiatric orthodoxy throughout the twentieth century normalized what it termed combat stress and battle fatigue as expected responses to the exhaustion of war best treated through the foundational doctrine of forward psychiatry—that is, psychiatry practiced on the frontlines. First developed in World War I, forward psychiatry emphasized treating soldiers as close to the frontlines as possible rather than evacuating them to the rear, thereby maximizing the likelihood of their return to duty.[31] Summarized by military psychiatry's well-known, if misleadingly culinary, mnemonic PIES, these principles emphasized *proximity* to the frontlines, *immediacy* of treatment, *expectancy* to return to duty, and *simplicity* of intervention.[32] Soldiers were given the proverbial "three hots and a cot"—the basic comforts of three square meals and a bed for a few days. Limited to sleep, food, sedation, occupational therapy, and physical training, treatment was designed to be brief and provide only short-term relief. Soldiers were expected to be in uniform throughout treatment to stay focused on their military role. Medicalized intervention was strictly discouraged, as treatment of the soldier as patient would foster malingering and unnecessary medical evacuation. Standard use of medications was therefore to be avoided.

The Vietnam War marked the first large-scale use of modern psychopharmaceuticals to treat psychiatric symptoms in combat.[33] US military physicians were provided a wide array of psychotropic medications, including newly available neuroleptic and anxiolytic tranquilizing medications and tricyclic antidepressants. The innovation of the use of tranquilizing drugs, particularly phenothiazines, meant that soldiers on the battlefield who previously would have required hospitalization or evacuation returned to duty. But following the war, US military interest in these medications quickly fell out of favor out of concern for the unknown long-term psychological effects of medicating stress reactions in combat. Critics also warned that it was dangerous to give soldiers medications that slowed their reflexes, a side effect that could increase the risk of being injured, captured, or killed.

The development of "cleaner," targeted psychiatric drugs in the 1990s—namely, Selective Serotonin Reuptake Inhibitor (SSRI) antidepressants—would reopen debate. Drawing on her experience in peacekeeping operations in Somalia during the early 1990s, Army psychiatrist Elspeth Ritchie was the first to propose a "psychiatric sick-call chest" for both psychiatric emergencies and for the chronic treatment of depression and anxiety. While Ritchie and others advocated for psychiatric medications to avoid damaging military careers and unnecessary removals from duty, skeptics warned that the safety of SSRIs in operational settings had not been proven.

Conservatism toward psychopharmaceuticals would persist into the late 1990s. Combat stress control in the Army during this period continued to emphasize nonpharmacologic interventions on the understanding that effective soldiers rely on their own psychological capacities, not pharmaceutical crutches, to rebound on the battlefield. Despite the meteoric rise of SSRIs in the US market and the development of a new array of second-generation antipsychotics during the 1980s and '90s, the documented use of psychiatric medications for the treatment of ongoing disorders in deployment would remain rare in US military psychiatry during this period.

The tide turned with the war on terror, reflecting the practical reality that the longest-running global conflict since the Vietnam War had stretched an already taut all-volunteer military force. In this context, psychotropic medications became an efficient means of helping soldiers handle extended war. But this turn also signaled significant transformations in institutional, cultural, and political attitudes toward soldier suffering during the period of the war on terror. For many Army officers who came of age during the post–Vietnam era, psychological distress was rarely discussed and certainly not prioritized. One NCO recalled of his time in the Army in the late 1990s, "If there was any mental health issue brought up it was quickly stifled. You'd be shunned, called names. You were told not to bring it up or they'd kill your career." To paraphrase the impression shared by several NCOs looking back on their careers, "mental health just wasn't a thing back then."

During the years of the war on terror, the Army would concertedly work to reform its institutional culture around mental health. Legislative and public pressure were key to demanding action. Accounts of veteran suicide and postwar struggles reported in the media and in Congress placed the psychological injuries of soldiers "center stage in the ways we talk about, digest, and engage with war and its consequences."[34] As Nadia Abu El-Haj has argued, the war on terror gave singular significance to the protection of military life and to the psychological trauma of soldiers in American understandings of war and its costs.[35] In this context, psychopharmaceuticals came to be publicly portrayed not only as an operational tool for troops under strain but as a moral necessity to safeguard the well-being of the soldier. Their use would become a salient, if deeply ambivalent, part of the Army's public articulation of humanitarian care for its own.[36]

These transformations were hardly seamless. Psychopharmaceutical treatment on the battlefield was highly controversial. Media accounts framed the "drugging of our warriors" as a symptom of the biopolitical exploitation of soldiers, the inadequacy of the US military's response to mental health issues, and the failures of the war on terror.[37] The idea of medicated troops also galvanized mainstream opposition to the war. A week after the war in Iraq had passed the four-year mark, Democratic Senator Barbara Boxer challenged the Bush administration on its failures in Iraq. "If you love the troops," Boxer said, bitingly evoking the prowar maxim, "you don't send them back to fight with post-traumatic stress disorder and a bottle of antidepressants."[38]

As debates in Congress and the media increasingly invoked the medicating of troops as evidence that the wars were misbegotten and that the Bush administration's policies were failing, psychopharmaceutical use also became a source of contention within the armed forces themselves.

Beyond raising broader institutional concerns about readiness and the quality of the force, controversy within the Army medical community centered on a proposed correlation between the rise in psychiatric medication use and increasing soldier suicide rates.[39] Reports have suggested a possible link between SSRIs—the popular class of antidepressants including Prozac, Zoloft, Paxil, and Celexa, which boost serotonin levels in the brain—and elevated suicide risk among young people. (SSRIs carry a warning label for elevated suicidality risk among adults under 25, the age group of many young military recruits.[40]) These medications, often combined with narcotic painkillers, were also implicated in a growing array of problems within the Army, including drug dependency and fatal accidents, sometimes from drug interactions. Psychotropic medication use further raised legal, ethical, and operational questions about soldier moral accountability, agency, and control while medicated.

As the controversy around military psychopharmaceutical use underscored, knowledge of what these medications might do in settings of war and how soldiers might use them was conjectural at best. As insights from anthropology and social studies of science remind us, technologies do not travel as stable objects. Rather, they must be "assembled and re-assembled in relation to particular ethical regimes and political projects."[41] Even drugs eminently familiar to American life must be actively remade in relation to the operational logics, ethical frameworks, and material settings of war making. They are what Andrew Barry has called "informed materials": they arrive at FOBs and combat outposts as medications familiar to civilian life, but they "have changing properties depending on their associations in everyday reality."[42]

Here is where psychopharmaceuticals are particularly instructive for the study of war and medicine. Anthropologists have richly documented the aftermath of war injury and trauma, including how medicine shapes the embodied, social, and political dimensions of postconflict military life.[43] Andrew Bickford has also highlighted the preemptive dimensions of military biomedical "big science," including research aimed at designing supersoldiers impervious to harm—effectively "kill-proofing" them before they ever reach the battlefield. Yet far less is ethnographically known about military medicine as it is practiced in and during war.[44] And while scholarly studies of military medicine have tended to focus on cutting-edge biomedical and technological innovations deliberately engineered to safeguard and enhance military life, we know comparatively little about forms of medicine that spill over into battlefield practice. What happens when pharmaceuticals routine to everyday life *become* battlefield medicine—and unintentionally so?

For at least initially, psychopharmaceuticals would be integrated into battlefield care in the war on terror, less in any planned manner than through reactive improvisation. As historian David Kieran has traced, Army mental health protocols were forced to respond quickly and reactively to postinvasion occupations of Iraq and Afghanistan that were never intended and for which the Army was unprepared. In an interview with Kieran, Secretary of the Army Peter Geren tellingly described the challenge as "changing tires on a bus going 60 miles an hour."[45] Indeed, the Army had to revise its deployment formularies early in the wars in no small part due to the unforeseen psychiatric medication needs of the National Guard and Reserve soldiers filling its ranks. Once these medications reached the battlefield, their uptake and lived effects were shaped as much by material, social, and operational contingencies as by clinical and strategic intentions.

When deployed, psychopharmaceuticals enter new regimes of value and economies of exchange and are incorporated into a wide range of official and unofficial technical, procedural, and embodied practices. They are used in unscripted ways as soldiers exploit the potential of pills in dynamic settings of risk, vulnerability, and violence. Even then, drugs can be fickle things. Their mutability owes much to the chemical nature of medication itself and the ambiguous and contradictory subjective and relational effects reported of psychopharmaceuticals more specifically.[46] Factors in deployment like irregular supply, variable prescribing practices, experimentation and sharing, and shifting operational demands can further shape the lived effects and social ecology of medication use, such that even routine medications can become unpredictable. Empire's chemicals shapeshift.

MEDICINE AT WAR

Stabilizing Empire tells a markedly different story than the one often told about the history of military medical innovation in war. This is decidedly not a tale of salvation on the battlefield. Wartime advancements—penicillin, the tourniquet, ultrasound, blood and plasma transfusions—have been retrospectively written into medical history textbooks as "game changers" and "magic bullets."[47] Such biomedical advancements, courtesy of the violence and wounding of battle, feature in what Jennifer Terry calls our "attachments to war," the affective attachments and technoscientific optimism that "may manifest as benefits or at least the hopes of getting something out of war."[48] Terry identifies a biomedicine-war nexus in which new forms of wounding provoke the continual innovation of rehabilitation medicine and prosthetic technologies. Psychopharmaceuticals in war, by contrast, shows military medicine in some of its most modest means and mercurial ends.

Sarah knows this well. She spent much of her second 15-month deployment in Iraq as she did her first, sitting in a highly secured SCIF on base.[49] A cryptologic linguist trained in Arabic, Sarah identified, translated, and analyzed communications and prepared classified reports to inform missions. It seemed only fitting that she would use Dungeons and Dragons taxonomy to explain to me the difference between cryptologic linguists and their human intelligence cousins, since the multiplayer fantasy game occupied much of their downtime while deployed. If human intelligence collectors were the bards, Sarah said, "then we're the wizards. Big towers, tons of information, super weird, and not allowed to talk about things."

Sarah took Ritalin for the first time when it was given to her in Iraq. Whereas during the Vietnam War, "pep pills" were freely distributed to soldiers embarking on reconnaissance missions and ambushes, stimulants came Sarah's way courtesy of a fellow specialist who had a prescription from the Army for ADHD and was willing to share.[50] The Ritalin was something their small team would take together during what Sarah called "surges"—escalations of intelligence-led missions that required them to move from 8- to 12-hour shifts, which, for Sarah, took place at night. During those upticks in operational tempo, their team rarely stepped away from the SCIF. Packaged meals known as mermites saved the crucial minutes it took to get to the chow hall and back, and trips to the bathroom were quick or uncomfortably deferred. Paired with vitamin supplements and energy drinks, Ritalin (the "go" pills) helped Sarah stay focused on her tasks at night, while the little baggie of trazodone given to her by a medic (the "no" pills) helped shut her down for a few hours of sleep during the day.[51]

But it was hardly ideal. Use of a fellow soldier's prescription medication is (technically) a violation of military law, and it ate away at their teammate's prescription supply.[52] The medication also had its drawbacks: Sarah said she had a hard time translating on Ritalin. Giving me a cursory introduction to the root and pattern system of the Arabic language, she described how meaning is encoded in the structure of words and how that structure is relational. "I feel like if you're halfway listening to somebody in Arabic," she explained, "you're probably getting a better reading than if you're trying to individually parse out every word." The kind of laser focus that Ritalin gave her interfered with how the language needed her brain to work; while it got her through those interminable night shifts, it compromised her ability to translate. The implications of this remained unspoken in our conversation. Instead, Sarah told me that where force protection and mission readiness are the goals, you do what you need to do to "get the job done." The rest, she implied, is collateral.

Sarah's account reflects the deep ambivalences, double binds, and damages of psychotropic medication at war. Soldiers like Sarah have cycled pills to "surge" in rhythm with round-the-clock missions, taking "uppers" to get themselves through nightshifts and "downers" to turn themselves off.[53] These are strategies of "high-strung desperation," as she tellingly described them: doing what you can with what you have to get by. While the Ritalin got Sarah through those night shifts, reliance on pills to "get the job done" also silently displaced the harms of medication use onto occupied peoples and places, where the consequences of mistranslations went unspoken.[54] Such are the telling instances when medicine does not redeem, justify, or undo the damage of war so much as compound its harms and obscure its risks. In these instances, war's destruction and medicine's effects comingle and displace each other; distinctions of therapy, enhancement, and harm fall away; and trade-offs, bought time, and getting by are the name of the game.[55] Sometimes, medicine undoes military empire from within.

. . . . .

Medicine, of course, is deeply familiar to the life of the soldier. Coerced and empowered by discipline, as Foucault formulated, the soldier is subject to any number of minute and technical compulsions.[56] The soldier is a biopolitical subject, not merely kept from dying but also aggressively made to live. Medicine is critical to that project.[57] Yet, it is worth noting that psychopharmaceuticals are distinct from other categories of medicine by their association with ideas of volatility. In the military, this perceived volatility rests in part with how psychopharmaceuticals signify underlying mental health disorder and thus, by extension, unfitness for war. (As one soldier bluntly put it, "'psychopharmaceuticals' has the word 'psycho' in it.") Given, too, the potential for adverse behavioral, emotional, neurobiological, and psychological effects noted of psychotropic drugs, these medications raise questions about drug effects and compromised soldiering in ways that antibiotics, statins, and vaccines, for example, generally do not.

High-profile military criminal cases have thrown a sharp light on the volatile associations of psychoactive medications in war. While defenses of crimes linked to the use of psychoactive drugs have rarely gained traction in military and civilian courtrooms, in a small but growing number of cases, lawyers are attributing their clients' behaviors to medications prescribed by the military. Consider the case of Robert Bales. In the early morning of March 11, 2012, Bales, then a staff sergeant in the Army, walked off the outpost where he was stationed in Kandahar and murdered 16 Afghans, including sleeping women and children, in two nearby villages. During his military trial and in the media speculation in its wake, questions were raised about whether the killings might have been "triggered" by Bales's use of several medications with psychotropic potential, including anabolic steroids, the sleep medicine Ambien, and the Army-mandated antimalarial mefloquine.[58]

The Bales case underscores a central argument of this book: psychopharmaceutical use on the battlefield has significantly shaped moral ideas of soldiering, norms and values governing the use of force, and the conduct of contemporary counterinsurgency war.[59] Through the consequences attributed to their chemical effects, the claims they enable around risk and benefit on the battlefield, and the terms they provide for judgments of what is right and wrong in war, psychopharmaceuticals have played an important though little-understood role in defining morality and virtue in the war on terror.[60]

At the center of how these normative ideas are defined and legitimated is a powerful construct: control. Constructs of self-control are not unique to the military or to contemporary iterations of counterinsurgency. Western concepts of the ideal self are built around the idea of an autonomous, rational individual capable of exercising self-control, an ideal that psychiatric illness is often seen to disrupt.[61] At the same time, coercive control, along with rhetoric and practices of emotional restraint, have been key to the production of masculinities and to the operation of power along lines of gender, class, and race.[62] Military institutions are known to submit individuals to hierarchical disciplinary structures predicated on emotional control. Recruits are conditioned to "master the external situation in which they find themselves through a process of gaining control over their own emotions"—a military ideal that is inseparable from its notion of masculinity.[63]

In the war on terror, "control" would take on specific doctrinal, strategic, technical, and ethical meanings. Counterinsurgency doctrine in the wars in Iraq and Afghanistan expected soldiers to practice what General Stanley McChrystal, then the commander in Afghanistan, famously called "courageous restraint"—the "discipline" and "courage" to refrain from firing weapons, even when feeling threatened, in order to minimize civilian casualties, while still reserving the right to use lethal force when necessary to protect the mission and themselves.[64] Soldiers were moreover expected to do so in occupied settings figured as inherently unstable and chaotic.[65]

Control thus brings into focus the normative disciplinary, technical, ethical, and biopolitical relationships to violence expected of soldiers in the wars in Iraq and Afghanistan. By condemning certain forms of (drug-induced) violence as arbitrary, wanton, and out of control, cases like that of Robert Bales parse and implicitly legitimate other forms of military violence as humane. Psychopharmaceuticals, then, have functioned as a powerful grammar in the production of the moralities of contemporary global liberal war. Their use has supplied a vocabulary and set of concepts through which transgressions that horrify Western liberal sensibilities are conceived and condemned, while simultaneously producing definitions of disciplined, reasonable, and just violence.[66] Constructs of soldier control are thus inseparable from liberal democratic fantasies that imagine the destructiveness of preemptive war can be calibrated and that harms to local civilians can be contained, because military violence and the soldiers who dispense it are restrained, deliberate, and "in control."

Where medicine promises stability while carrying with it the potential to destabilize, control is closely tied to constructs of risk. Risk plays a central role in how psychopharmaceutical use and its effects are embodied, managed, and imagined.[67] Risk takes multiple forms in relation to medicine and war in this book. Military providers and command objectify and stratify risk to maximize operational and strategic outcomes, while teams and units continually assess the nature of risk in relation to individual and group performance. Soldiers, too, forge norms and values concerning what is acceptable while medicated—or working alongside someone who is. Critically, the intensive labor of risk management among providers, command, and soldiers that I ethnographically trace in these chapters is not about the risk to Iraqi and Afghan lives as such or even primarily about the protection of soldier well-being. Rather, it is above all about the strategic objectives of counterinsurgency.

It follows that I do not take constructs like risk, control, stability, or counterinsurgency as self-evident reflections of medical or political realities but rather as part of what Derek Gregory calls a "military dispositif": a "heterogeneous assemblage of discourses and objects, practices and powers distributed across different but networked sites," which, in the case of military psychopharmaceutical use, blends the ethical, operational, psychiatric, and political.[68] *Stabilizing Empire* examines how concepts and practices of control and risk operate in liberal security regimes and contemporary counterinsurgency doctrine and in the biomedical fantasies of securing life through medicine, in which psychiatry plays an uneasy role. This, then, is an ethnography of what happens when medicine is harnessed to stabilize those who would stabilize nation-states—medicine that, as Sarah and others in this book remind us, is itself untamable in its uses and effects. Psychopharmacy in the war on terror, I argue, both materializes the characteristic volatility of imperial overreach and illuminates fantasies of chemical corrective—a dialectic I call *in/stability*, and which frames my approach in this book.

IN/STABILITY

In its most familiar form, *in/stability* reflects the everyday language soldiers used when talking with me about who was mentally "stable" enough—and more often, who was considered too "unstable"—to carry out the work of war and occupation. Soldiers' ideas about in/stability often reflected masculinist, classed, and imperialist ideas of who is capable of exerting control, and who requires subjugation. At the same time, the term "stability" is pervasive in the language of the military medical community. It functions as the key clinical and administrative concept by which military medical providers evaluate and officially document soldiers' readiness to deploy while on psychotropic medications.[69]

My use of *in/stability* also foregrounds the concept as an organizing principle of US militarism in the twenty-first century. "Stabilization" and "stabilization operations" are relative newcomers to the lexicon of military strategy, having seen tremendous growth during the war on terror. The concept of stabilization and the specific policies enacted under its name during the war on terror normalized the role of military power in the transition of states and were mainstreamed under the term "stability operations." Reflecting a wider securitization of development and aid spheres and peace-support intervention, stabilization is premised on a logic of control and on the idea that "failed" and "weak" states compromise national and global security. These techniques were predicated in part on Orientalist constructions of occupied Iraq and Afghanistan as inherently chaotic and pathological spaces in need of domestication.[70] In the case of Iraq, for example, US and coalition forces sought to control territory and people by systematically dismantling Iraq's existing political and economic structures and enacting divide-and-rule tactics that rendered everyday life highly precarious, coercive, and destructive, as Hayder Al-Mohammad, Omar Dewachi, Kali Rubaii, and Nadia El-Shaarawi have documented. The consequences for Iraqis have been lethal.[71]

In/stability, then, has mattered in a multitude of ways to counterinsurgency doctrine and military institutions in the war on terror: as a logic of administering territories and populations, a framework of global security, a form of military embodiment, and a means of governing the minds and bodies of soldiers. But *in/stability*, as I use it, does more than point to a coincidental convergence of language. First, it emphasizes the shifting configurations of pills, people, weapons, information, infrastructure, strategy, and terrain that shape the use and effects of psychopharmaceuticals in contexts of war and occupation. These more-than-human assemblages, as Sarah and Nate both know well, can be mercurial, even volatile.

Second, by ethnographically tracing how chemical efforts to stabilize imperial power are themselves deeply *unstable*, often to deadly effect, my use of *in/stability* exposes the illusory promise of the military psychopharmaceutical solution.

In/stability identifies an imperial and counterinsurgent fantasy of mastery and enforced order over occupied territories and populations, a fantasy that is uncannily mirrored in military control of soldier mental health: in institutional policies administering medication use, in military medicine's intensive management of the risks posed by soldier behavior and drug effects, and in soldiers' own efforts to regulate their conduct in relation to the drugs they consume. In drawing this parallel, I take inspiration from Begoña Aretxaga's insight that the state is not simply the product of rational technologies but a "subject of excess" in which fantasy plays a central role in the materialization of political life, the structuring of power relations, and the enactment of state violence and technologies of terror.[72] My inroad into these fantasies in the war on terror is the key role granted to biomedicine and the "psy" sciences in the dream of providing global security, order, and stability, and of realizing control through drugs.[73]

To be clear, I am not arguing that a more stable US military empire would make for a more secure world. Nor does my use of *in/stability* casually insinuate that military personnel and veterans are "unstable"—a harmful stereotype that both stigmatizes those who must live under its shadow and severely constrains our understanding of war's consequences.[74] While the experiences of individual soldiers, officers, and veterans feature centrally in this book, this is decidedly not an ethical analysis of military psychopharmaceutical use or a critique of the Army medical community or its providers. It is also not an ethnography of soldier mental health and suffering.[75] Rather, it is a study of the condition of US imperialism in the twenty-first century as illuminated through medicine. It is an account of the fantasies conjured and the volatile formations of pills, people, weapons, and tactics produced in practice, when securitized, imperial, and biomedical ways of apprehending the world converge. *In/stability* appropriates the language of US empire and reflects it back upon itself, turning an ethnographic lens onto its conceits, and ultimately, onto its nervous, anxious state.

THE OFFICIAL, THE TACIT, AND THE AMBIGUOUS

A study of military psychotropic medication use may provoke a desire for numbers. Is the US Army "drugging our warriors," as reporters have suggested?[76] Are militaries "dishing out" antidepressants to today's troops, as one British retired major told the *Telegraph*?[77] Satisfying this desire for numbers is tricky, first and foremost because data on military psychopharmaceutical use has been highly elusive in the wars in Iraq and Afghanistan. Little is known about the use of different therapies for the management of what the US Army collectively refers to as "mental and behavioral health conditions" in deployed settings. Even less is known about the authorized and unauthorized use of psychopharmaceuticals for reasons beyond the treatment of these conditions.

Psychopharmaceutical use has been notoriously difficult to track in theater. DoD record-keeping on the distribution and use of these medications in deployment has historically been lacking and likely underreports medication use. Additionally, in the war on terror, psychotropic medications were often prescribed outside of mental and behavioral health encounters, circulated through informal practices that escaped regulation, and were rarely accessed at fixed locations. Particularly in what the DoD calls "far-forward" locations, little or no retrievable documentation of care is available. As in American life more generally, in the war on terror, mental health diagnoses and treatments were cut loose from the control of psychiatry, with the majority of psychopharmaceuticals prescribed not through mental and behavioral health providers but through general providers like physician assistants.[78] They also entered deployed settings through informal routes, sometimes in packages mailed by family and friends or through prescriptions obtained by private sector providers. Once in theater, they were often shared, experimented with, and traded.

Even official numbers are limited. To date, most of the research on psychopharmaceutical use among active-duty military personnel has been conducted before or following deployments. The few published studies on psychopharmaceutical use in deployment offer snapshots but, again, fail to capture informal practices. In one large study describing prescribed treatments by mental health providers for over 1,300 treatment-seeking military personnel deployed to Iraq, medication was the most prescribed treatment but was often combined with recommendations for counseling or behavioral modification. Antidepressants were the drug type most frequently recommended across all diagnostic categories.[79] Another study of soldiers assigned to a brigade combat team in Iraq found that SSRIs came second to sleep aids as the most prescribed medications. Benzodiazepines were prescribed, though rarely, for short-term management of acute anxiety.[80] As with civilian use, military providers prescribed psychotropic medications for both indicated and off-label use, including for a variety of reasons besides mental health conditions, such as headaches, smoking cessation, and pain. Insomnia was the most common initial complaint for military personnel referred to mental health.[81]

Other numbers give clues to the growth of military psychopharmaceutical use over time. Tricare Management Activity, the division of the DoD that manages health care services for the military, reported a nearly 700 percent increase in the number of psychoactive drugs prescribed to military personnel between 2005 and 2011—this despite a steady reduction in combat troop levels beginning in 2008.[82] Data from the military's electronic health record suggests that 80 percent of reported mental health encounters and 81.5 percent of psychotropic medication prescriptions occurred in military operations carried out in Iraq, compared to 20.2 percent and 16.7 percent respectively in military operations in Afghanistan.[83] One could also speak in terms of the billions of dollars of taxpayer money raked in by pharmaceutical companies through lucrative contracts to meet these medication needs. For instance, a 2010 report found that between 2001 and 2009, the Defense Logistics Agency spent $1.1 billion on psychiatric and pain medications.[84]

As suggestive as these numbers may be, this book remains agnostic on further quantifying military psychopharmaceutical use. One reason for this is that psychopharmaceutical access and use varied widely over the course of the war on terror. Unsurprisingly, access to psychopharmaceuticals depended on factors such as timing, location, infrastructure, and a soldier's military occupation and daily duties (the two not necessarily—or often—one and the same). Demographic shifts in the armed forces, continually fluid DoD policy, and pendulum swings in the military medical community's acceptance of psychopharmaceuticals over the span of the wars added to this variability. Numbers offer snapshots, at best.

But it is also here, in the face of the varied and often-elusive ways these medications were accessed and used, that anthropology stands to be especially instructive. Ethnographic methods can illuminate how the availability, uptake, and lived effects of medication were shaped by specific and situated infrastructural, operational, and clinical factors on the battlefields of the war on terror; at the same time, these methods can situate these factors in relation to political, ideological, and cultural fields that extend beyond the battlefield. And notably, while aspects of psychopharmaceutical use in deployment have been elusive to the surveillance and tracking mechanisms of military data systems, interviews opened spaces in which soldiers shared experiences of all kinds about their own psychopharmaceutical use and that of others. These were experiences known through direct observation but also through tacit knowledge.

Consider Alex. As a light-wheel vehicle mechanic deployed to Iraq in 2006, Alex maintained and fixed vehicles, regularly went on convoys to Baghdad in search of repair parts, and was assigned observation-post duty over a highway running through Fallujah. As his platoon's motor sergeant, Alex was also responsible for the training, welfare, and morale of his junior soldiers—duties that demanded a different kind of eye for detail. Alex told me he could infer a lot about the mental health of his soldiers by tracking their movements. Soldiers might need to arrange to get themselves on convoys to pick up medication or to meet the brigade psychiatrist at a larger base. "It would be, 'Hey, someone needs to head to Baghdad,' or 'Somebody needs to head to Bagram,' and we'd have to arrange a flight for them or get them on a truck," he told me. "So, you started picking up on what was what." There were other ways of figuring out who needed looking out for. When Alex conducted hooch checks—inspections of soldiers' sleep and work areas—opened drawers and dumped shave kits revealed which medications were being taken and by whom. He made mental notes of it all. The signs were everywhere, if you were properly attuned to them.

Stabilizing Empire centers the skill of soldiers like Alex to read deployed military life for medication use and effects. Officers and enlisted soldiers alike develop experiential, sensory, and intuitive ways of knowing when psychotropic medications are present in deployment and in the lives of fellow soldiers. For me, the anthropologist, this often meant listening for what went unsaid. To take one example: soldiers frequently assumed that I would accept their assertions about widespread medication use or, say, a buddy's experimentation with (another buddy's) trazodone, at face value. Many suffered patiently through my persistent follow-up: "But how did you *know*?" I asked this question not to test the veracity of their claims but out of an epistemic curiosity. *How* did they know what they knew about medication use in deployment? Over time, it became clear that I had tapped into social and embodied aspects of deployed military life that were unknown to me—spaces where intimate cohabitation and mutual reliance lent themselves to forms of direct and tacit knowledge about others, both socially intimate and distanced. Tacit knowledge is fueled in no small part by an active rumor mill—what some call the PNN, or Private News Network—which works overtime in deployed life. Not unlike high school gossip, the PNN is not always reliable, so it demands discriminating use; but it can also generate credible and clutch intel.

This orientation to the tacit foregrounds military personnel and veterans as "participant observers" of empire—analysts of the institutions of war and regimes of imperial power of which they are a part.[85] It also emphasizes the relational and corporate aspects of psychopharmaceutical use among soldiers. Elsewhere, I have theorized this social landscape as a form of "medication by proxy," a term I use to highlight the dispersed locus of psychopharmaceutical effects in contexts where medication use often has direct implications not just for the individual but for the team and unit.[86] The term also plays on the adjacent idea of proximity to emphasize the spatial, material, and sensorial ways soldiers become attuned to the presence and use of psychotropic medications by peers and teammates.

While attending to tacit knowledge, my analysis also makes room for the ambiguity that often accompanied what felt implicit. Alex, for instance, might have felt certain about which of his soldiers were taking medication, yet rarely did he know what those medications were or what they did. Precisely because soldiers actively observe behavioral and performance change and evaluate advantage and risk in relation to substances taken, I did not predefine for my interlocutors what "counted" as a psychopharmaceutical. Instead, soldiers and veterans were invited to elaborate on any medications they observed to have behavioral, emotional, neuropsychiatric, or psychological effects. Within that space, soldiers often felt committed to what they *knew*. What they knew, however, was almost always attended by the displacements, ambivalences, and ambiguities that can proliferate in corporate settings that are defined by performance and shared survival, as much as by dissociation, distancing, and silence.

In this sense, my attention to the tacit also underscores how the military quietly permits certain activities and behaviors as it gives precedence to military practicality over things like regulations, standard operating procedures, and official policy. It recognizes how military institutions and military leadership often avert their gaze from inconvenient realities—to maintain a buttoned-up exterior, yes, but also because willful ignorance often has collateral benefit.[87] Take, for example, the former Army recruiter who half-joked about repeating the same mental health screening question ad nauseum to a recruit until he received the answer that entailed a clean bill of health, allowing the recruiter to fulfill his quota.[88] Or consider the ways soldiers tacitly view pills as tools to be entrepreneurially hacked, often to violent efficacy.

Tacit knowledge and its ambiguities also shaped the research process itself. In the classificatory schemes of many I spoke with, I am a civilian. I am also an academic and a researcher. (One soldier joked that as all these things—and an Asian woman to boot—I couldn't be further outside the military).[89] At the same time, upon learning that I was an anthropologist, many presumed a certain kinship. Anthropologists, a National Guardsman once remarked with unblinking sincerity, had become great friends of the military in recent years—a comment he anchored in the fact that some anthropologists had been involved in the Army's Human Terrain System.[90] Another was interested in my take on human nature and warfare, having versed himself in the writings of Napoleon Chagnon. Throughout the research, I spent considerable time explaining that there are many kinds of anthropology and many kinds of anthropologists and that I wasn't "that" kind. Others assumed that, as a researcher interested in psychopharmaceuticals, I must be studying "soldier mental health." Early in my fieldwork, a colonel caught wind of my project and left me a voicemail saying he could get four hundred soldiers in a room the next day to take my survey. I politely declined. (What survey, I would never know.) I found myself having to carefully disabuse people of these misrecognitions—those tied up in anthropology's historical complicities in US imperial projects, as much as in the clarion call to action commanded by military mental health research.[91]

While I found myself working through my interlocutors' assumptions about me, I also had to work through my own about them. Some of my most deeply set ideas about the US military have been shaped by the inheritance of familial memories of violent displacement and encounters with US soldiers from my parents' childhoods in the Philippines—memories that, in the context of the long, turbulent, and complicated history of American (and Spanish and Japanese) colonization, occupation, and war, both heroized and demonized the US military.[92] In interviews, institutional kinship mattered more than history, as soldiers and veterans almost always asked if I had family in the military. (As it happens, I do: an in-law retired from the Air Force and another who deployed to Iraq and Afghanistan.) This fact seemed to make me somewhat familiar. It vetted me to some degree. For others, our tenuous, temporary connection and my "outsider" civilian status may have made me easier to speak with. But there were clear limits. *Stabilizing Empire* emerges in these relational spaces of in-between, where both the tacit and the ambiguous shaped possibilities for what might be known, felt, and told.

SCOPE OF THE BOOK

The research for this book is based on fieldwork conducted over four years, beginning with pilot research in 2016 followed by fieldwork between 2018 and 2021. Until March 2020, interviews and focus groups were conducted in-person in North Carolina, with a small handful of interviews in Virginia. Research also included archival research in the Maryland and Washington DC areas, ethnographic observation at national military and VA health care conferences, and discourse analysis of over 1,500 pages of documents accessed through a Freedom of Information Act (FOIA) request. Over 130 individuals participated in semistructured interviews and focus groups. Following the onset of the Covid-19 pandemic, research switched entirely online. Remaining interviews—roughly the last 20—were primarily with military health care providers, and the switch to virtual interviews enabled me to widen my geographic scope.

This book thus derives in significant part from interviews and accounts shared retrospectively of experiences that, in some cases, were a decade or more in the past. In their own temporal distancing from the events they described, many of my interlocutors gained new space to critically reflect on their experiences and the role of medicine in war. I write about the accounts that they shared in a way that tries to contextualize everyday environments of military pharmaceutical life and war making. While the observations shared by my interlocutors allow me to describe a kind of para-ethnographic setting, I was not immersed in a sustained way in environments and practices of pharmaceutical use. This distinction carries clear limits, not least that these accounts derive from my interactions with interlocutors in the narrow context and frame of research-driven interviews. At the same time, the interviews afforded insights into the heterogeneity and complexity of military psychopharmaceutical use across the span of the wars—insights that may not otherwise have presented themselves.

The evolution of this project was significantly shaped by the adept contributions of research assistants, several of whom are veterans of the US military and one of whom was in my home university's ROTC program at the time of the project.[93] Working and collaborating with these research assistants meant that the project shifted and evolved in ongoing dialogue with them as coanalysts of the complexities and contradictions of military institutions and their moralities and of global US power. Each of them has enriched this project in their own way.

This book is Army focused. During the war on terror, the Army would lead all other military branches in polypharmacy use of psychotropic, opioid, and central-nervous-system-depressant medications, with data from 2016 suggesting that approximately one in seven active-duty Army soldiers was on multiple concurrent medications.[94] Perhaps unsurprisingly given this trend, the US Army also led all branches and coalition forces in its role in ground combat operations, contributing, in the military's unit of accounting, 1.5 million personnel-years to Iraq and Afghanistan deployments between 2001 and 2011, compared to less than 1 million for the Navy, Marines, and Air Force combined.[95] The Army also led the programmatic transformation of mental health care on the battlefield during the war on terror, with Army research reforming DoD policy and clinical practice.

All participants at the time of interview were US Army active duty, National Guard or Reserve, or Army veterans. They represent a wide range of Army occupations, deployment experiences, and career trajectories. Nearly two-thirds were enlisted only, and about a quarter were officers only.[96] This is a "Big Army" study: about 90 percent of participants were conventional Army, with the remaining 10 percent in Special Forces. They were roughly equally distributed as far as location of deployment: a third each having deployed to Iraq only and Afghanistan only and the remaining third having deployed to both Iraq and Afghanistan. The average number of deployments among participants to either Iraq or Afghanistan was 1.77, with the highest number of deployments to Iraq or Afghanistan for a single participant being seven. (The highest number of deployments anywhere for a single participant was 22). Their deployment histories ranged across the chronological expanse of the wars: the earliest deployment among participants to either Iraq or Afghanistan was 2002 (Afghanistan); the most recent were in 2019 (Iraq and Afghanistan).[97] Given that psychoactive medication use has potential implications for peers and teammates, the recruitment criteria invited Army personnel and Amy veterans who had either themselves personally used or observed the use of psychopharmaceutical use by another while deployed.

Stabilizing Empire proceeds in six chapters. Chapter 1, "Buildup," lays out some of the transformations that enabled the normalization of psychopharmaceuticals on the battlefield in the wars in Iraq and Afghanistan. Just as SSRIs take time to build up their chemical effect in the body, psychopharmaceutical use in global counterinsurgency required its own kind of military buildup: the development of an ever-evolving web of official guidelines and policies, the maturation of military infrastructure in Iraq and Afghanistan, the accumulation of experiential knowledge and clinical practice in theater, shifts in concepts of soldier suffering and its management, and the expansion of global supply chains. This buildup would only be possible with protracted war and occupation. Treating mental health as a chronic condition on the battlefield was thus both a result and a possibility of chronic war itself.

In an era of chronic war, the occupation Army confronted unprecedented demands in sustaining what counterinsurgency strategy called "constant presence" in Iraq and Afghanistan. While chapter 1 details the buildup of military force, chapter 2, "Chronic," examines how this protracted commitment of military force over time and space impacted the US military's recruitment and retention strategies. It traces the ambitious task envisioned for pharmaceuticals in addressing the accumulated, embodied dilemmas of waging forever wars and returning the same soldiers to the same battlefields.

Chapter 3, "Stability," turns the lens from soldier mental health as a manpower problem to soldier instability as a strategic liability in the campaign to win hearts and minds. More than simply probing the parallels between the mental stability of soldiers and the stabilization goals of US military operations, this chapter considers what is at stake in military efforts to link the two. In the war on terror, soldier stability became the very ground on which the stabilization of occupied nations was imagined to rest.

In chapter 4, "Supply," I follow the material flows of pills and tablets across the infrastructure of war and occupation. Psychopharmaceuticals are commonly taken as daily medications and thus require ongoing logistical commitments and a continuous supply chain. Tracing these pharmaceutical flows illuminates the material requirements of sustaining the people and operations of empire. It also reveals interruptions in circulation and the ways soldiers make do in these gaps.

The last two chapters engage the experiential dimensions of military psychopharmaceutical use, considering the individual and intersubjective ramifications of chemical stabilization in war. Chapter 5, "Reaction," attunes to the uncertain and often volatile alignments of people, infrastructure, technology, weapons, and tactics that psychopharmaceuticals in war draw into working arrangements. It examines ideas and practices of risk management around medication use from the perspectives of military leadership and medicated soldiers and their nervous peers. It also considers the politics of death that practices of risk management produce. Chapter 6, "Encapsulate," is an ethnography of suicide prevention on the battlefield; it details what efforts to stabilize military life look like in war when psychopharmaceuticals fail. The book concludes with reflections on the prospective role of psychopharmaceuticals as US military planners envision future conflict.

1 Buildup

When a bottle of pills, carried in a rucksack, wound its way up a mountainside in the Korengal Valley in 2007, a young platoon sergeant named Andrew was there to meet it. The hand-off happened when Andrew pulled the doc aside to chat over a smoke. "He didn't smoke," Andrew would later recall to me, "but he'd dip with you, 'cause he was a good guy like that." On his second deployment in four years, the first during the 2003 invasion of Iraq, the infantryman was feeling rough around the edges. Every foot patrol, every interaction with the lieutenant who got under his skin had become a test in control. Andrew confided to the doc about the anger inside him, anger he worried would combust. He opened up, and in short course, the doc opened his rucksack. "Whereas the rest of us have ammo and water and food," Andrew tells me laughing, "he had a ruck full of pills."

Years later, some details are hazy. Andrew can't recall if the doc had been a psychiatrist or a psychologist, though he assumes the former because of the pills. Other details he remembers acutely. The moment the doc pulled the drugs out of his ruck is one of them. Like a magician pulling a rabbit out of a hat, Andrew pantomimes the moment for me, diving his tattooed arm into an invisible bag slung on his shoulder and tossing me a pretend bottle of medication. Joyful disbelief and mild concern play on his face. With the Celexa, "it was just like, 'Here's an energy drink and a cigarette.' Just like, 'Oh, hold on, try this.' Same thing." Same thing but not quite, since unlike energy drinks, by military policy antidepressants require that the provider initiate a medical profile. Andrew remembers the doc placing a three-month supply in his hand and wishing him luck. He doubts that the Celexa made it onto his medical record. After all, "it was literally on the side of a mountain in Afghanistan."[1]

Andrew jokes at the unexpectedness and ease of it all but also says that he considers himself lucky. It was a fortuitous convergence, getting the meds that day, one even more extraordinary for the fact that Andrew was stationed at an installation the Army would describe as "remote." Nestled in the high mountains of eastern Afghanistan near the border of Pakistan, and part of a tributary system of the Pech River, the Korengal valley resisted counterinsurgent military occupation and its attendant flow of things during the war on terror. Engineering in the valley was notoriously difficult. Steep mountains, thick forests of pine, and loose shale challenged US military efforts to establish its presence during a campaign that began in 2004 and ended with the US withdrawal from the valley in 2010. The infamous Restrepo outpost, for instance, had to be built mostly by hand because the hills were too steep for heavy equipment.[2] Soldiers slipped up the hilltop at night and frantically dug shallow trenches under the cover of dark. Over several weeks, they gradually chipped away at rock, which they threw into bags and Hesco barriers, to create walls and fighting positions. Supply was constricted; most trucks couldn't make it into the hills. Getting water, food, and gear to hilltops required helicopter lifts or infantry soldiers carrying it up on their backs.

What, then, did it take to get a bottle of Celexa to a hilltop in eastern Afghanistan and into Andrew's hands? In one sense, this is a patently practical question, one about how the things of empire reach its farthest corners. In the case of a bottle of Celexa, the answer has to do with how pharmaceuticals cross landscapes of US military power and capital. Medications enter military formularies courtesy of lucrative contracts between the DoD and pharmaceutical companies and course through a vast military and commercial logistics network to reach across an expansive US global basing system.[3] The provisioning of mental health care in the form of pills to soldiers in Iraq and Afghanistan required, in military jargon, the "mature" infrastructure that enduring occupation provided the time to build: the sprawling FOBs, combat hospitals and clinics, military pharmacies, transportation routes, and teams of circulating mental health care providers tasked with traversing them.[4] When the system worked, it could deliver a bottle of Celexa to logistically remote locations on the counterinsurgency battlefield. In this sense, Andrew's experience on that hilltop represents a limit test in the collaborative material reach of profit, medicine, and empire.

Read in yet another light, to ask how a bottle of antidepressants reached a soldier on a hilltop in Afghanistan is to ask a broader question about the cultural transformation of mental health and its care in war and the new importance accorded medication in that transformation. So figured, this question queries how the post-9/11 US Army shifted its approach to the age-old dilemma of soldier stress on the battlefield, breezing well past military psychiatry's twentieth-century focus on expected reactions to war—namely, combat stress and battle fatigue—toward the broad provisioning of outpatient mental and behavioral health care in the war on terror. The routinization of medication treatment for mental health in war could only come with significant material and discursive transformations, on and off the battlefield.

This chapter examines some of the transformations that enabled the normalization of psychopharmaceuticals on the battlefield during the wars in Iraq and Afghanistan. I frame these transformations as forms of *buildup*—a term with military and medical meanings. Just as SSRIs take time to build up their chemical effects in the body, psychopharmaceuticals could only "work" in global counterinsurgency through a corresponding military buildup: the development of an evolving web of official policies; the maturation of military infrastructure in Iraq and Afghanistan; the accumulation of experiential knowledge and clinical practice in theater; shifts in concepts of soldier suffering and its management; and the expansion of global supply chains to feed the pharmaceutical needs of empire. Such a buildup was only possible through protracted war and occupation. Treating mental health as a chronic condition on the battlefield was therefore both a consequence—and possibility—of chronic war itself.

These dynamics suggest that war and medicine may play to the same tempo. But if the term "buildup" commonly assumes steady accumulation,

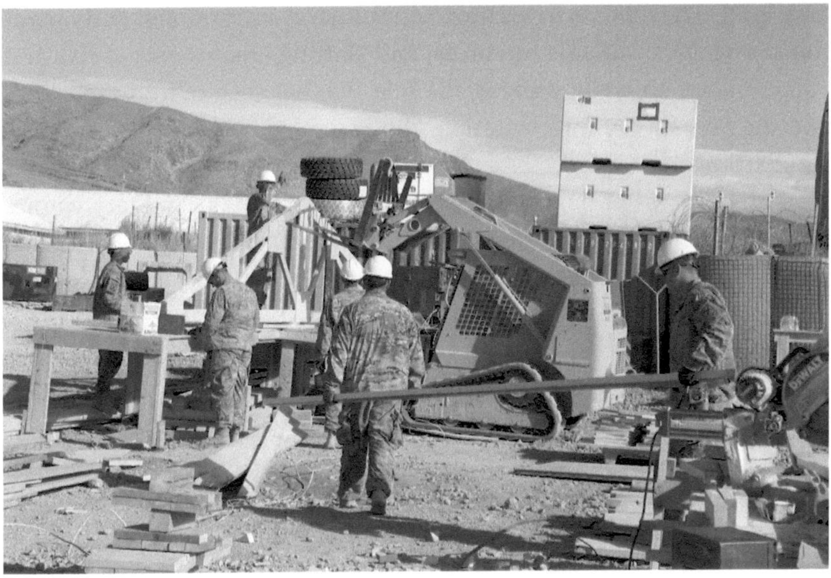

Figure 1. 1151st Engineer Company building B-hut living quarters on FOB Lightning in Afghanistan. Photograph by SPC Charles Willingham, via DVIDS.

in fact, military buildup ebbs and flows across time and space, responsive to changing public sentiment and military strategy and variable across the landscape of war and occupation. Likewise, psychopharmaceutical use was highly uneven across the time-space of the war on terror. Indeed, as Andrew's experiences at the COP reveal, little was obvious, straightforward, or settled about pharmaceutical buildup in war. For one thing, access to and steady availability of medications on the counterinsurgency battlefield were hardly seamless. A few weeks after beginning on the Celexa and just when the medications were starting to "kick in," Andrew was moved to a new location. The junior soldier saw no follow-up and didn't know how to orchestrate another meeting with the doc. It became clear there was no refill coming. So, he simply ran out.[5]

Taking my cue from Andrew, in this chapter I approach buildup as a tentative and unstable project, in which soldiers, officers, and military care providers alike had to continually work and rework psychopharmaceuticals into settings of war and occupation in the effort to make them take hold. They did so in relation to multilevel institutional and operational demands, variable resources, and shifting assessments of risk and vulnerability, all while walking the fine line between official guidelines and the necessity of improvisation. While guided by a tangle of policies, standard operating procedures, and the high-level strategy of war planners, the process of buildup reveals that the making of military empire ultimately comes down to practices, norms, and values forged in situated and contingent circumstances. Medicine is no exception.

MASTER OF HIS OWN ANXIETY

While psychopharmaceuticals are now routine across many settings of US life, there was nothing inevitable about their use on the battlefield. Indeed, a story of the buildup of psychopharmaceuticals in war could be told as a history of ambivalence, or at least, of stops and starts. One version of such a story might begin with the Vietnam War, the first major global conflict to see the use of modern psychopharmaceuticals for the treatment of psychiatric symptoms in combat. With the development of psychopharmacological agents beginning in the 1950s, the US military became interested in the potential of medication in returning soldiers to duty and reducing psychiatric casualties of war, an ambition that has guided military psychiatry since the field's inception. US military psychiatrists and primary care physicians in Vietnam were among the first to be routinely trained in the use of neuroleptics, anxiolytics, and tricyclics.[6] The tranquilizers prochlorperazine (Compazine) and chlorpromazine (Thorazine) were widely used to treat symptoms of combat stress and battle fatigue. Army physicians commonly used prochlorperazine—also a powerful antiemetic and antidiarrheal drug—for the treatment of upset bowels understood to be a physiological symptom of anxiety.[7] Anxiolytics—namely, chlordiazepoxide (Librium) and diazepam (Valium)—were also used for less severe psychiatric casualties and for alcohol detoxification.

The use of these medications in theater was controversial. Psychoactive medications were extensively prescribed to soldiers during the Vietnam War, but their risks and benefits were not tracked.[8] A limited survey conducted in 1967 showed that military psychiatrists tended to prescribe psychotropic drugs in heavier doses and for longer periods of time than did military primary care physicians but that they also tended to be less convinced of their efficacy in theater.[9] Major tranquilizers were known to decrease alertness and motor skills. Critics also warned that psychopharmaceuticals could impair a soldier's ability to integrate emotional experiences and thus cause long-term harm and that soldiers traumatized by battle might be unable to make a reasoned decision to consent to taking medication. Retrospective accounts have suggested that the use of psychopharmaceuticals during the Vietnam War was in the service of military objectives at the expense of the needs of soldiers and may have contributed to the development of PTSD.[10]

Standard use of psychiatric medications in the military soon fell out of favor after the Vietnam War and remained uncommon for the treatment of ongoing disorders during US military operations through the '80s and '90s. The initial US Army field manual (FM) 8-51 on combat stress control, published in 1994 and updated in 1998, focuses on triage and nonpharmacologic treatments aimed at normalizing and minimizing combat stress.[11] Despite the advent and popularity of second-generation antidepressants, including SSRIs, beginning in the late 1980s, field manual 8-51 maintains a highly restrained approach to psychopharmaceuticals. The word "medication" occurs 25 times in the 255-page manual and is used mainly in reference to stabilizing agitated soldiers in emergency situations, a practice for which the manual provides some guidelines but which on the whole it clearly discourages, particularly for those soldiers expected to resume duties. Little guidance is otherwise given on the role and dispensing of psychopharmaceuticals.

This conservatism is justified along multiple lines in the manual. Medication use may produce behavioral changes that confound the clinical picture, making it difficult to assess whether a soldier can return to duty. Medication may also impair readiness and pose risks to others. Beyond these concerns, pharmaceuticals are framed as interfering with another vital process: soldiers' ability to participate actively in their own recovery.[12] The field manual warns that reliance on medication can undermine nonpharmacologic treatment "based on helping the soldier master his own anxiety himself."[13]

This ideal of the effective soldier as master of his own anxiety is rooted in the principles of forward psychiatry. Forward psychiatry was first devised in World War I and today remains the standard intervention in US military psychiatry for what is now called combat stress reaction (CSR). As its name implies, key to the strategy of forward psychiatry is keeping troops "forward"—that is, as close to the front lines and integrated in their units as possible so that they maintain the expectation of returning to duty. Intended to reduce so-called evacuation syndrome and malingering, forward psychiatry aims to normalize stress experiences in combat and keep rehabilitating soldiers' sight trained on the inevitability of their return to the battlefield by keeping them "in, or near the fight."

A central tenet of forward psychiatry is the avoidance of pathologizing expected stress reactions, premised on the recognition that normal individuals will inevitably experience transient symptoms in response to combat. Drawing on the experiences of US ground forces in World War II, a handbook on combat psychiatry published by the US Army Medical Department emphasizes that the normalization of symptoms is critical to the goal of returning soldiers to duty. "Management consists in pointing out to the soldier that these sensations represent a normal response to combat," the handbook states. "Then the soldier must return to duty, either immediately or after a few hours of rest at the aid station." Managing the soldier's expectations is vital: "Neither he nor the physician should expect that he will be relieved of the symptoms, since they are merely the normal autonomic response to fear." "The soldier," the handbook asserts, "must learn to live with it."[14] In expecting the soldier to learn to live with it, forward psychiatry has emphasized brief and nonpathologizing restorative and convalescent treatments. Medication for the long-term management of symptoms is to be avoided, since it risks solidifying the soldier's perception of being sick and thus unfit to return to duty. By strictly avoiding the patient role, forward psychiatry seeks to mitigate manpower loss and prevent the development of long-term psychiatric disorder.[15]

This long-held conservatism toward medication, evident still in the 1994 US Army combat stress control field manual and its 1998 update, makes the shift in the subsequent 2006 field manual so striking. In the years following the 2003 US-led invasion of Iraq, the Army mental health community revised the field manual based on changes to Army doctrine and recommendations emerging from the US's first sustained conflict in over three decades. The 2006 Army field manual on combat and operational stress control reflects a subtle yet significant shift in the acceptance of psychiatric medication use in theater: medication was now permitted to treat those with reemerging symptoms of a previously diagnosed mental disorder and those newly diagnosed on the battlefield.[16]

Far Forward

It was in this doctrinal context that Captain Hanes expressed a measured yet definitive enthusiasm for the role of psychotropic medications in keeping the deployed soldier deployed. I met him one gray December morning at a state military headquarters in North Carolina, having arrived early enough to get lost in the building's labyrinthine hallways and partitioned offices and still make it to our appointment on time. Captain Hanes's office is dark and the door is shut, so a chair is magically summoned from a nearby conference room and placed for me by a warm, humming Xerox machine, along with coffee in a Styrofoam cup. He arrives 15 minutes later, to gentle chiding from one of the office staff for making me wait. I joke that the old Army adage to hurry up and wait must be true, which cracks a few smiles.

Captain Hanes's office is spare and functional. A few three-ring binders and reference manuals rest at the edge of his desk, and framed diplomas and certificates line the walls. The room is otherwise dominated by large white boards with numbers: tallies of soldiers going through soldier readiness processing (SRP), the administrative and medical process for preparing soldiers to deploy, with a handful of names in red under a column labeled "no go." I can tell he has a packed schedule today, from the incessantly ringing phone that he mostly picks up but sometimes diverts to voicemail. With little prelude, he jumps into sharing with me some of his reflections and experiences as a former Behavioral Health Officer (BHO) in multiple locations in Iraq during a recent deployment, as well as his work developing the psychological readiness program that operates in support of the North Carolina National Guard.

As we broach the topic of psychopharmaceuticals, Captain Hanes first distinguishes what he calls the more common "eyes wide open" cases—in which soldiers already on medication are approved to deploy while continuing on their medication "on the front end"—from those in which medications are newly prescribed in theater. While emphasizing the conservative use of new prescriptions in deployment, Captain Hanes also acknowledges that something like an SSRI can be a critical tool to retain a soldier who might otherwise be unnecessarily evacuated. That might mean seeing a soldier at an aid station, where a provider like a physician assistant (PA) may be able to prescribe from a limited formulary and, ideally, be able to monitor the soldier and document them as stable on the new medication.[17] Alternatively, the provider might arrange for medications to be moved to the forward location where the soldier is stationed. If this is not possible, or if the issue is acute, a soldier may be transported further "back" to a larger installation "where there's more assets for stabilizing the soldier," after which they can be "pushed back forward." The need to keep soldiers in place and the utility of medications in accomplishing that task, quickly became evident in the early years of the conflicts when the military medical community found that soldiers who left theater for mental and behavioral health reasons were very unlikely to return to duty. Rates of return fell precipitously as patients moved further out along the evacuation chain.[18]

The tradition of forward psychiatry joins us like a third presence in the room. "As the BHO who goes forward," Captain Hanes explains, "we go, we take 3,100 forward, my job is to keep 3,100 there. Do everything you can do. We move forward into wherever they're at and try to treat in place, because if we treat in place, the chances are they stay soldier." "You pull them away from their unit," he cautions, "they start turning into patients. It just changes the mindset." Captain Hanes's description of the principles of forward psychiatry is textbook. Yet, in sharp contrast to forward psychiatry's traditional nonpharmacologic approach, Captain Hanes and other military providers I would later interview repositioned medication as a key tool to enabling soldiers to remain with their unit and "stay soldier."

At the same time, Captain Hanes emphasized the risk calculus that comes with new medication, when the provider and military command must consider "the mission of the soldier and how crucial that soldier is to the mission."[19] So, "if it's an O5 who is the battalion commander," he tells me, "we're going to do everything we can—right?—just because of his position, to support him, to keep him there." Though, Captain Hanes adds, even with an "E-2 who is not critical to the mission," it can be worth it to try to keep the soldier in place with medication. Sending even a junior soldier home unnecessarily or prematurely can have negative ramifications for their mental health. "Sending someone home can be like a free fall," Captain Hanes warns. "Because it's just a real sense of not accomplishing what you set out to do. There can be a lot of internal and external negative effects for somebody who gets returned." Far from leading to pathologization and patienthood, medication is now seen as key to maintaining soldiering—and to realizing full selfhood on the battlefield and off.

Interestingly, advocates like Captain Hanes have promoted the use of psychopharmaceuticals as a revitalization of forward psychiatry's core principles. The lack of true "rear" areas that allowed for military personnel to be safely treated and stabilized away from the frontlines in the wars in Iraq and Afghanistan meant it was all the more essential to treat mood and anxiety disorders in situ.[20] By this logic, the relatively easy availability of medications through a combat operational stress control (COSC) team, a battalion aid station, or a division mental health (DMH) section would enable more troops to remain mission capable without leaving station and, in many cases, without dismissal from operational roles.[21]

Captain Hanes's logic reflects what the military medical community itself describes as a revolutionary shift in the use of psychotropic medications as definitive forward treatment in the war on terror. But it also signals a major transformation in what constitutes mental health and its care in war, from forward psychiatry's near-singular concern with combat stress to the broad provision of full-spectrum mental and behavioral health care. Indeed, psychopharmaceuticals in deployment can even enable projects of self-realization, as Captain Hanes envisioned. These shifts, however, have not been uncontroversial. How to account for this apparent pendulum swing from the medication-free soldier as master of his own anxiety of the 1990s to today's medicated soldier as a self-actualized person? Any attempt at such an account must look beyond top-echelon military strategy and planning to the ways the buildup of psychopharmaceuticals in theater accumulated through reactive improvisation, experiential knowledge, and a certain opportunism in the war on terror.

DRIFT

Despite the strategic planning that the evolution of military policy would suggest, the buildup of psychopharmaceuticals in the wars in Iraq and Afghanistan was in part the consequence of a series of accidents and stopgaps. Much of this related to the unanticipated challenges of gatekeeping—namely, the creep of standards and practices of psychopharmaceutical use and outpatient mental health care common to American life into the military corporate body and, by extension, into theater. The rise of battlefield psychopharmaceuticals, then, was less the result of premeditated, high-level military strategy than a matter of drift.[22] Once in theater, psychopharmaceuticals would appear as the solution to a wide range of occupational, interpersonal, and operational problems. Their uses and applications proliferated.

Gatekeeping of mental health and psychopharmaceutical use begins at the point of military enlistment. During the war on terror, applicants who were currently taking psychotropic medications or had certain psychiatric diagnoses including major depression, bipolar disorder, or psychosis were typically disqualified from entering the military.[23] Waivers were sometimes granted if the individual had been off medication for a period, if their condition was stable, or if there was a low risk of recurrence. But once in the Army, soldiers could be diagnosed and prescribed psychotropic medication by military health care professionals. In some cases, they sought care "off the books" from civilian providers, outside the knowledge of the Army.[24]

In the early years of the wars in Iraq and Afghanistan, military psychiatrists were caught unprepared by the medication needs of their soldiers, an issue they attributed to the large proportion of National Guard and Reserve soldiers in their ranks. In 2004, President Bush took an unusual step to plug the hole in troop deficits, calling up 37,000 members of the National Guard and Reserve.[25] By 2005, they accounted for nearly half of the total army in Iraq.[26] In a 2007 publication, three military psychiatrists writing about their deployments in the early years of the war in Iraq describe being caught unprepared by the needs of a changing army. The increased reliance on National Guard and Reserve soldiers "meant that the Army was receiving personnel who were treated according to civilian community standards rather than military readiness standards concerning prescriptions for SSRIs, atypical antidepressants, and antianxiety medications."[27] "If a psychiatrist had to contend only with new-onset disorders, then a limited formulary would suffice," they write. "However, soldiers may deploy with a wide range of medications and present in theater only as they are about to run out of medications."[28] The authors propose an expanded and diversified psychiatric formulary to maintain supplies for reserve force soldiers already on psychopharmaceuticals at the time of deployment. National Guard and Reserve soldiers were quickly identified by providers as having brought in variable civilian standards that contributed significantly to initial pharmaceutical supply challenges.[29]

The military medical community thus explained the unexpected turn to psychopharmaceuticals in the war on terror through what I have elsewhere described as a discourse of "pharmaceutical creep." This discourse blamed an overmedicated civilian society for spreading psychopharmaceutical use into the military corporate body and, ultimately, onto the battlefield.[30] Pharmaceutical creep emerged as a distinct clinical, operational, and logistical supply concern for military providers in the wars in Iraq and Afghanistan, while resonating with long-standing anxieties about soldier quality and fitness.[31] The finger-pointing at National Guard and Reserve soldiers is significant. Unlike full-time, active-duty soldiers, reserve force soldiers are part-time personnel who maintain nonsoldiering occupations and reside off military installations, though they may be deputized to active duty and deploy. These reserve military forces are therefore "social and organizational amalgams—they are soldiers and civilians, they are outside yet inside the military systems, and are invested in both spheres."[32] Pharmaceutical creep courtesy of reserve military forces thus raised the specter of military corporate body contamination, stoking concerns for compromised gatekeeping at a time when the US military, and the Army in particular, faced continuing struggles to meet recruitment targets.[33] The medication use among troops that would take deployed providers by surprise would come to symbolize the declining quality of recruits more generally, while highlighting the disproportionate lack of readiness among Army reserve forces, in particular.[34]

But the reasons for the failure to plan for psychiatric medications early in the wars arguably go far deeper. They reflect what historian David

Kieran observes was a broader unpreparedness by the US Army Medical Department (AMEDD) to anticipate the mental health needs of its active duty and reserve soldiers in so-called wars of unknown duration. After the Vietnam War, the US military would turn away from insurgency warfare to focus on building capacity to fight conventional war against potential Soviet aggression in Europe. In lock step, AMEDD prepared itself for the likely mental health fallouts of a brutal but brief war with the Soviet Union. As Kieran notes, while Army researchers did take combat stress seriously in the '80s and early '90s, "they developed combat stress protocols modeled on notions of battle fatigue that originated in the early twentieth century, largely forgot any lessons that Vietnam might have offered, and focused instead on the war the United States thought—or perhaps hoped—that it would fight."[35] By the war on terror, AMEDD was neither prepared for protracted war nor expecting to have its soldiers deploying while already on medications for depression, ADHD, and anxiety.

While providers were initially caught off guard, supply challenges were quickly identified. The deployment formulary—the reference list of medications approved for use, which enables standardization and stocking during military operations—expanded apace to contain a broad spectrum of antidepressants, sleep aids, and stimulants, categories of medication specifically noted by military psychiatrists as lacking.[36] This formulary was frequently reevaluated at quarterly meetings held by military pharmacists, at which providers were allowed to make suggestions for additions or substitutions. With time, several options for resupply of medications became available in theater. DMH units were generally located at Level II aid stations with access to medications, and COSC units often had relationships with local unit medical clinics. COSC units could also establish medical resupply chains with medical logistics units. Psychiatrists played a central role in maintaining communication with resupply sources and reporting utilization trends, which enabled medical supply officers to anticipate and maintain supplies. Combat Support Hospital (CSH) pharmacies at large, fixed locations providing more comprehensive care—like Balad Theater Hospital and the 28th Combat Support Hospital in Baghdad—began collecting information on prescription requirements and stocking chronic medications for soldiers in their area, while units were instructed to provide detailed listings of their soldiers' chronic medication needs. This

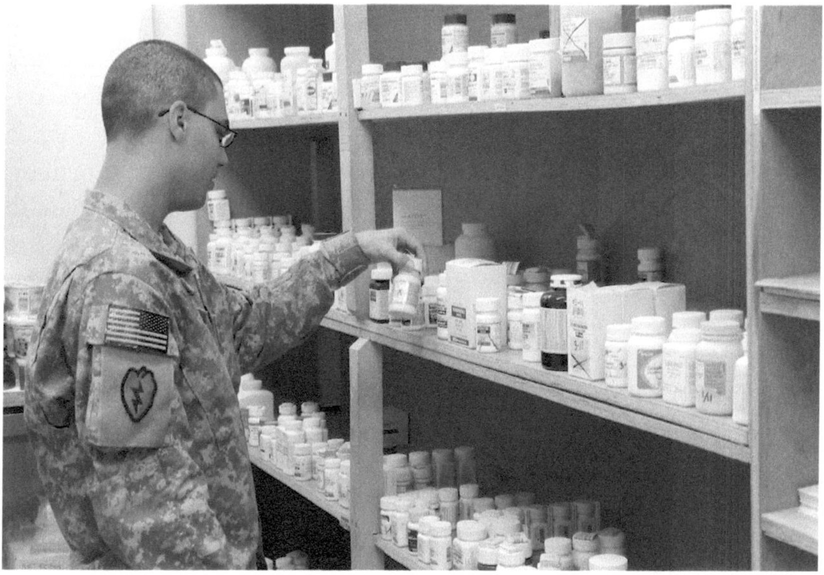

Figure 2. Restocking medication shelves. Photograph by SGT Brandon Bolick, via DVIDS.

requirement would eventually lead to a major reengineering of the deployment process to ensure that prescription requirements were captured in a clinical database during predeployment processing before soldiers even set foot in Iraq and Afghanistan.

But even when pharmaceuticals became more readily available, military providers had little guidance for how to administer them on the battlefield. Following the Vietnam War, the Army lost, abandoned, or destroyed documentation that included records pertaining to the provision of military psychiatric services, and AMEDD made no effort to develop a historical summary of psychiatry during the war.[37] Even though psychoactive medications were known to have been widely used during the conflict, little institutional knowledge would be passed on. No reports on utilization rates or guidelines for the use of psychotropic medications were published from the Persian Gulf War, likely because of the lack of prolonged combat exposure and because stress-control practice continued to emphasize triage and normalization.[38]

Experience started to accrue with peace-keeping deployments in the 1990s, but knowledge shared was largely piecemeal and sparse. In a rare publication providing a rationale and decision-making process for a deployment formulary from this period, Army psychiatrist Elspeth Ritchie was the first to propose two broad categories of emergency and maintenance medications.[39] Reports from a year-long peacekeeping mission to Bosnia-Herzegovina also mention the use of psychotropic medications in outpatient visits, indicating a nascent shift toward mental health provision in overseas military operations that more closely resembled garrison-based mental health care.[40]

Even then, clinical guidelines specific to deployment would remain desperately lacking. It was not until 2006 that the DoD released, for the first time, a memorandum outlining the restrictions and minimum health deployment criteria for service members with diagnosed psychiatric conditions, including those on medication treatment.[41] Prior to this policy, military psychiatrists did not have clear regulatory guidance for deployed psychiatric care or which mental health conditions or medications would render a soldier nondeployable. And while intended to bring clarity, the memo left much to the military provider's clinical judgment and the needs of military command. If a condition developed in theater, for example, providers were instructed to take a variety of factors into account, including work duties and possibilities for monitoring and follow-up, but were provided no specific criteria for doing so.[42] With the exception of the stipulation that "psychotic or bipolar disorders are considered disqualifying for deployment," the memo stated that "there are few medications that are inherently disqualifying for deployment for all military occupational specialties, to all potential operational locations, and at all times during the conduct of operations."[43] The memo thus codified an informal practice that placed on individual military providers the responsibility to use their own judgment, in coordination with military command, to decide who could deploy and who could remain deployed on which medications, on a largely case-by-case basis.[44]

While such policies were intended to provide straightforward regulatory guidance, actual practice proved complicated. Two military psychiatrists who deployed to Afghanistan within a year of completing their residency painted their experience of being "thrust into the breach" through a litany of scenarios they were not expecting, given official guidelines. "Regardless of whether a certain disorder makes a soldier non-deployable per regulations, you will see patients with that disorder (and sometimes taking the requisite anti-psychotic medication) while deployed," they write. "A psychiatrist may see service members who were previously hospitalized for suicidal thoughts or behavior, but deployed via a command waiver, with medications that are difficult to refill in such an austere environment."[45] Policies governing deployability could quickly become insufficient for clinicians seeing soldiers who shouldn't have deployed in the first place or who were permitted to deploy on medications that were difficult to refill in theater. Policy was not keeping up with reality.

MENTAL HEALTH IN REAL TIME

While little institutional or experiential knowledge existed at the start of the wars concerning the battlefield use of psychopharmaceuticals, the wars themselves would see the continuous rollout of real-time data on military mental health. This development would play a significant role in influencing public sentiment, transforming Army culture, and evolving concepts and practices of mental health treatment on and off the battlefield. Typically, it takes years and often decades after combat before researchers examine the mental health impacts of war. However, as troops were mobilizing to Afghanistan and Iraq in 2002 and 2003, respectively, Army researchers built on experience gained during the Bosnia and Kosovo deployments to initiate comprehensive plans to study the impacts of war on soldiers. Recognizing that few studies had yet to examine mental health problems and health care utilization proximal to the time of war, they sought to provide real-time data to inform policy, programs, and training targeting the mental health of military personnel as well as their families. This steady looping of data, analysis, and implementation would shape the broader setting in which psychopharmaceuticals would come to be harnessed as part of the larger toolkit addressing the impacts of mental health on mission readiness. If the medication needs of soldiers initially caught deployed military psychiatrists and military medical policy planners by surprise at the start of the war on terror, operational research psychologists and epidemiologists, by contrast, were poised from the outset to study the war's unfolding psychological and neurological effects.

With the onset of the war in Afghanistan, researchers at Walter Reed Army Institute of Research (WRAIR) initiated a major effort in 2002 to measure the mental health impacts of the war. The research program, called "Interventions to Enhance Warfighter Psychological Resilience," helped to establish the need for real-time data to predict rates of mental disorder, assess and develop tools for psychological screening in deployed troops, and to develop interventions to support psychological adjustment to the demands of combat and improve resiliency. Using tools such as population-based health care data systems, epidemiological surveillance, and anonymous cross-sectional and longitudinal surveys, Army researchers worked directly with military units to produce ongoing assessments that would inform policy change in real time, establishing new methodologies to conceptualize, quantify, and manage population-level mental health on the battlefield in the process.[46] This "metrification" of troop mental health would be made possible by integrated electronic databases available after the Persian Gulf War.[47]

War was in continuous feedback, generating data that could be rapidly analyzed and fed into implementation. Initiated in 2003, the large-scale epidemiological surveillance study, known as the five-year land combat study, used anonymous surveys of over 50,000 military personnel in combat infantry brigades serving in Iraq and Afghanistan to assess mental health and well-being before, during, and after deployment. Just a year after the study was launched, data from some of the first units to return from deployment had been analyzed and published in the *New England Journal of Medicine*, providing the first systematic overview of the mental health of soldiers and Marines involved in combat operations in Iraq and Afghanistan. Data from this study would also be presented in multiple congressional testimonies and supported another key initiative that would develop serial, anonymous epidemiological assessments of mental health of troops during deployment on a near yearly basis, known as the MHAT studies.

Beginning in 2003, Mental Health Advisory Teams, or MHATs, were chartered by the US Army Surgeon General to assess the mental health status of soldiers. Each MHAT conducted comprehensive mental health surveillance of deployed US military personnel, offering a "proactive" examination of mental health in combat deployments. As a result of these findings, the Army would revise its combat and operational stress control doctrine and training and devise ratios of mental health professionals to troops to optimize distribution and access to treatment throughout theater. The ability to now monitor the prevalence of mental and behavioral health concerns and to identify emerging threats to soldier mental health would expand the realm of responsibilities for military mental health care providers. Indeed, as military strategy in Iraq shifted from ground warfare to stability operations and once theater mental health assets established the fundamentals of their jobs in a combat environment, providers' roles began to expand into specialty services not typical of combat psychiatry, including forensic and administrative psychiatry services.[48]

Real-time data would also reach the American public, fueling concern for mental health struggles among soldiers and veterans as the wars wore on. The war on terror would see deeply conflicting notions about the nature of mental health in combat. In the tradition of forward psychiatry, the Army and VA sought to reassure the American public that stress disorders were normal, treatable, and transient reactions to abnormal circumstances—but accounts in the media and in Congress framed soldiers' mental health problems as persistent, severe, and fundamentally abnormal.[49]

Media coverage also brought the practices of military mental health care providers in theater under heightened scrutiny. In May 2006, *The Hartford Courant* ran a series of investigative journalism pieces under the headline, "Mentally Unfit, Forced to Fight." One article in the series recounted stories of soldiers prescribed medication in deployment who later committed suicide. Antidepressants and other psychotropics, the authors suggested, were being prescribed in theater too liberally, with insufficient surveillance and follow-up—and this despite FDA warnings that these drugs can increase suicidal thoughts. They described military doctors treating combat stress symptoms and sending some soldiers back to the front lines after rest and a three-day regimen of medication, despite evidence that it typically takes several weeks for the prescribed medications to begin working. In response to a Congressional directive, just months after this series was published, the DoD released the 2006 memo providing its first policy guidance for the deployability of soldiers on psychiatric medications.

Real-time surveillance of troop mental health was critical to the buildup of data—as well as of public scrutiny—that would guide the standardization of psychopharmaceutical use on the counterinsurgency battlefield. Little of this would have been possible, however, without the material buildup of the landscape of war and occupation.

CARE IN THE FOBSCAPE

The accrual of data, the development of clinical guidelines and policies, and the growth of deployment formularies would all come with time. But the practical use of psychopharmaceuticals on the battlefield would also require the infrastructural buildup of occupied Iraq and Afghanistan that shifting military strategy demanded and time enabled. It required the development of "mature infrastructure," in the military jargon, most notably in the form of an expansive network of built-up installations and a spread of embedded providers circulating across the counterinsurgency battlefield. This buildup would facilitate both the material provisioning of psychopharmaceuticals and their broad role across the scope of full-spectrum mental and behavioral health care.

While historically, the Army had drawn support from activities located on Allied bases or from US bases established in host countries, that strategy would shift in the war on terror. With the initial invasion of Iraq in March 2003, Kuwait served as the major "staging area" for US-led forces as units prepared to cross the border into Iraq. But as US military strategy shifted to counterinsurgency and nation-building operations by May of the same year, the US Army Corps of Engineers and private contractors began a massive construction effort to house and sustain an occupation Army. Built-up installations known as Forward Operating Bases, or FOBs, provided the framework and network for the US military presence and operations in Iraq and Afghanistan, distributing US forces among the population while providing a relatively secure position "situated literally on the battlefields."[50] Thus, while used to support tactical operations, FOBs would also have operational and strategic implications.[51] The

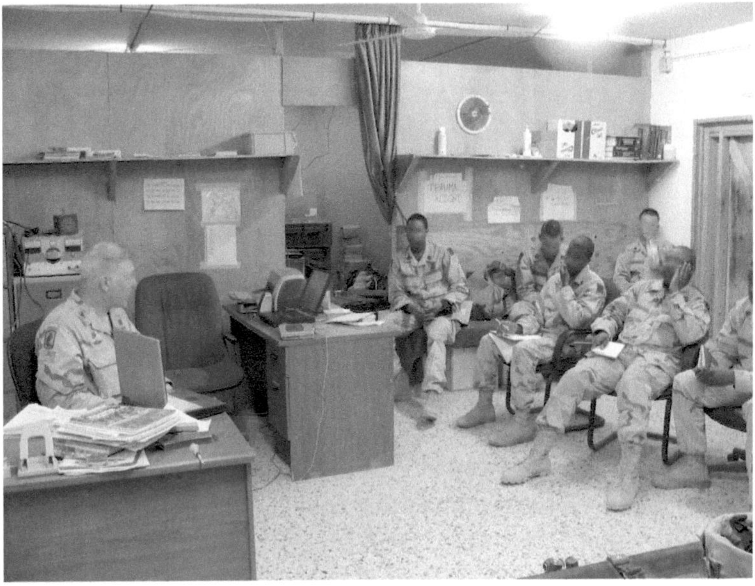

Figure 3. Combat stress control conducts a mental health maintenance class at FOB McKenzie in Balad, Iraq. Photograph by US DoD, via DVIDS.

construction of combat outposts, or COPs, served to further extend the "FOBscape."[52] Situated miles from a supporting FOB and typically occupied by platoon-size elements for brief periods of time, with units constantly rotating back and forth between the COP and supporting FOB, COPs were intended to provide a further "constant presence," while allowing for agility. Together, FOBs and COPs strove to provide continuous maintenance, transportation, logistics, and medical and personnel support over the expeditionary expanse of US military war and occupation.

Conditions at FOBs varied greatly. At one extreme, huge "super-FOBs" such as Bagram Air Base north of Kabul in Afghanistan and FOB Al Asad in Al Anbar Province in western Iraq boasted air-conditioned sleeping and work trailers, as well as an array of franchise fast-food chains, coffee shops, and internet cafés. In general terms, FOBs provided housing logistics and support areas where munitions and supplies were stored and vehicles could be maintained and repaired and locations from which operations could be launched. They also provided a relatively permanent and secure location where mail could be received and transferred, soldiers could retire to beds, showers, and warm meals at the end of the day, and medical care was provided.

The maturation of infrastructure would help transform mental health care on the counterinsurgency battlefield, enabling the shift from forward psychiatry as triage and nonpharmacologic treatment for combat stress to mental health care including treatment more consistent with outpatient psychiatric practices. Care in deployment would thus increasingly mirror soldiers' expectations of outpatient mental health care in garrison, facilitating the slippage to treatment for a broad range of mental and behavioral health concerns. The built-up environment of occupation would have direct impacts on how care took shape and how it was delivered. For example, what would eventually become a relatively robust tele–behavioral health system allowed soldiers in remote locations or at installations without dedicated mental health care services to video chat with providers without either party needing to travel.[53] Telehealth would only be possible with the dedicated bandwidth and established network capacity of a "mature" battlespace.

Mature infrastructure reshaped not only how care was accessed; it also reshaped the problems for which soldiers sought and received care and the treatment that military health professionals provided. In the wars in Iraq and Afghanistan, COSC teams of mental health providers offered prevention and intervention to soldiers, with the primary intent of returning them to battle. In keeping with the tradition of forward psychiatry, one of the central principles behind COSC has been to maintain a nonclinical approach to managing soldiers with combat and operational stress reaction, or COSR. The Army uses COSR like its combat stress predecessor: as a subclinical diagnosis understood to be a transient reaction to the cumulative stresses of military operations, with the expectation during the war on terror that over 95 percent of service members experiencing COSR would return to duty.[54] Yet reports suggest that during the first years of the wars, the average number of new psychiatric contacts rose disproportionately higher than the average number of new combat stress contacts and that military providers may have been more willing to use medication to treat combat stress and thus convert what would traditionally have been a new combat stress contact into a psychiatric one.[55] Why were COSC personnel treating—and likely diagnosing—psychiatric conditions on the battlefield?

The reasons for this slippage were likely multiple, but certainly infrastructural. As war and occupation persisted, the provisioning of combat stress care in more built-up military environments would lend a new "feel" to the services provided. Three high-level medical officers writing about their experiences during the Iraq War report that living and working conditions for soldiers improved considerably beginning in 2005, with direct impacts on outpatient mental health practice. During the invasion of Iraq and in its immediate aftermath, "soldiers (including mental health personnel) lived and worked out of tents for the most part, using burnout latrines, field-expedient showers, and meals, ready-to-eat."[56] As the US-led invasion became a long occupation, US forces fortified bases, supply routes, and staging areas, leading to an expansion of FOBs to accommodate an occupation Army. As climate-controlled trailers and buildings with electricity and running water replaced tents, this transformation would alter the provision and perception of mental health care for both soldiers and providers, where "working in buildings instead of working outside the same tent where one lives lends itself to a *more clinical feel* (my emphasis)."[57] As the infrastructure of occupation literally hardened, services provided under the umbrella of combat stress became more akin to what soldiers would have experienced had they sought mental or behavioral health care in garrison or through a civilian provider—indeed, these interactions would feel "more clinical." Combat stress treatment in war increasingly resembled mental health care at home.

For COSC personnel, who were trained to normalize stress responses to combat and were unprepared to handle psychiatric disorders in theater, this slippage raised fundamental questions at once practical and epistemic. Are COSR and psychiatric disorders always categorically different? Might they sometimes overlap in symptoms and treatment? Should documentation for the treatment of a behavioral health diagnosis or psychiatric disorder be different from documentation for COSR? COSR, by definition, is situational and should be treated as a temporary reaction using brief, restorative interventions. It typically requires no documentation, with notation in the outpatient treatment record reserved only for those with more severe, yet normal, stress behaviors. By contrast, many

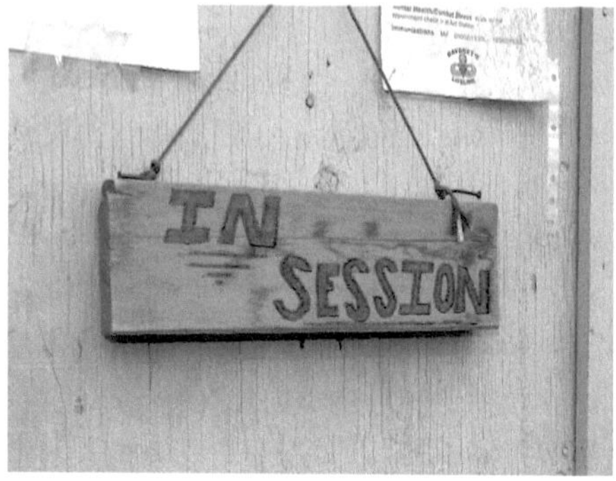

Figure 4. Weathered "In Session" sign outside Combat Stress Control at FOB Fenty in Afghanistan. Photograph by CPT Monika Comeaux, via DVIDS.

psychiatric disorders are considered chronic and may require ongoing management and documentation. COSC personnel, furthermore, were officially told they must consider "behavioral health diagnoses that resemble COSR but defer making the diagnosis" to "preserve the Soldier's expectations of normalcy."[58] Their emphasis should be on triage and stabilization, not long-term treatment. What should be the role of medication in addressing these distinctions? These were questions military providers would have to navigate in the course of their daily work and in the absence of precedent.

The slippage toward psychiatric diagnosis in this context can be seen in the case of adjustment disorder and acute stress reaction. Adjustment disorder has been reported as the most common psychiatric diagnosis among military personnel in the wars in Iraq and Afghanistan and the most commonly diagnosed mental health disorder among active-duty military personnel.[59] Both adjustment disorder and acute stress reaction are mental health conditions that occur in response to stressful events and may cause emotional distress and difficulty in everyday functioning. Like COSR and acute stress reaction, adjustment disorder is also defined as transient and less severe than other mental health diagnoses like PTSD and major depression. It also shares with COSR the notion that it can be a normal, if maladaptive, response to a stressor. But as a psychiatric diagnosis, adjustment disorder can imply different modalities of treatment and have potentially different implications for the soldier's medical record and duty limits. Whereas adjustment disorder can be caused by a less severe stressful event, such as a relationship breakup or a change in jobs, an acute stress reaction is typically understood to be caused by a severe or traumatic event. While not a psychiatric diagnosis recognized in the Diagnostic and Statistical Manual, or DSM, acute stress reaction can evolve into what the DSM does recognize as acute stress disorder.[60] If specific symptoms of acute stress disorder worsen beyond one month, the condition may progress to PTSD. A stepped care approach for acute stress reaction in the military includes detection and assessment, followed by behavioral intervention, and medication intervention to help manage debilitating symptoms and prevent progression to PTSD.[61]

Several mental health professionals and general providers told me that COSR is essentially synonymous with acute stress disorder, while others said that COSR was on the "same spectrum" as—and, for one PA, nearly synonymous with—adjustment disorder.[62] In the epistemic slippages between COSR, adjustment disorder, and acute stress reaction, medication often served an ambiguous role.[63] In the case of COSR-cum-acute-stress-disorder, the diagnosis of acute stress disorder likely offered military providers a practical way to begin definitive treatment—often with SSRIs or short-term benzodiazepines—within the constraints of circumstance and time that characterize deployment and thereby to mitigate progression to PTSD.[64] While in the case of adjustment disorder, treatment criteria prioritize psychotherapeutic and supportive counseling interventions, military providers have used medications to alleviate specific symptoms like anxiety or sleep problems, a practice likely supported by the psychiatric nature of the diagnosis itself. Treatment possibilities in this space of slippage and constraint would have to be navigated on a case-by-case basis, in an institutional and clinical context that increasingly expected providers to be full-spectrum in their care.

The infrastructural buildup of war and occupation were vital to shaping the care provided and expected. But the buildup of battlefield psychopharmaceuticals was also facilitated by shifts within the military itself, including the Army's efforts to destigmatize mental health care within its ranks. The post-9/11 Army would actively work to reform its institutional culture around mental health through a series of initiatives focused on improving access to confidential treatment, promoting a culture of support, and normalizing mental health discussions through leadership engagement. A critical part of this normalization has been the expectation that, in global counterinsurgency warfare, anyone and everyone is a potential stress casualty.

OCCUPATION STRESS

Military psychiatry has utilized a variety of terms over its long history to capture the expected responses of soldiers to the stress of combat.[65] During World War I, the British psychiatrist and anthropologist W. H. Rivers described a type of neurosis suffered by soldiers that he attributed to a form of repression, suggesting that soldiers would attempt to mentally withdraw from the adverse stimuli of war.[66] By World War II, the generic term of "war neurosis" would be replaced by "battle fatigue" or "combat fatigue," which would remain important concepts for US Army physicians during the Vietnam era.[67] Battle fatigue remains in use today in discussions of what US military medicine now calls "combat stress" and "combat-operational stress." In February of 1999, DoD Directive 6490.5 mandated the use of the term "combat stress reactions" to describe the "acute emotional disorder long recognized by military commanders and physicians."[68] The term was ultimately expanded to COSR after requests by the Navy, Marines, and Air Force to recognize that military personnel are just as vulnerable to stress reactions during peacetime as they are during combat.

The expansion to COSR is significant. In the war on terror, it suggested that anyone—be they a cook stationed exclusively on a FOB or an infantryman who left the FOB daily—was susceptible to stress. This was in part because combat support troops, who were often colocated with combat troops, could be tasked with tactical missions or could be vulnerable to mortar attacks, even if they never "left the wire." But the concept of COSR also suggested that stress in enduring war and occupation was not only combat-related: it was now formally understood to be interpersonal, occupational, and environmental.[69] Soldiers and providers offered me examples: stress might appear in the deployed young private who leaves his small rural Midwestern town only to be suddenly immersed in an unfamiliar cultural environment. It could emerge from trying to manage a dissolving marriage from afar or from dealing with toxic military leadership

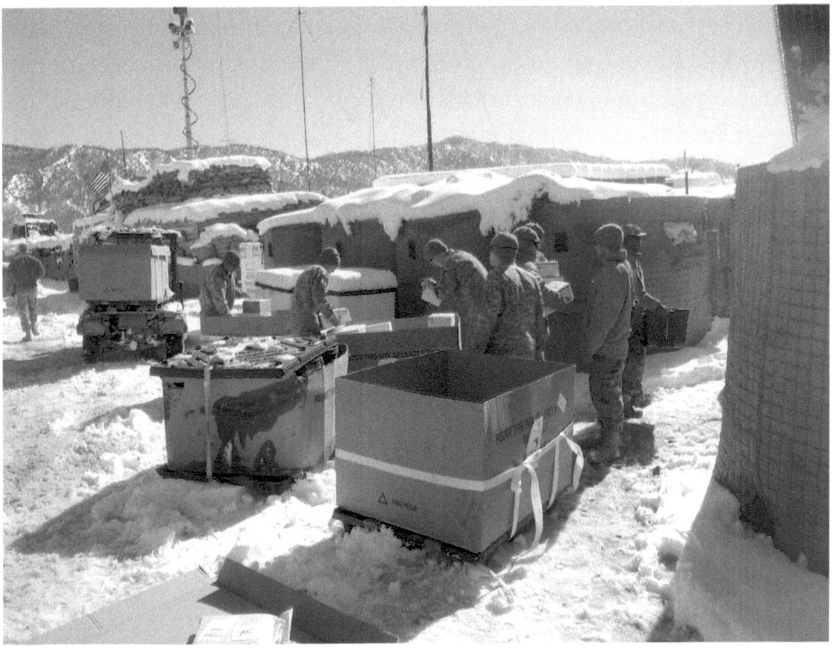

Figure 5. Sorting mail at COP Zerok in East Paktika Province, Afghanistan. Photograph by PFC Brandon Rickert, via DVIDS.

in the form of an overbearing platoon sergeant. As Army psychologists Brett Moore and Greg Reger write, "COSR is a more inclusive term. . . . Everyone is a potential stress casualty, hence the appreciated addition of 'operational' in the designation."[70] COSR thus offers a revealing, albeit medicalized and depoliticized, lens on "occupation stress" in two senses: stress inherent to military work as a professional occupation and stress associated with being a force of imperial occupation. This expanded framing signals an emerging recognition within the military community that it is not combat alone that produces injury, but occupation as well.

While the term generally hadn't entered the vernacular of the lower enlisted ranks at the time of this research, COSR was ubiquitous in the parlance of providers and military leadership. The concept of COSR officially recognized the idea that stress was expected regardless of one's occupation and location in the war on terror and that it should be "business as usual" for military personnel to seek assistance in dealing with it. As the idea that anyone could experience COSR became mainstream among clinicians, psychopharmaceuticals often played an operationally definitive yet clinically ambiguous role, critical to keeping soldiers in place and maintaining the mission, while linked to diagnosis in ways that could be quite variable from one provider to the next.

Javier spoke extensively with me about how psychopharmaceuticals could be used to ease soldiers through expected stressors in theater. We were one month into the Covid-19 shutdown and speaking by Zoom, both of us balancing the interview with childcare on our respective ends—Javier cautiously optimistic that successive episodes of Sesame Street might hold his three-year-old's attention, and me regularly interrupted by my four-year-old's mounting inquiries about when I would be ready to build Legos. There's a mutual generosity in our shared circumstances as we check in about the other child's waning patience.

Javier is articulate and sharp, with an acerbic wit. His thoughtfulness as a clinician is evident as he walks me through diverse examples and cases from his 2013 deployment to Afghanistan in crystalline, complex detail. Javier tells me he was relatively comfortable with prescribing psychopharmaceuticals in theater but emphasized that he would only do so if it were "truly clinically indicated."[71] He relied on consultations with his psychologist colleagues for diagnosis and, at least unofficially, their medication suggestions—advice along the lines of, "a little Celexa is going to help overcome the anxiety in this case" or "a whiff of a beta-blocker will help in that one." But even with the psychologists providing their input, as the primary care PA, it ultimately came down to Javier to do the risk stratification and recommend to military command whether a soldier of concern could stay in theater or should be medically evacuated. A multitude of dynamic considerations went into making any single recommendation.[72] Fortunately, the guidelines were "perfectly vague enough to allow you to navigate them within reason," said Javier.

These medications, he told me, were ultimately important because they could help the stressed soldier "conquer the deployment." "We're trying to keep people in theater and a lot of times we're keeping them in theater because it's the best thing for them," said Javier. "The worst thing you can do is put them in the Army's medical system or send them home as though,

'You can't hack it, you can't hang. You've got to go home.' That's the worst thing you could do." Reflecting a long-term view of mental health beyond the deployment, Javier asserted that "the best outcomes are the people who you helped, and you kept in theater, and they went home with pride and maybe they stayed in the Army, maybe they didn't, but they did really well knowing that they've made it through." He went on to clarify, "I'm not talking about the guy who'd sleep for one hour a night, not eating, talking crazy about hurting himself. I'm talking about the kid who is away from home for the first time in his life and he's freaking out. Understandably. It's a steep learning curve trying to learn the job and get along with his peers who are older and more mature than him." That kid was the one you wanted to keep in the fight, and psychopharmaceuticals could help, Javier explained. Let that kid "win their fight safely," and "that just became part of their story, part of the testimony of their life."

But while medication could help win the fight for the generic kid soldier struggling to adjust to deployment, overprescription and overreliance on psychopharmaceuticals were real problems, Javier said. Pills often became the convenient solution to all kinds of issues in theater. While listening to him, I think of the law of the instrument: if all you have is a hammer, everything starts to look like a nail. Javier told me that overreliance on medication happened most frequently with patients who were referred by command. Javier was pointing to the two ways soldiers come to the attention of military mental health care: through what is called "voluntary-" or "self-referral" and through "command-referral"—the latter referring to when commanders identify a soldier for mental health evaluation. Despite the neat binary, treatment for mental and physical health in the military happens along a spectrum that blurs elements of forced or coerced intervention to more agential forms of care-seeking, quickly exposing the limits of conventional concepts like barriers to care and stigma in the dynamics of military health care access. In the military institutional context where health is fundamentally tied to performance and medical channels can serve as administrative means for the temporary or permanent removal of a soldier, Javier told me that interpersonal and occupational problems can quickly be made into medical problems. A frontline supervisor, for example, might have issues with a soldier for any number of reasons and refer that soldier to see the doc for mental health in order to expedite their removal.

Javier recalls several cases where he had to push back against command and assert that the nature of the problem was not medical; but often in those cases, the supervisor referring the soldier "would just keep applying stress until it became a medical issue. They just make life so miserable for the person to where it does become a clinically significant adjustment disorder or depressed mood from this toxic environment." At that point, the problem moves "out of the realm of just an occupational problem" to become "a psychiatric problem for which medications are clinically indicated." And sometimes, it's all because of a "personality thing," Javier said, shaking his head. "But that's the military," he tells me. "You're stuck." But that's also the military tasked with occupation, I think to myself. "You're trapped in this environment that is not ideal for you, and you can't leave," Javier says. "You can't leave."

. . . . .

As a newly recognized asset in the work of forward care, psychopharmaceuticals became a critical tool in military psychiatry's objective to stabilize soldiers and keep them in place during the war on terror. Pills were used to enable soldiers to continue to fight, seize, and hold territory; they were also used to ease interpersonal problems in the workplace and the stress of being far from home and help the young soldier standing in his own way. As we've seen in this chapter, the normalization of psychopharmaceuticals on the battlefield required discursive and material shifts in the concept and treatment of soldier mental health. The pharmaceutical solution, however, would not have been possible without the time and military buildup of enduring war and occupation.

The developments tracked in this chapter underscore how the buildup of psychopharmaceuticals in theater unfolded less as the product of strategic planning than as a response to multiple, overlapping diffusions: soldiers deploying with unknown medication needs, the dissemination of real-time data on soldier mental health into the US public sphere, the expectations soldiers brought for outpatient mental health care in theater, and the spread of psychotropic prescribing practices and mental health care into general medicine. This was a buildup resulting from drift more than from any blueprint on the part of the Army or its medical planners.

But once in theater and later routinized in military policy and standards of care, psychopharmaceuticals opened opportunities for providers, soldiers, and military command alike to leverage them for a myriad of operational, clinical, and personal ends. First among these opportunities was addressing the embodied dilemmas and recruitment challenges of chronic war.

2 Chronic

> Time may be the ultimate arbiter of success: time to bring safety and security to an embattled populace; time to provide for the essential, immediate humanitarian needs of the people; time to restore basic public order and a semblance of normalcy to life; and time to rebuild the institutions of government and market economy that provide the foundations for enduring peace and stability. This is the essence of stability operations.
>
> *Stability Operations Field Manual 3-07*, iv

> We advertise that we can go anywhere in the world in 18 hours and destroy anyone. So, we've got to pay for it.
>
> Special Forces soldier

Sergeant First Class Wright peers through the wraparound windows of the large conference room where I am waiting alone, like a goldfish in a bowl. That he is in his Army combat uniform (ACU) in a public library in the middle of the day causes no one to blink an eye in this military town. I give him a tentative wave. After confirming that he's in the right place, Wright enters, lanky, tall, with a thin mustache, and enveloped in a haze of cigarette smoke. He must have snuck a quick smoke before walking in.

We've only just met, yet Wright wastes little time before he is cracking jokes with me about, of all things, death. Death is his life, after all—at least since 2005, when he reclassed from communications to mortuary affairs. He's been in the Army long enough now to have two careers, having just hit his 18-year mark. When I ask him how he came into mortuary affairs, he quips with a straight face, "I've always been interested in it." The longer story is that he joined the military before September 11, 2001. At the time, he was told, "We don't really need anybody to do that job." That would change soon after Wright began basic training and the towers fell. Cracking a boyish smile, he tells me, "When it came time to re-enlist, I was like, 'Hey, can I get this job now?'" Wright seems intent on making me find humor in the work of war death. When not peppering our conversation with corny funerary puns, he regales me with mortuary hi-jinks, like the time he hid in a display casket to scare the chaplain. Finding lightness, he seems to be instructing me, is also part of the work of war death.

Wright and his team, after all, have been tasked with "processing" war's literal remains, to use his term. Despite the jokes, there is a stark materiality to how he talks about what war metabolizes. Telling me that he processed 365 cases during his 2008 Kuwait deployment alone, he describes the bureaucratic routine with an economy of words: "Someone is killed. Their body is taken to the hospital. They're pronounced dead. Then they're brought to us. We're the ones that sit there and inventory everything." That includes the possessions on the body, often good luck charms and mementos carried in pockets. He remembers pictures, letters from family. There was also the pilot who put a nickel in his flight suit pocket for every flight he completed. Wright counted 25. "We had to inventory them all."

Wright's career has spanned two simultaneous protracted wars and includes five deployments over two continents. Over that time, he has learned as a team leader what to do to endure the grind and to help his team perform the endless day in and day out of embalming, dressing, casketing, and all else that (recognized) war death necessitates. For Wright, this has included protecting his soldiers by removing them from cases that might be, in his words, "triggering." Like the time he excused the one soldier on their team who had kids so she wouldn't have to see the bodies of the Iraqi children who had been killed in a school bombing. Or the time in Korea when Wright pulled out the private whose dad had beaten him up as a kid so he wouldn't have to handle the case of the six-month-old whose soldier father, in frustrated rage over her incessant crying, had thrown her across a room. Such is the relational labor Wright has done over the span of two long wars to keep on keeping on—a kind of intimate labor both necessitated and made possible by enduring war. To keep *himself* keeping on has required multiple medications, among them, Wellbutrin, Prozac, and Ambien for sleep. Wright has been given as many diagnoses over the past decade: generalized anxiety disorder with PTSD symptoms, depression, and adjustment disorder.

In a time of chronic war, the occupation Army in the wars in Iraq and Afghanistan endured unprecedented demands in the goal to provide constant presence. This chapter considers the accumulated embodied dilemmas of waging America's forever wars and the ambitious task asked of medicine to resolve them. The previous chapter tracked some of the discursive and material processes that contributed to the mainstreaming of psychopharmaceutical use on the global counterinsurgency battlefield. It situated the routinization of medication treatment for soldier mental health in relation to the buildup of US military presence and the consequent expansion of the occupation Army's needs. This chapter considers what the protracted commitment of military force over time and space meant for the US military's recruitment and retention strategies during the war on terror and the role of psychopharmaceuticals as a modest tool to, in the words of the Army Medical Department, "conserve the fighting strength." It considers what happens when war becomes chronic and medicine is charged with keeping soldiers grinding on and processing that which war reaps, as Wright has done for nearly two decades.

With the US all-volunteer military stretched thin by prolonged and repeated deployments in the war on terror, psychiatric medications—as well as their not uncommon counterpart, opioid-based medications—became a practical means of returning the same soldiers to the same battlefields. The psychopharmaceutical solution framed the limits of the US empire as a problem of human endurance, channeling pills through the cumulative "churn" of repetitively mobilized and demobilized military life.[1] To understand how psychopharmaceuticals would become a tool of chronic war is to first ask how the problem of what the military calls "force sustainment" unfolded for US military leadership, policymakers, and planners in the decades leading up to and throughout the war on terror. By many accounts, it came down to a problem of bodies.

BODY PROBLEM

During the 1990s, as part of the post–Cold War drawdown in US military forces and a congressional cut in military spending, the US Army lost more than 205,000 soldiers, reducing its total active force by over 30 percent.[2] Beyond the budgetary goal, the Army wished to avoid a "hollow force"—low-quality, poorly trained recruits and undermanned units—a critique the Army suffered after the Vietnam War.[3] The push for a scaled-down, streamlined, "flexible" US military would be cast during the war on terror in the language of business-style efficiency savings under Secretary of Defense Donald Rumsfeld, who sought to modernize and transform the US military by relying heavily on corporations, military contracting, and the privatization of military jobs.[4]

But the reduction in forces converged with an increase in military missions, which grew a staggering 300 percent during this same period.[5] Sustaining an all-volunteer force for both overseas operations and homeland security and doing so at an increasing operational tempo, or OPTEMPO, would emerge as one of the preeminent concerns for military leaders, policymakers, and planners beginning in the first years of the wars in Iraq and Afghanistan.[6] Unexpected heavy demands of sustained ground combat depleted military manpower and equipment faster than they could be replenished, and shortfalls in recruiting took their toll on a military that in many ways remained designed for containing a Cold War threat—not for exerting full-spectrum dominance around the globe, as the Pentagon was envisioning.

As the wars dragged on—and with the reinstatement of the draft being too controversial—the Army leveraged multiple strategies in the face of its numbers crisis. Financial incentives were upped to entice potential enlistees, and thousands of recruiters were added. The Army relaxed standards to meet recruitment demands by increasing the age limit for recruits from 35 to 42 and permitting more recruits to score on the low end of the acceptable range for standardized aptitude tests. Attrition was reduced by permitting soldiers who would have otherwise been discharged to stay. The Army also allowed more recruits with criminal records, including felony convictions.[7] While the military routinely grants waivers to take in recruits who have low aptitude scores, medical problems, or criminal records that would otherwise disqualify them from service, the number of Army and Marine recruits needing what the military calls "moral waivers" for felonies and serious misdemeanors more than doubled from 2003 to 2006.[8] While the Army characterized the changes as reasonable and well within quality standards mandated by the Pentagon and Congress, they amounted to the permitted enlistment of thousands of prospective recruits who would have been rejected in the past.

The Army's decision to loosen standards came amid calls from the House Armed Services Committee to investigate accusations made by some Iraq War veterans that, nearing the end of their enlistments, they were made to choose between reenlistment or an Iraq deployment. A sergeant at Fort Carson, who served nearly a year in Iraq, reported to *The New York Times* that, rather than reenlist, he would risk the chance of being reassigned to a unit bound for Iraq. "I can understand we're in a war, and extraordinary things happen in war," he told reporters, "but the Army is moving the goal posts on me."[9] "Stop-loss" policy, which permitted the involuntary extension of a soldier's active-duty service beyond their original end-of-term-of-service date, continued to move the goal posts further down the field.[10]

More than a problem of numbers alone, the Army's recruitment challenges also raised concern for soldier quality and the reshaping of the Army as an institution. Explanations for rising Army suicide rates reflected anxieties about how the prolonged wars were compromising institutional culture. The 2010 *Army Health Promotion, Risk Reduction, Suicide Prevention Report*, also known as the Red Book, associated rising suicides to institutional erosion and the decline of Army standards stemming from fighting a multifront global war. The Red Book argued that as the wars went on, Army leadership was retaining substandard trainees and increasingly tolerating crime and substance use among its force, promoting a culture of "permissive complacency."[11] The report warned that "as a result of the protracted and intense operational tempo, the Army has lost its former situational awareness and understanding of good order and discipline within its ranks."[12] These concerns pointed to a deep institutional crisis, in which the strain of prolonged conflict was not only depleting the Army's numbers but also undermining the very values and standards that had long defined its identity.

If the Army needed bodies, it also knew that those it had could not be squandered. The wars in Iraq and Afghanistan saw an unprecedented pattern of prolonged and repeat deployments across the US Army. Data from 2009 showed that about 40 percent of current military members had deployed more than once, with over a quarter of a million having served more than two tours.[13] Once the military effort known as the Iraq troop "surge" began in 2007, with President Bush ramping up deployments by sending 30,000 additional American troops to Baghdad and Al Anbar Province, the Army extended deployments from 12 to 15 months. It was a decision made by the US Chief of Staff Peter Shoomaker, "with the intention of helping soldiers and families set expectations for a long deployment rather than confront an unexpected extension."[14] Additionally, rest time between deployments—what the military refers to as "dwell time"—was shorter than established policies. Both regular and reserve components of the Army saw a notable downward trend in the length of dwell time over the first decade of the wars, with the Army at one point deploying units to Iraq for 15 months with a 12-month dwell-time between deployments.[15] The Special Forces community generally operated on far tighter cycles, with deployments typically lasting six months, followed by six months of dwell time, with special mission units far exceeding these rates.[16] The impacts of reduced dwell time on the health and readiness of the force became such a focus of concern that in 2011 the Army initiated a two-year dwell cycle. Speaking before Congress in 2009, Vice Chief of Staff of the Army Peter Chiarelli warned against the "increased deployments, short dwell-time, and insufficient recovery times for our soldiers, their families, and our equipment." "It is a resilient force. It is an amazing force," Chiarelli said. "But I have to tell you, it's a tired and stretched force."[17]

. . . . .

Paul knows the Army's body problem all too well. He is what the military would call a careerist—25 years in the Army, and freshly retired when we met in early 2020. Having first enlisted as a 67 Romeo, an Apache helicopter crew chief, Paul was later commissioned to become a military intelligence aviation officer. By all accounts, Paul had had a sterling career evidenced by a string of promotions. But his body had trouble keeping up. "A helicopter is a machine that, when it's up in the air, is trying to pull itself apart. Ten thousand parts, just trying to fly apart—but you have to maintain control and fly it," is how Paul described it. That pulling apart, that's what happens to your mind and body, he told me.

When I met Paul on a drizzly afternoon, he looked like he was wearing ill-fitting body armor under his raincoat. It turned out to be a bulky three-ring binder: over 800 pages of records and documents he had compiled, with the help of a paid veteran consultant, to substantiate his application to the VA for disability benefits. As he recounted how he had been worn down over the course of his military career, he would periodically flip through the hundreds of pages, as if the documents made real his experience, rather than the other way around. The documents account for diagnoses and countless medical procedures, among them PTSD and multiple invasive back surgeries. What the pages don't fully account for are the many drugs—psychotropic medications, as well as opioids—that Paul has taken over the years, some more carefully documented than others but all to keep himself from flying apart.

At first, it was his sciatic nerve, and from there, degenerative disc disease. Paul turned to the flight doc for medications to manage the pain. "Spine was sitting bone to bone, and whenever you're flying and you're yanking, and you're banking as hard as you can," he describes to me, "all those g-forces just pull on you." Over the years, Motrin gave way to Flexeril and Celebrex which eventually gave way to hydrocodone, oxycodone, and valium—drugs considered disqualifying for pilots because of their effects on alertness, cognition, coordination, and reaction time. "I was doing oxycodone since 2003 while flying," Paul tells me. "And I look back now and that's crazy. I was literally one of those military members that was just, 'Hey, I hurt.' 'Here's some oxy to continue our mission and we'll see you in three or four days.' And that became an addiction." Paul says his back surgery in 2007—a three-level fusion—opened the door to what he freely admits became opioid addiction. "Imagine 120 pills and 30 valium and the doc saying, 'See you next month,'" he recalls, with a shake of his head.

Paul was moving between so many different locations during those years that the flight doc "couldn't control whether you were up or whether you were down." Sometimes they were taking off and landing from such operationally remote locations during his Kuwait, Afghanistan, and Iraq deployments that they were having to do their own assessments. Who was going to say they weren't good to go?[18] "We had a habitual relationship with the ground commander who we were assigned to," Paul said. "And you've got ground guys that are rough, tough—guys in Bradleys—just, just gritty."[19] As the pilot coming in from outside, Paul had to be ready to play. "You can't be all nice and clean and fresh. You got to live with these guys. You've got to be like them. You've got to be embedded with them. I never thought twice about not flying." The drugs kept him going, even when his foot was dragging across the flight line: "I was riding high."

Riding high meant falling would be steep. That fall came in 2013 when Paul deployed to Saudi Arabia. It was a prestigious, one-year State Department gig as a training advisor to the Saudi Army, the kind of deployment that people like Paul only get from years of proving their worth. While there, his small team was housed in a gated community with three-story townhomes designed, as Paul described it, "to be fully Americanized inside." "I was still popping pills at that time," Paul tells me. Then, one night, he began seeing cats—a lot of them—inside their townhome. "Unfortunately, I told the wrong person," he says. Hours later, Paul was in a locked ward in Qatar; from there, Germany, Walter Reed, and then back to Fort Bragg. "It's hard to swallow sometimes," Paul reflects of the end of his career, "because everything is taken away from you."

RE-CYCLING

In the rub of vertebra against vertebra and in the years of heavy medication use, Paul knows the wear and tear of two protracted wars. Given the demands to keep a stretched force in place across the time-space of the war on terror, medication could often present as a solution—or at least a Band-Aid—for a range of recruitment and mission-readiness challenges. While psychopharmaceuticals drifted into the military body in initially unplanned ways at the start of the wars, they came to appear as an opportune tool in efforts to stabilize and sustain a strained force as the wars wore on. Now, soldiers like Sergeant First Class Wright and Paul could be patched up and sent back, not uncommonly with diagnoses and on medications that would have disqualified them from military service from the start.

But this is not a straightforward story about medicine and the biopolitical exploitation of soldiers. As Paul himself says, "I never thought twice about not flying." The chemical push is normalized by multiple dimensions of military institutional culture, including the masculinized hierarchy of martial violence—here, the valorization of the rough and tough "ground guys" understood to be close to the action—that made it impossible for Paul to admit he wasn't good to go.[20] It is also bolstered by financial realities. Soldiers need to deploy to keep their jobs and advance their careers; depending on the circumstances of the deployment, they might also be eligible for special and incentive pay.[21] In Paul's case, even temporary disqualification from flying could mean not receiving flight pay. Coercion and complicity can be close kin, particularly when practical necessity takes over and willful ignorance is effortless. The chemical push that can come to shove, then, is not medical alone.

For the most part, though, prior to the war on terror, military medicine and military psychiatry had not operated with the intent of treating so that soldiers could deploy again. A soldier like Paul or Sergeant First Class Wright, for that matter, would likely not have been permitted to return to war. Following the Vietnam War and until the war on terror, PTSD had been seen as an unfortunate fallout of war that veterans suffered from and that the VA dealt with. The Army "was neither prepared to treat nor interested in treating PTSD."[22] The attitude of the Army medical community was, as Army psychiatrist Carl Castro asserts, "if someone has PTSD, we will just kick them out of the military."[23] But as the wars in Iraq and Afghanistan dragged on, the military increasingly kept and sent the same troops back. Military psychiatry and the broader Army medical community were initially ill prepared for what this meant or how psychopharmaceuticals would feature in this re-cycling. The protracted nature and recruitment shortages of the war on terror raised new clinical, operational, and ethical questions around what it would mean to repeatedly deploy soldiers, including those diagnosed with psychiatric disorders.

In that setting, it was not uncommon for the push to mission readiness to take precedence over policy. In the words of the 2006 DoD policy guiding medications on deployment, "it is the responsibility of the Service member to report past or current . . . mental health conditions . . . and associated treatments, including prescribed medications." But in practice, over half of soldiers with mental health conditions were failing to fulfill self-reporting requirements.[24] This underreporting had collateral benefit to an Army facing recruitment issues. As one Army psychologist reflected on his time working within the headquarters of a deployed unit, "What I quickly came to realize was that the practice of relying on known inaccurate self-reported data—whether tacitly condoned or not—unmistakably benefitted our military leadership.'" In an institution obsessed with regulation compliance, willfully ignoring potentially disqualifying mental health conditions and related medication use "had become so widespread in certain units as to become almost an open secret."[25]

If this open secret was a way to keep numbers up, it also kept soldiers employed. This practicality was not lost on military leadership and was folded into arguments in favor of medication use. In a 2011 editorial for *Time,* Elspeth Ritchie, a former Army psychiatrist and top advocate for mental health inside the Office of the Army Surgeon General, wrote, "Remember in this era of high unemployment, service members want to keep their jobs, and deployment is part of keeping your job and getting promoted. Staying behind for three months because you have had your sertraline switched to fluoxetine—both very safe and common antidepressants, also used for the treatment of PTSD—is not good for unit cohesion, or promotion."[26] While medications may have protected jobs, arguments like these did double duty to justify further stretching an already overextended force.

The relative discretion of medication compared to other therapies would also have its appeal to soldiers. Being able to access these medications through a nonpsychiatric general provider further obscured the nature of care—and thus the nature of the soldier's problem. Mirroring patterns familiar to US life more broadly, in the war on terror, psychopharmaceuticals including mood and anxiety disorder medications and sleep aids have commonly been prescribed outside of mental and behavioral health encounters by general medical providers like PAs and nurses. Despite reporting lower comfort levels with prescribing psychotropics and less knowledge of common psychological symptoms, complications, and treatments, general providers sympathized with suffering soldiers, which contributed to their desire to provide definitive care through medication.[27] In an institutional setting in which mental health carries stigma and potential implications for one's career and where it may be more acceptable to report physical symptoms than emotional ones, soldiers often prefer seeking care through their general provider, even when that same provider might encourage them to seek assistance from outpatient mental health.[28]

Major Nowak, an Army PA who deployed to Afghanistan in 2013, shared with me his take on this. "There's the stigma," he told me. "They don't want to be known," he said of the soldier seeking help with mental health. "If they come see me, it could be because they have a hangnail, a cough, a backache, or I could be helping them through some depression." Their peers wouldn't know the difference. "But as soon as you go sit in the little metal box," Major Nowak told me, referring to the COSC clinic building, "everyone knows: 'Oh, he's talking to the crazy people.'" The frequency and regularity of appointments matter, too. While going to sick call or having one or two irregular appointments with the doc can be easily written off, standing appointments can quickly raise the eyebrows of teammates.

Concerns to hide treatment reflect a long-standing ambivalence toward mental health in the US military that is grounded in its ideal of masculinity. While the post-9/11 Army has actively sought to reshape its institutional culture around mental health, there persists a pervasive feminization of mental health concerns and a perception of mental health care as unnecessary for strong, self-reliant "real men." Ambivalence toward mental health treatment is also shaped by the nature of the administrative power that military providers wield. In the military, being sent to or seeking out mental health care is described as going "off to see the Wizard," a reference to the titular character of the novel and film *The Wizard of* Oz, who has the presumed power to send a lost girl back home to Kansas from the mystical land of Oz. Whether commanded by superiors or voluntarily sought, going "off to see the Wizard" is seen as stigmatizing and potentially career-ending, since the Wizard has the power to make the soldier "disappear" from their unit and send them home.[29]

Medication that can be prescribed by general providers has been advantageous to what the military calls "stealth" mental health care, enabling soldiers to access treatment while avoiding the unwanted scrutiny of peers.[30] It has also opened more space for treatment outside the administrative purview of mental health providers. In keeping with forward psychiatry's normalization of stress responses on the battlefield, the use of psychotropics by general providers in the war on terror typically focused on the management of symptoms rather than diagnosis. The coding system used across military health operations can further obviate accounting of diagnosis. Particularly when forward-deployed, providers in the wars in Iraq and Afghanistan often lacked regular access to the Armed Forces Health Longitudinal Technology Application (AHLTA), the DoD's electronic health record system. Even when they did, they did not uniformly code for psychiatric and psychological conditions. Many general providers were also commonly known to utilize V-codes, which denote situations or circumstances that are not psychiatric disorders themselves but may have clinical and operational relevance, to avoid diagnostic codes from the ICD or DSM, which could imply more serious issues in a deployed environment.[31] In some cases, military providers would miscode a diagnosis to protect the soldier from potential harm to their career, stigmatization, or discrimination.[32]

As one PA put it, "We all tend to be a little more conservative because once we start diagnosing people, the shot clock starts for that person to prove they are getting better and can maintain functionality." What this PA calls conservatism certainly did not preclude the use of psychotropic medications. For example, several PAs reported using SSRIs like fluoxetine, sertraline, and citalopram to address depressive and anxiety symptoms, while documenting no DSM or ICD diagnosis or documenting a COSR or the time-limited psychiatric diagnosis of adjustment disorder.[33] Treatment that doesn't rise to the level of psychiatric diagnosis has great appeal for soldiers in an institutional context where documentation of a physical or mental health condition can have significant implications for being deemed incapable of performing duties as defined by military standards. At the same time, the prescription of psychopharmaceuticals by general providers provoked deep ambivalence, with the military mental health community praising the possibilities for definitive forward treatment while simultaneously criticizing overreliance on medication by their general provider colleagues. For their part, general providers saw few options due to the constrained resources of deployment, especially for problems they understood to be rooted in the wars and their high operational tempo—issues far above their pay grade.

OPTEMPO

Chief Warrant Officer Greene had the distinction of counting the most overseas deployments of any soldier I'd met up to that point: 11 total, spanning three decades. Greene's deployments are a microcosm of the spread of US military involvement post–Cold War, beginning with a tour in the Balkans in the late 1990s, Honduras in 2001, eight to Iraq and Afghanistan, and, most recently, one to the horn of Africa. Like Paul and Sergeant First Class Wright, Greene was a careerist, having put in 22 years, and he was close to retirement when he came to meet me in my office in Chapel Hill. Solidly built, sporting a stubble beard and North Face gear from head to toe, Greene looked like he had stepped off the pages of an outdoor apparel catalogue.

Greene tells me he grew up in a military family and that the Army was the only way to move up and out. There was just one hitch. "I have a bit of a rebellious streak in me and a problem with authority," he says, grinning. "The Army let me choose my job, so I chose the Army." Friends from high school had joined shortly before Greene and sold him on the intelligence field. Greene liked that the intelligence field offered small ways to rebel in an authoritarian institution. "This job? You get to wear civilian clothes. You don't have to shave. It's a cool job to have," he recalls his friends telling him. "I was like, 'That's me.'" He chose to train as what the military calls a counterintelligence (CI) special agent, or 35L.

The Army defines the job of a 35L in less sartorial terms than did Greene or his friends. The work of the counterintelligence special agent is, by the Army's posture statement, to "conduct investigations, collect and process forensic and physical evidence to identify and detect foreign intelligence and international terrorist threats, and plan the appropriate countermeasures to neutralize them."[34] From counterespionage to covert action, CI special agents are expected to seek as much assignment diversity as possible to advance their careers. Greene described this diversity to me. "When I'm deployed, it varies greatly, so I can be doing anything from being out in the field talking to local nationals and sources of information, trying to locate high value targets, to sitting in staff meetings and advising the commander on how to screen the local nationals working on our FOBs." A 35L must be able to switch channels quickly and continuously. "One day I might be in Nairobi at the embassy in a suit, and two days later, I might be in Somalia at an austere location, in North Face pants and a tee shirt," he recounted. "So, my duties are really varied."

Greene's career has meant frequent deployments—averaging one every two years, each anywhere from five to 16 consecutive months —with limited true dwell time in-between, since, as Greene laments to me, even time at home can be so packed with trainings that he's never actually *at* home. And even when he is, he's too wound up to do things like help with his kid's math homework or make dinner with his wife. In a time of full-spectrum dominance, when soldiers like Greene are tasked with "identifying and neutralizing" potential threats of many kinds, military life has meant continual high performance and agile shapeshifting even when at home. If it was g-forces that literally pulled Paul apart, for Greene, it's what he colorfully called the "mind fuck" of high OPTEMPO special mission assignments. As Greene described it, "I could be in a firefight and in a tick, I can be back at my house. Seventy-two hours earlier, I was staring at the body parts of a suicide bomber and now I'm sitting in my living room, having a beer."

Anthropologists and other scholars have illuminated aspects of militarized embodiment, bringing careful ethnographic attention to experiences of disability, injury, and vulnerability.[35] Attending to the push and pull on soldiers like Greene is significant, too, highlighting what it takes to *endure* over the long term of protracted war and to be a vector of force domination around the globe. Such analyses can help diagnose US imperialist ambitions as a project to colonize time and space and bring into focus the unstable place of medicine in getting people to fight, neutralize, and occupy, on a global scale.

Medications can reset ideas of the "normal" in these circumstances. "It's super hard to come down after Adderall performance," Greene notes of the off-prescription use of the stimulant he observed among members of the counterintelligence community and Special Forces teams he worked with. Where gaining an edge wherever you can is both valued and tacitly encouraged, optimizing drugs like Adderall can normalize higher levels of performance as the new business as usual. "Your teammates come to expect that high performance of you now. There's a level of expectation that you have to meet, and in this community, if you don't meet expectation, you're gone. You're black-balled, so to speak." Soon, that high performance comes to be expected, even necessary, across other domains, too. Adderall is now in arm's reach "to focus on whatever it needs to be. Maybe it's that I need to focus on my kid's baseball game this weekend, some project I'm working on at home, or I need to focus on this class I'm taking for training."

Medicine can also be harnessed to synchronize military bodies to the tempo of war-making and its institutions.[36] It's not only the use of sleep aids to help adjust soldiers like Greene to the cycle of missions done under the cover of darkness or the antidepressants he worries are being "blanketed," in his word, across the cadre of senior guys like him as they hope to eke out enough time to hit their 20-year mark.[37] There's that, to be sure. But there's also the continuous cycling of mobilizing and demobilizing—of being there and then being back home on your living room couch, 72 hours later—that has its cumulative effects.

For this, Greene tells me, he has found something promising. The US Army has shown interest in a procedure called stellate ganglion block, or SGB. Used since the 1940s by anesthesiologists to relieve pain, the procedure involves inserting a needle into a bundle of nerves located near the base of the neck and injecting a local anesthetic that temporarily blocks signals to the cervical sympathetic chain, part of the nervous system that regulates "fight or flight" reflexes. Growing evidence suggests that SGB may offer a fast-acting treatment that may "reset" the parasympathetic nervous system of service members with severe or chronic PTSD.[38] The anesthesia itself wears off after a few hours, but the effects of the procedure, experienced within minutes, last several weeks to months. How exactly SGB works remains unclear. Nevertheless, for troops cycling through deployments, SGB appeared as the gold standard of biological treatment for those able to access it.[39] Special Forces soldiers, who typically deployed far more often than conventional Army units in the war on terror, were particularly keen to access SGB. With many having seen upwards of double-digit tours and as little as a handful of weeks' dwell time at home between deployments, the itinerant temporality hit these soldiers and their families particularly hard. Fast acting and long (but not too long) lasting, SGB was used by soldiers to "come down" quickly from deployments, wearing off just in time to deploy again.

By way of a timely "reset," SGB offered a chemical adjustment to frequent deployments, one appealing to soldiers like Greene who may be wary of overmedication and the stigma or career-compromising threat of psychiatric treatment.[40] "It basically re-zeros you," Greene describes. "It sends you back to the baseline of your fight or flight response." Prior to the SGB treatments, Greene found himself constantly "switched on," constantly "on edge," even when home. "My wife noticed that weeks before I would deploy, I wouldn't be home. I'd be physically there, but mentally, I'd already be across the pond." The SBG worked just efficiently and long enough that Greene could maximize his time feeling present with his family. Even then, he is hardly Pollyannish about it. "It's a Band Aid on an arterial bleed," he smirks.

If the time-space of full-spectrum dominance has demanded high operational tempo for some military personnel, chronic war produced embodied dilemmas of another order for others. Asking what prolonged war demands is to consider not only countless combat tours and high-tempo assignments but also the boredom, monotony, dull repetition, and felt futility of being an occupation Army. For soldiers who deployed with expectations and untested desires for "seeing action," sitting behind a desk all day or being bunkered in encapsulated "little Americas" wore them down in other ways.[41]

GROUNDHOG DAY

In the 1993 film *Groundhog Day,* local television weatherman Phil Connors (Bill Murray) is stuck reliving the same day, over and over again. Cynical and frustrated by years of reporting on mundane events, Connors is sent to cover Groundhog Day in Punxsutawney, Pennsylvania, with his producer, Rita Hanson (Andie MacDowell). The duo gets stuck in Punxsutawney because of a snowstorm that Phil, ironically, failed to predict. At his bed and breakfast the next day, he awakens at 6:00 a.m., the radio alarm blasting the opening lyrics of Sonny and Cher's epochal, "I Got You,

Babe." So begins the replaying of yesterday's Groundhog Day. Phil relives this day repeatedly over the course of the film, and only he is aware of it.

Groundhog Day is a familiar film reference in soldiers' descriptions of the day in and day out of life as an occupying force in Iraq. Morten Ender has noted the film's ubiquity in how US soldiers dramatize the mundanity of everyday existence in describing deployment experiences in Iraq. "In this sense," Ender writes, "there was routine, monotony, and boredom in their activities. Each day was similar to the day before—sometimes off the Forward Operating Base but always on, with an unbearable heat, tan-colored vehicles, similar meals, the same people, and predictable, and hopefully uneventful, days."[42] Ender notes that the film also featured in reportage of the Iraq War. In a *New York Times* opinion piece, "'Groundhog Day' in Iraq," columnist Thomas Friedman describes an uncanny familiar in Rumsfeld's talk about the battle for Fallujah and how it echoed Bush's declaration of a "mission accomplished" after the 2003 Iraq invasion.[43] Friedman writes, "the 'déjà vu all over again' battle for Fallujah only reminds me that I still have the same questions I had before the Iraq War started." Tongue firmly in cheek, Friedman advises his ambivalent self: "So lay off. Shut up. Watch Fox. Wave flag. Visit a red state. Don't ask how the US got into this fix. Shut up. Lay off. Watch Fox." *Groundhog Day* thus lent a potent metaphor to descriptions of both soldier experience and US military strategy at a time of chronic war.

Soldiers had much to say about the boredom and monotony of daily life—specifically, daily life on the FOB, and how it could wear on you. You woke up to Groundhog Day each morning, one soldier stationed at FOB Fenty in Afghanistan told me. "It was mostly just waking up, eating, gym, eating again, sleeping, and start the same routine over and over again." It is sometimes said by, and more often assumed of, soldiers who were stationed at built-up FOBs that they missed "seeing the action." As one soldier said of his Iraq tour, "I was over there as a warrior who was not doing any kind of warrior stuff. I wasn't, you know, doing any missions. I was just on the base doing nothing." By the mid-war years, FOBs were typically fortified by concrete barriers and guard towers and provisioned with amenities like hot meals, hot water for showers and laundry, and recreational facilities. For at least some soldiers, they enabled what amounted to the closest thing to a nine-to-five desk job in war.

The presumption that military personnel in so-called combat support roles rarely, if ever, leave the relative safety of a built-up FOB has generated a playful but pejorative lexicon of terms. "Fobbit"—a combination of "FOB" and "hobbit"—is prominent among them and is meant to evoke the comforts-loving, peaceful, hairy-footed homebodies of J. R. R. Tolkien's world.[44] The figure of the fobbit stages a culturally resonant divide between those who can remain "inside the wire" and may be reluctant or afraid to leave the FOB and those who must go "outside the wire."[45] The experience of war and occupation as Groundhog Day—as boring, predictable, and mundane—thus offers a revealing view onto the hierarchical politics of military institutions that prioritize combat as the grounds of "real" experience.[46] Significantly, the experience of war as Groundhog Day is also the secured experience of encapsulated US military life as an occupying force.

Even then, soldiers found, or invented, ways to bide time on the FOB. New hobbies were picked up and old hobbies were rediscovered. Attempting to learn a few chords on the guitar or harmonica was popular, soldiers told me of their buddies, often with a roll of their eyes. And with internet access and laptops and online shopping services able to deliver to practically every corner of the world—or at least those with Army Post Office (APO) addresses—one could easily buy passing, if esoteric, distractions. One soldier told me he picked up wood burning during his deployment and made a bunch of amusing signs that he gave to his friends. (The best hobbies, after all, are those that entertain both you and others.) Everyone worked out at the gym both to distract themselves and stay in shape—two, even three times, a day. Pirated TV shows and movies, gaming on PlayStation, playing Monopoly—ideally with real cash to gamble with—or just sitting around, bullshitting, were easy ways to kill time. One infantryman, whose mother inexplicably included an industrial roll of tinfoil in a care package, recounted with amusement the wardrobe of clothes, undergarments, and hats he and his buddies made of the 2,000-foot cache. Some, aspiring for promotions or bold enough to plan for the future, invested time in more practical ways, by taking online classes and working toward a degree, for example, as Imani did during her 15-month deployment to Iraq. As a human resources specialist, she stayed on the FOB and "never left my bubble," something the mother of three was grateful for. Most of

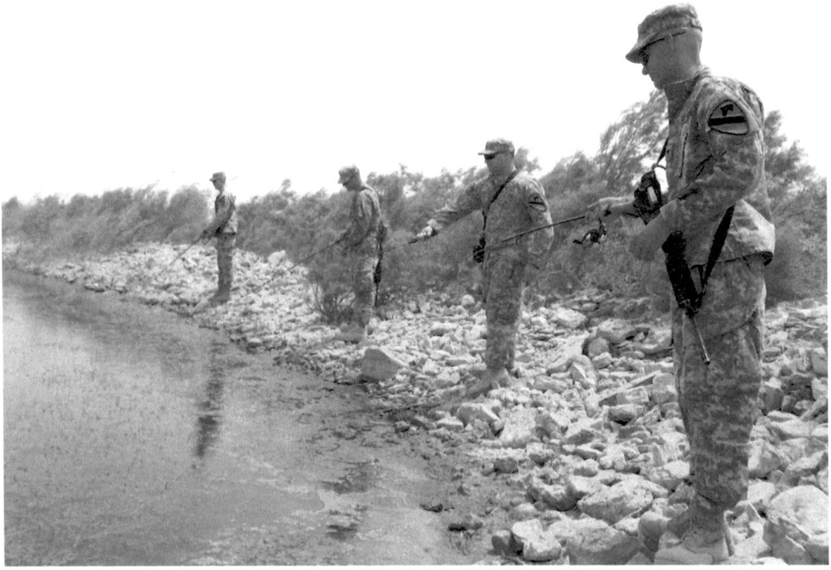

Figure 6. Enjoying fishing in a pond built by the Army Corps of Engineers at COB Adder in Iraq. Photograph by 1LT Justin Hackett, via DVIDS.

her night shifts were spent preparing casualty reports. When things were slow or she was bored, she studied for her distance learning courses and online shopped on a laptop provided free through eArmyU, mostly for her three kids back home, and then, as her deployment was coming to an end, for clothes for herself.[47] "That's mostly how I kept myself busy," she told me. "Studying, online shopping, and daydreaming."

Military boredom is hardly a new phenomenon.[48] The "enduring inner enemy of soldiers at all times," boredom has long been of concern to military leaders who see it as a threat to mission success, morale, and discipline.[49] Nate, a medic, mused that half his efforts on the COP were dedicated to preventing his guys from doing something dumb to themselves when they got bored. "It's constant boredom," he described of deployments, "and then you've got a bunch of boys trying to find something to do." I can barely wrap my head around the stunts he recounts: hurling throwing stars of unknown origin at one another, tasering one another out of curiosity, and daring one another to eat anything from chunks torn off

C-4 bricks to scorpion stingers. Mix that with general levels of dehydration and the Hydroxycut taken to "get ripped," and "it's just a cocktail for disaster."[50] Medications were not off limits. "Anything that can bring the slightest bit of happiness—even if it's Lexapro, mirtazapine, or citalopram—they'd crush it up and snort four or five," Nate recounted. Chemicals of all kinds can become improvised and experimental means less to optimize, cure, or even induce pleasure than to alter the flow and tenor of experience.

While military boredom is not new, the phenomenological conditions that FOBs made possible were in some ways unique to an occupation Army that was at once expeditionary and bunkered in the war on terror. While soldiers in previous conflicts have generally had to move to rear areas away from the frontlines for safety, rest, and recuperation, fortified FOBs in the wars in Iraq and Afghanistan kept soldiers on the battlefield; yet their home-away-from-home conditions, 24-hour internet connectivity, and relative refuge created new unforeseen challenges for soldier morale and mission readiness.

Some providers told me that FOB life could be detrimental to mental health, exacerbating the potential for adjustment disorders among young soldiers already facing the challenges of deployment. Army psychologist Major Hansen, the commander of a COSC detachment that served 35,000 troops in Afghanistan, said that FOBs drove a deep wedge between expectation and reality. "You expect to go to Afghanistan and do everything that you trained to do in the Army. And then when you get there and you're on the FOB, sitting there looking at a computer screen, it's not the most exciting thing in the world," he explained. "Having a lot of downtime in that sense was really hard for a lot of soldiers." One PA similarly averred that 90 percent of the mental and behavioral health challenges he saw among his soldiers were adjustment disorders due to "people showing up with preconceived notions of what life is going to be like and it does not end up being like that." In some cases, Major Hansen would try to work with a given soldier's chain of command to get them connected with what he described as "opportunities and meaningful activities," like manning the guard towers. Breaking up 12-hour shifts to get more soldiers in the towers, even for four or five hours, could break up the monotony of a desk job. Little things like this, Major Hansen told me, could get these soldiers feeling one step closer to war.

Constant Presence

Fortified military life in the war on terror also brought with it unprecedented electronic interconnectedness. Beginning immediately after the invasion of Iraq, the military sought to provide an internet connection to troops, who were siphoning bandwidth from military networks for access. Seizing an opportunity, enterprising Iraqi businessmen set up internet kiosks. The fiber optic infrastructure on which they relied, however, did not survive the invasion, opening the way for a small Virginia-based company named Segovia to contract with the DoD to provide satellite broadband internet access across the Iraq theater.[51] With the Segovia contract, Voice over Internet Protocol (VoIP) phone capability was added to broadband services on FOBs. This meant that soldiers could now keep—and were often expected to maintain—daily, or even minute-to-minute, contact with concerned family. (Compare this to the fact that telephone calls, while possible, were extremely rare during the Vietnam War.) With internet available in living quarters on some FOBs, soldiers could buy into continuous broadband in their rooms, adding webcams on laptops while instant messaging with longer lists of contacts.

As Leonard Wong notes in a study of how communication technology on FOBs reshaped soldier life, increased interconnectedness could create new types of stressors for families and military personnel, intensifying the tempo of worry and concern, while also placing increased demands on communication upkeep. For instance, instant message, which often includes a presence awareness feature, can indicate if a person on a user's contact list is currently online and available to chat. "In other words," Wong writes, "a wife can look at the computer screen to check if her deployed husband is back from a mission and online."[52] The quality of communications also changed, permitting a new depth and level of interaction that had not been possible with written letters or even email. "Soldiers are handling problems, dealing with issues, and getting involved emotionally in real time."[53]

While soldiers were careful not to relay worrisome information, family members often unloaded their problems on soldiers. Hearing about even little things could be taxing to soldiers who wanted to let spouses air stress and annoyances but could do little from a distance. In trying to convey

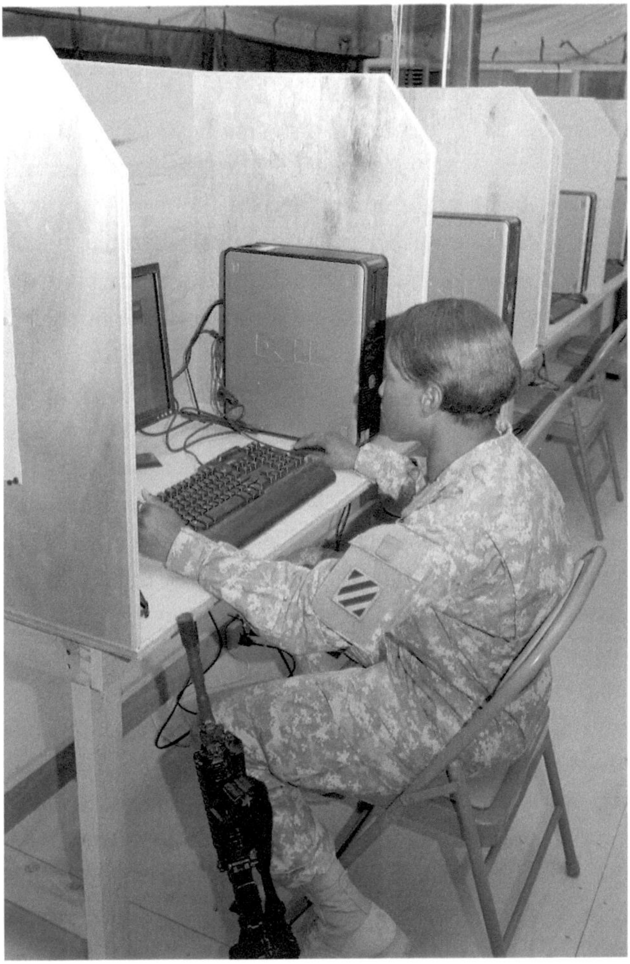

Figure 7. Distance Learning Center at FOB Kalsu in Iraq. Photograph by SPC Amanda McBride, via DVIDS.

to me how continuous communication with home can wear on deployed soldiers, Javier, a former Army PA, shared a personal example from a domestic deployment several years prior. "One night, my wife called me, just irate," he recalled. "The pilot light went out on the water heater. And she's like, 'Why aren't you here to fix this?'" "There's nothing I can do about this," he told her over a tense phone call. "'If you want to yell at me over the phone, and unload some stress, then so be it. But otherwise, I think you should go out and light the pilot light." The next day, the plywood on the porch fell. Javier received a text: a photo of the fallen plywood and an angry face emoji. "Life goes on in your family while you're deployed. All the things that you were supposed to be there to do, your family's mad at you for. Nothing I can do about it. Everybody knows it's not your fault. But it doesn't mean you're not mad and you're not frustrated by it."

As soldiers shared in the emotional burden of the everyday rhythms and daily dramas of home life, some found comfort in the regularity of communication. But more often, soldiers told me it added stress to their time away. Family matters bled onto the battlefield, weighing on their minds when focus was essential. Sergeant First Class Alvarez told me communicating with his family on deployment was his Achilles' heel. "If I have distractors such as my family bickering about whether I talked to them or not, or my wife arguing with my mom, or my dad treating my wife like crap, that's going to be the priority in my mind and that's a problem." Alvarez decided to "shut them out" so he could remain focused. He stopped communicating with them entirely in the last weeks of deployment. Radio silence.

For some, FOB life, with its enclave-like existence and ties to home, could worsen the stress of deployment. Sitting behind a desk all day could play mind games on soldiers who had expectations and ambivalent hopes of seeing war beyond bunkered life. Boredom, monotony, perceived futility, and domestic dramas beyond soldiers' control became the playground for all kinds of demons, especially when they had little else but time on their hands.

. . . . .

While military futurism pursues ever-more sophisticated and invasive strategies to transcend the limits of the human body, psychopharmaceuticals offer a comparatively modest means of reconciling the dilemmas of time and space during an era of US full-spectrum dominance. As the all-volunteer force faced its perennial body problem—now manifested across multiple theaters and protracted conflicts under the banner of a global campaign against terrorism—psychopharmaceuticals presented a modest solution to stabilize soldiers in place and return them to those same conflicts. The embodied dilemmas produced by endless war and its pharmaceutical fixes materialize in this chapter as vertebra rubbing against vertebra, thick binders of paperwork, and the contortions of being at war one day and drinking a beer on your living room sofa the next. But for an occupation Army in it for the long haul, these dilemmas also took the form of boredom, mind-numbing monotony, and the struggle to tend to life and relationships as if you were home.

Modern military psychiatry has long sought to mitigate the psychiatric casualties of war. In the war on terror, psychopharmaceuticals became essential both to addressing acute recruitment shortfalls and to stabilizing the fighting force. As the next chapter will show, however, mental health care, including the use of psychopharmaceuticals, was also closely tied to battlefield ethics and soldier conduct in the wars in Iraq and Afghanistan. In a doctrinal context that cast soldiers as agents of nation-state stabilization, soldier *instability* would emerge as a strategic and operational liability in counterinsurgent campaigns aimed at winning hearts and minds.

3 Stability

Howell does a few quick calculations in his head, flicking up fingers from a balled hand to keep track. He pauses at a provisional 500, revises upward, and lands at 600. That's the number of missions he estimates he participated in over the course of his 12-month tour in Afghanistan from 2011 to 2012. Stationed at a combat outpost near the border of Pakistan, the young private was one of about 60 soldiers composed of a platoon of military police, or MPs, and another platoon of infantry soldiers who, together, were responsible for an operating area that would typically be covered by a battalion of up to 1,000 soldiers. Stretched thin across a vast terrain that they were tasked with aggressively patrolling and controlling, their platoon ran two, three, sometimes four missions a day—an unrelenting level of activity, or high OPTEMPO, as the military calls it.

Most missions involved jobs Howell never predicted he would be doing as an MP. But they had been seriously shorthanded, so you did what you were asked and figured it out along the way. Howell knew enough not to be surprised by the surprises or intimidated by the tasks he hadn't exactly been trained to do. He recalls his father, who deployed to Afghanistan in 2002, advising him to "stay flexible, and be ready for anything." Such is the nature of forever war that a father and son could share the same battlefield, a full decade apart. The advice proved prescient. Adjustability and learning on the job were the name of the game. As Howell tells me with a shrug, "We all just kind of plugged and played."

For many of these missions, Howell was a gunner. From up in the turret of a Humvee, he observed and helped map areas of the thousands of natural caves that lattice Afghanistan's mountains along the Pakistan border. On the way back, his squad would enter the caves and crawl through the connecting network of *karezi,* ancient irrigation tunnels designed to collect water seeping from beneath stream beds and aquifers, some of which dip as far as 100 feet below ground. Their job was to search and clear the tunnels of weapon caches and people who might be hiding or sleeping in the caves—suspected Taliban leveraging these convergences of ancient technology, geology, and terrain to their advantage. Their squad also did frequent night missions, sitting up in the mountains or down in riverbeds where they would wait for "enemy movement." "We wouldn't always engage them; a lot of times we would just watch for recon gathering and turn that intelligence over to higher echelons," he explains. Howell saw the recon gathering to be as critical as the combat: "You know, 'cause we realized that we've been in this war for so long, there has to be something more to it other than just attacking the bad guys when you see them."

Other times, the young private, then in his early 20s, would be out "making contact with villagers," a phrase, I would come to learn, Howell means quite literally. Howell's squad was tasked with traveling to villages to collect biometrics data: fingerprints, iris scans, facial structure data, and DNA swabs.[1] When I ask him if that work was difficult, he does what I am learning is one of his characteristic shrugs. It wasn't necessarily *technically* difficult, he responds, with a hint of impatience at my apparently facile question. I take that to mean that he found it simple work, running the handheld platform and touching fingers repeatedly to screens. Though he admits that getting DNA samples could be a bit tricky, even with the help of translators to explain and move the process along, and to make sure their squad "respected local customs." "We didn't collect data from the women, and none of it was really cultural violations," he adds as if in assurance, though of what and for whom, I'm not entirely sure.

The biometrics data collection was generally easy work if you could get it, Howell tells me. But it also depended on which soldiers were out there

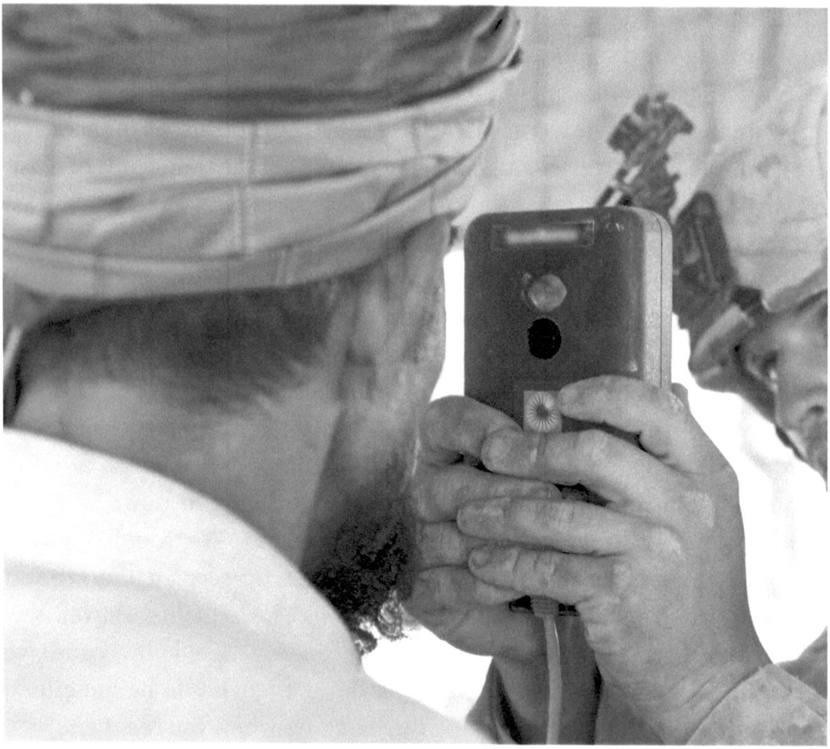

Figure 8. Scanning the iris of an Afghan man at a checkpoint in Helmand Province, Afghanistan. Photograph by Lance Cpl. Jeremy Harris, via DVIDS.

with you. Some were less predictable than others. He paints me a scenario. "Let's say we're going into five different villages today and we're going to walk around, let people touch us. Because they do. They want to poke you and check out your gear, especially if you're carrying weird stuff," Howell says. But the poking hardly went one way, I think to myself. Howell goes on. "They're a very touchy-feely kind of people over there. It doesn't mean anything to them. And you've got to deal with that. People are going to touch you, kids are going to run up and pull on your stuff, and you've just got to watch." It's the kind of situation where you wouldn't want a soldier next to you with an itchy trigger finger. Now throw medications into the mix and things get even more dicey. "What if they have major mood swings or aggression because they ran out of their medication a few days before or had their medication switched?" Howell says, his eyes growing wide. A recipe for disaster. Best for everyone that those guys stay behind on the COP. Swap them out with someone else.

Scholars have argued that contemporary counterinsurgency should be understood as a regime of biopower that has sorted and classified life, designating certain types as monstrous and thus life that must be killed and designating others as valued life made to live.[2] As the conflicts in Iraq and Afghanistan wore on, US military doctrine would shift "from catastrophic techniques that damage and destroy life to providential techniques that repair and improve life."[3] The much-publicized turn to counterinsurgency strategy in the war on terror promised an ostensibly better and more "humane" way of defeating the enemy, supplementing bombs and bullets with cultural knowledge and psychological tools.[4] This shift placed strategic importance on protecting local civilians from injury and death and mitigating the harm when civilians were killed or injured.[5] As Army General Stanley McChrystal wrote in his 2009 tactical directive for coalition forces serving in Afghanistan, "We must avoid the trap of winning tactical victories—but suffering strategic defeats—by causing civilian casualties or excessive damage and thus alienating the people."[6] Counterinsurgency strategy in the war on terror and its claim to the moderation of violence would set the terms for the campaign to win hearts and minds. As Howell suggests in his reflections on who you kept back at the COP, psychopharmaceuticals would occupy a contradictory place in this campaign.

Chapter 2 examined how the Army's "body problem" drove reliance on medicine to repair soldiers and return them to the battlefield. This chapter shifts the focus from soldier mental health as a manpower issue to soldier instability as a strategic and political problem for counterinsurgency doctrine. As a crisis of mental health took shape within the Army in the war on terror, real-time mental health surveys of deployed troops began linking the problem of unstable soldiers to unethical behavior on the battlefield, including "unnecessary" and "excessive" harm to noncombatants. Framed in the normative terms of battlefield ethics, concerns about soldier instability recast mental illness as a strategic liability, one that was narrowly defined by its potential to erode the support of local populations.[7] The figure of the unstable soldier thus emerged as a central threat to stability operations, undermining claims of control, constraint, and the humane moderation of violence. In this context, psychopharmaceuticals played an ambivalent role, used to stabilize soldiers' behavior and their relationships to violence, even as they signaled—and sometimes exacerbated—the very instability they were meant to control.

In tracing how soldier instability featured as a strategic and political liability for counterinsurgency in the war on terror, this chapter identifies multivalent meanings of *stability*. For Howell and soldiers like him, counterinsurgency strategy meant carrying weapons and knowing when and when not to use them, but it also meant collecting swabs, heeding culture, and "making contact" with villagers. In spanning the distinction between what the military calls lethal and nonlethal capabilities, wide-ranging military activities like these have been collectively mainstreamed under the term "stability operations." Stability operations aim to create compliant, "market-friendly" states by aligning the governing systems and institutions of postwar societies with international norms and the market economy against the "destabilizing forces" of government collapse, criminal networks, and humanitarian emergency.[8] The concept of stabilization and the specific policies enacted under its name during the wars in Iraq and Afghanistan enshrined development and political administration as responsibilities of the Army, coequal to war fighting.[9]

But stability is not the preserve of military strategists alone. Stability is a key clinical and administrative concept by which military medical providers evaluate and officially document the readiness of soldiers on psychopharmaceutical medication to deploy overseas. Soldiers also commonly use the terms "mental stability" or just "stability" to describe and assess everyday emotional, behavioral, and mental states. In our conversations, soldiers told stories about the stable soldiers they knew, and even more about the unstable ones, in ways that merged ideas about personality, performance, and pathology. The stable soldiers, I was often told, were reliable and predictable; they were known entities who didn't change much between home and deployment. For some, stability was seen as a relatively inherent trait that a soldier came into the Army either blessed with or not, depending on factors like family upbringing. Others told me that stability eroded with successive deployments. It was not only the violence of war that threatened to undo one's mental state and unsettle the nervous system: even unfamiliar physical environments and cultures could do the same, as implied in Howell's description of "touchy-feely" Afghan villagers who tested his control. Still others said that soldier stability, defined as being unflappable in a firefight, accrued with the hardened experience that comes with multiple tours.[10] Stability, then, was read as a marker of time and exposure—whether to combat, multiple deployments, or childhood stressors—but in ways that were layered and sometimes contradictory. As Howell's account suggests, it could also be used to articulate more specific relationships between mental disorder, medication use, and the controlled application of violence.

In the war on terror, then, *stability* operated as a key term among soldiers, military mental health experts, and military strategists alike. But rather than simply tracing the structural parallels between soldier stability and the stabilization goals of US military operations, this chapter examines what is at stake in military efforts to bind the two together. Soldier stability became the very ground on which the stabilization of occupied nations was imagined to rest. What does it mean when the stability of nation-states and that of the soldiers tasked with stabilizing them are understood as fundamentally entwined, each poised at the edge of *dis*order? How do psychopharmaceuticals figure within this field of uncertainty, and what role do they play in the pursuit of control through medicine?

FRAGILE STATES

In 2008, Lt. Gen. William Caldwell, who helped author the US Army's keystone doctrinal field manual for the conduct of stability operations, appeared on *The Daily Show with Jon Stewart*. Caldwell was then commander of the Army's Combined Arms Center at Fort Leavenworth, Kansas, his predecessor none other than David Petraeus, author of the Army's counterinsurgency manual and main implementor of the doctrine in Iraq. Caldwell appeared on the liberal comedian's satirical news program to talk about the newly released field manual. Stewart playfully kicked off the interview by tapping a copy in front of him and charging the lieutenant general for writing a "very dull" field manual. Suggesting he was bored by "the nonlethal stuff," Stewart scoffs, "Where's the zazz?"

Stewart's comedic misrecognition of what an Army field manual "should" be feeds the message Caldwell had been sent to deliver: the Army is undergoing a major makeover. This is the "new" Army, whose role is made to appear benign, even beneficent, and whose focus is on stability operations—tasks and activities that, as the field manual itself reports, will ultimately contribute more than the Army's traditional bailiwick of combat operations.[11] But it is Caldwell's description of what stability operations demand of today's soldiers that puts the field manual in practical perspective. "These men and women, these young men and women, they're out there today, they're able to look at a situation that we never could have envisioned, and take and apply their resources, their energy," Caldwell tells Stewart. "One minute they're drinking tea with a sheikh, the next minute they're over surveying where they're going to put a well in, the next minute they're taking sniper fire from some insurgent and they're returning fire, and the next minute they're over here figuring out whether they're going to put another road in."

Caldwell's vision of today's soldier requires that they possess more than the clenched fist. As described in the *Stability Operations Field Manual 3-07*, penned by Caldwell and his coauthors, it requires the "culturally astute" soldier who can adapt "to nuances of religion, ethnicity, and a number of other considerations essential to success."[12] This is the "soldier as governor," who can influence events and circumstances normally outside the bounds of the military instrument of national power and is flexible, adaptable, and resourceful in a fluid battlespace and ever-shifting communications and media landscape.[13] This is also the soldier required of counterinsurgency warfare as a biopolitical project. Rather than targeting the figure of the networked insurgent alone, the eventual US military response in the war on terror, as laid out in the Petraeus doctrine, would target the entire population as an "unstable collective of future friends and future enemies that contains an ever present potential to become (counter)insurgent."[14] In seeking to isolate and undermine support for insurgents, counterinsurgency strategy would center psychological and cultural tools to win "popular support." It would also mark a new confluence between warfighting, governance, and development that would task soldiers to be nation builders as well as warriors.[15]

Much was made by the US military of the "counterinsurgency turn" as a revolutionary and gentler way of embodying force. This was, in part, a

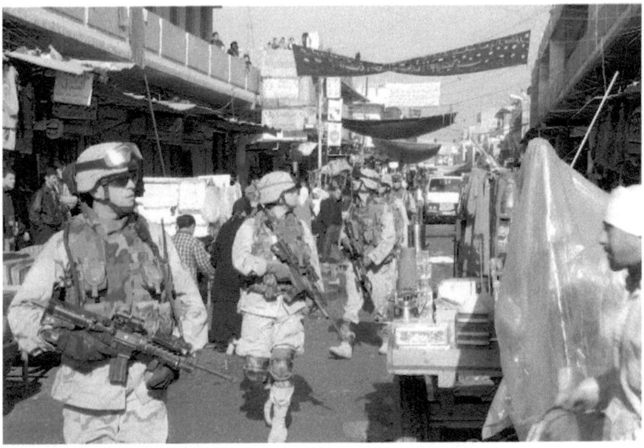

Figure 9. Soldiers patrol a market in Mosul, Iraq. Photograph by SPC Adam Sanders, via DVIDS.

response to the fact that the actual conduct of the war on terror had proven sobering. In 2004, leaked photos brought abuse and strategies of abjection used against detainees in American custody at Abu Ghraib prison to the attention of the American public. A year later, on November 19, 2005, in what came to be known as the Haditha massacre, a group of US Marines killed 24 unarmed Iraqi civilians, sparking what would become one of the largest war-crime investigations in the history of the United States.[16] While the public information campaign around counterinsurgency was intended to restore belief in the virtue of the wars, revelations like these raised ethical, legal, and political questions in the American media and in Congress about the capacity of soldiers to do the work of stabilization; it also raised questions about the legitimacy of the wars themselves, questions the military would come to narrowly cast in the normative, apolitical terms of soldiers' mental and behavioral health.

These questions would gain institutional salience with the release of the 2007 MHAT study, the Army's fourth real-time assessment of the mental health of deployed military personnel that would be released just a year before the publication of Caldwell's *Stability Operations* field manual. MHAT IV was commissioned with the request to investigate combat ethics and did so through survey questions and focus group discussions. Its findings stunned the military community. The results indicated 35 percent of surveyed personnel screened positive for any mental health problem.[17] They also suggested an association between mental health issues and what the study framed as unethical behavior on the battlefield.

For the first time since the MHAT program was started in 2003, the MHAT IV assessment included survey questions about what the military terms "battlefield ethics." The MHAT IV found that soldiers and Marines who screened positive for mental health problems and high levels of anger were twice as likely to report engaging in unethical behaviors than those who did not screen positive. These behaviors included modifying or ignoring Rules of Engagement, damaging and destroying private property, and insulting and physically hitting Iraqi noncombatants "when not necessary."[18] The findings of the MHAT IV consolidated an association between unethical battlefield conduct and mental health problems, an association further confirmed by the findings of MHAT V the subsequent year.[19] The mental health of soldiers had featured as an operational worry for the strength of the force during a time of prolonged war. With the release of the MHAT IV and V, it also came to the Army's attention as a concern for battlefield ethics and military strategy.[20] Recommendations included incorporating battlefield ethics into all behavioral health counseling and anger management classes.

MHAT IV and V understood soldier mental health in relation to normative ethical and legal failures involving the use of force among civilian populations, especially where Rules of Engagement (RoE) were violated or insufficient. RoE are directives designed to restrict soldier conduct in war by delineating the parameters within which force may be used and what actions are allowed under the law of war. In military parlance, RoE "may appear in various forms, linked to various levels: strategic, operational, and tactical."[21] With respect to the latter, the military gives soldiers discrete RoE about when and what kind of force is authorized; for example, what type of weaponry is allowable, the targets that may be attacked, and the circumstances in which lethal force may be used. The Pentagon saw RoE as crucial to the stabilizing goals of counterinsurgency doctrine in the war on terror. Adherence to RoE and a broader "mindset" of the use of force that is "discriminating," "appropriate," "measured," and "proportional" were meant to ensure that troops employed "the right tools correctly with mature discernment, good judgment and moral resolve," thus minimizing the collateral damage to civilians and property identified as critical to the success of counterinsurgency and stabilization operations.[22] The MHAT findings appeared to indicate that by contributing to the indiscrete and unmeasured use of force, soldier mental disorder and "excessive" anger were grave liabilities that threatened to drive local civilians into the arms of insurgents.

Diagnosed with depression and anxiety three months before his first deployment to Iraq, Sergeant First Class Davis knew firsthand how the threat of mental instability appeared to others around him. In keeping with destigmatization efforts in the post-9/11 Army that encouraged open discussion of mental health by senior leadership, the senior NCO and former drill sergeant told me he tried to normalize mental health for his own soldiers by being candid about his own experiences. It had been an uphill battle. "There is still misunderstanding among some leaders that people who require any kind of assistance behavioral health–wise are unstable," Davis explained. That instability carried specific risks in the biopolitical project of counterinsurgency. "They felt that them having, you know, bullets and regular access to a weapon and things like that, were they going to shoot themselves? Were they going to shoot a bunch of civilians because they're unstable?"

Soldier mental health and psychological injuries of war have featured centrally in the ways Americans talk about and engage with war and its consequences.[23] As Kenneth MacLeish has noted, "Emotional investment in soldiers' wounded psyches has long been a part of the anxiety, fantasy, concern, and alarm with which American civilians regard those who fight and die in their name."[24] These investments powerfully animate the moral economy of military suffering for the injured who return from war, but they also extend to political and military fantasies of control and stabilization. As Davis captures in his comments about perceptions of mental instability among senior leaders, the link made between soldiers' fragile states and the fragile states of occupied nations not only further cemented soldiers' psyches in the DoD agenda; it legitimated soldier mental health as a concern for national and global security. Importantly, the problem of unstable soldiers for the US military was not so much the risk they posed to Iraqi and Afghan lives as such but rather the biopolitical and strategic risk these soldiers posed to a counterinsurgency mission that understood civilian lives as "a means to an end rather than an end in themselves."[25]

At stake in linking soldier stability to the stability of nation-states are liberal democratic fantasies of control: fantasies that the destructiveness of preemptive war can be calibrated and that local civilians can be protected from harm because both military force and the soldiers who wield it are restrained, deliberate, and disciplined. In the wars in Iraq and Afghanistan, the imperial and counterinsurgent logic of enforcing governance over territory and population was mirrored in the regulation of soldiers' use of force. Such regulation entrenched imperialist violence, as US counterinsurgency techniques reproduced Orientalist constructs of occupied Iraq and Afghanistan as inherently chaotic, irrational, and pathological spaces in need of domestication.[26]

Within this vision of the struggle for control, the unstable soldier—the kind Howell describes needing to leave back at the COP—posed a specific kind of risk: the "bad" actor incapable of "good" disciplinary, technical, and biopolitical relationships to violence in a doctrinal and political context that demanded "courageous restraint" and in a setting cast as inherently chaotic.[27] This was the soldier who, for any number of reasons, lacked or had lost control and discernment in the use of force.

The illusion that war can be more humane if soldiers are in better control of themselves and those they govern reflects what Kali Rubaii calls a "less-than-lethal paradigm" leveraged by the US military, which rebranded preemptive war as benevolent and less deadly. As Rubaii argues, in parsing degrees of lethality and framing calibrated violence as saving lives, minimizing deaths, and avoiding killing, "extreme US military coercion worked alongside liberal democratic values" in Iraq to placate US popular perception and "minimize the political power of death and dying on the global stage," while disseminating nonkilling forms of extreme harm in the process.[28] Concepts of soldier stability and control reinforce this paradigm, casting the problem of violence in preemptive war as a problem of calibrated dominance and mastery, not of politics.

DAMAGE CONTROL

As the military mental health community was making the association between the troubled mental health of deployed soldiers and unethical battlefield conduct, soldiers like Matt had to work through these knots without it all coming unraveled. They did so in the course of their daily work and through signs they read in the behaviors of their teammates over time.

Matt recalls when he knew things were falling apart. The former Special Forces engineer with 13 years of military service and five combat tours to his name told me he could read it in his teammates. For many of those deployments, Matt served as part of an Operational Detachment Alpha, or ODA, a small, versatile, and highly trained 12-man Special Forces team that travels and works closely to execute, in his words, "sensitive tactical operations." ODAs are touted by the Army as "quiet professionals" who operate in "autonomous environments," or what Matt described as "a self-sustaining, holistic unit that can go anywhere in the world and conduct operations."[29] ODAs are designed to be "a highly functional, cross-trained team when they're working correctly. We all do each other's jobs." It was in this context of mutual reliance, shared performance, and cosurvival that the team grew concerned that two of their own were getting "too close to the line too often."

The ODA's multiple, back-to-back tours had gotten these two teammates "overheated," Matt explained. On several occasions that Matt did not detail for me, they overstepped what he euphemistically referred to as "the line." "There's an interesting balance you have to have to control your adrenaline and control your ability to go out and execute with high levels of precision and anger and cruelty that's necessary to the situation," said Matt. "But there's a clear line there that delineates when you step over." "When you do," he warned, "that's when you start getting into war crimes, things that are beyond the scope of even what uncivilized men do."

When I asked Matt to clarify what he meant by "the line," he paused, then recalled the laminated pocket card of RoE he always carried on his body.[30] While formally deferring to the technical specifications of international law symbolized by his pocket card, in fact, Matt described the capacities needed to negotiate "the line" by blending official and tacit ideas of appropriate force. He referenced the legal category of war crimes while basing judgment in the use of force not in rational calculation or precise definitions but rather in embodied feelings, intuitions, and assumptions about the "anger and cruelty that's necessary to the situation."[31] Normative arguments have often attributed the ambiguity soldiers report in the use of force in counterinsurgency to the ambiguity of RoE themselves. But Matt's description of control suggests that soldiers generate their own values, practices, and norms of stability in war.[32] They intuit and produce boundaries where counterinsurgent violence tips from appropriate to excessive. They do so through the interpretation of official rules, the enactment of technical practices, the cultivation of perceptivity in relation to teammates, and affective judgments in the use of lethal force. Even as they care about and insist on normative distinctions like RoE and the clarity of "the line," these distinctions are not purely rational calculations of an autonomous agent but distinctions that are felt, intuited, and tacitly known.

Consider what Matt described as the "gut feeling" the team had when someone was close to too far gone. "Look," he told me, as if about to own up to something, "we're all freakin' crazy. Every one of us out there. If you're not a little bit of a psycho then you're not doing your job right." If so, how do they know when it's time to intervene, I asked. "We're all crazy," Matt reiterated, "but we also know what our baseline of crazy looks like."[33] Matt physically marks a hypothetical baseline for me, placing the edge of his hand on the table in front of us. "Once you have that baseline, and you get guys who start going a little further and further away from it and staying there," he tells me, shifting his hand closer and closer to the edge of the table, "that's when you're like, 'Hey, we've gotta pull you back in now.'"

Matt was not alone in asserting the need to be "crazy" in the right way in war. Nor was he the first person to scramble relationships between madness, war, and suffering for me. Soldiers who had served in the combat arms commented about needing to be "a little bit suicidal," "crazy," or "psycho" to risk your life to kill others. While seeming to reinforce American stereotypes of war and madness figured in the stereotype of the "crazy vet," these assertions in fact turn the tables on the traditional economy of war suffering: it's not that war produces madness so much as *requires* it.[34] "Crazy" in war could be good. Indeed, it could be lifesaving and, by some accounts, the only way one gets the job done. The right kind of crazy means you're willing to "run at bullets," as Matt put it, and sometimes that's exactly what the mission requires. But there's also a line. Getting too close to it too often could be a sign of too much crazy in the wrong way.

Matt and the team's understanding of "good" and "bad" forms of crazy blended psychiatric norms, ethical reasoning, and operational efficacy with medical solutions. In cases where soldiers had drifted too far into the territory of "bad" crazy, the team would turn to medication treatment to course correct. "If we had people starting to flirt with that line, we would try to interdict with drugs," Matt stated, as if the approach were perfectly self-evident. In the case of the two "overheated" soldiers, Matt and the rest of the team eventually confronted and convinced them to ask their PA about medication. The two were eventually placed on SSRIs.[35] The use of medication to recalibrate soldiers' relationships to lethal force is predicated on a fantasy of the titration of violence through precision medication, wherein SSRIs "do not act upon the person as a whole but are targeted precisely to correct a specific anomaly."[36] Where the "bad" kind of crazy presents as a behavioral potential that can be externally modulated and chemically controlled when self-regulation fails, medication comes to be seen as a tool to correct the imbalances of brain, behavior, and team.[37]

In the shadow of MHAT IV, soldier psychiatric and behavioral deviance came to be read as a problem of battlefield misconduct that jeopardized the strategic success of counterinsurgency. In that framing, psychopharmaceuticals provided a practical means of restoring soldier stability while also supplying the moral terms through which soldiers *produced* the edges of legitimate violence. For Matt and his team, medicating behavior they defined as crossing the line helped authorize "good" violence as controlled and moderate—sufficiently humane so as not to compromise the inherent humanity of soldiers by drawing them toward what "uncivilized men do."[38] Matt's account suggests how soldiers may instrumentalize medication to titrate "excess" violence, while reinforcing the moral authority of the ostensibly controlled violence they "normally" perform.

For Reynie, self-control in the use of force was vital to how he trained his soldiers as an infantry officer and how he deciphered which soldiers had fallen off the edge. In our conversation, he linked the capacity for self-control to the shift to counterinsurgency strategy in the wars in Iraq and Afghanistan, a shift he experienced as an infantry officer. He recalls wondering at the time: How does one now recondition soldiers, taught to shoot on sight, to become a police force? "We had to get people out of what they'd been trained to do," he told me. "Because what are you trained to do? See the enemy, you shoot the enemy. That's what we do. It's our job. Search for things and destroy." The transition to counterinsurgency and stabilization operations—what Reynie summarized as a transition from a Department of Defense to a Department of State–led objective—meant recalibrating soldiers to learn to hold their fire, to "try things out in a different way."

Drawing on the language of psychological operations, Reynie described the kind of soldiers he needed. "I needed people who could walk through a town, and high-five little kids, and talk, and communicate with anybody and everybody. That's what I needed," he told me. "I needed people who were good at building rapport, and good at communicating. Behavior change was the goal." At first, I think Reynie is referring to the goal of winning hearts and minds, but in fact, he's referring to changing his soldiers' behaviors. Soldiers, he continued, had to be able to make that "switch" from "hard, stone faced, steely eyed, barrel-chested killing machine" to "chill, happy, smiley, 'Hey, how you doing?'" Sometimes that meant the soldier taking off their helmet or slinging their weapon. "We're not looking to be big and mean as we're talking to people. We're trying to get them to be honest."

This was a challenge for the surge Army, Reynie told me frankly. "We took the dregs of society, gave them guns, and taught them to kill." I'm reminded of the Army PA who once told me that when you're serving from the bottom of the pot, all you're going to get are the burnt bits. As tours got longer and the wars dragged on, the Army started granting moral waivers, which permitted soldiers to enlist with one or more of a list of otherwise disqualifying situations, including prior criminal convictions and history of drug abuse.[39] "Look at the amount of moral waivers and the kinds of people we let into the military to have a number so that brigade could deploy," Reynie says, shaking his head. "I love my boys. I will love my boys until the end of time," he went on to say. "But they are not the best human beings on the face of the earth. They're good kids. They mean well, but I'm not letting them date my daughter, you know?"[40]

In that context, mental health issues among his soldiers were not issues per se, since according to Reynie, "we all have something wrong with us." What ultimately mattered to him as a leader was the capacity for control in the moments it mattered. "Even I have mental issues," Reynie said candidly. "The question is: Are they going to affect me?" He raised the issue of medication. "My concern with my soldiers that were on medication was

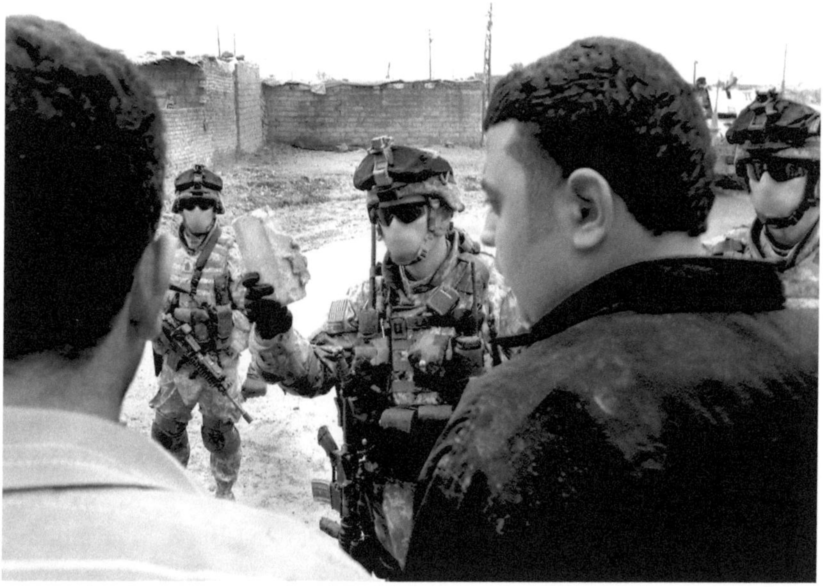

Figure 10. Confronting adults about brick throwing by children. Photograph by SSG Russell Klika, via DVIDS.

how well did they control the side effects? How in control are they? Mentally, how accustomed are you to medication and your dosage? Everyone shows side effects. For me, it was, how well can you control that?" When I asked Reynie to explain what it means to be in control, he talked about anger. "It's okay to be angry; everyone gets angry. I'm sure the Dalai Lama gets angry," Reynie mused. As a soldier, though, "you need to find that right level of anger that motivates someone to do something that they wouldn't normally do. But it's not okay to be angry 24-7."

Like Matt, Reynie spoke of a world of norms, values, and intuitions that he characterized as unique to the combat arms. To find another entry into that world, I asked him what he and his NCOs would look out for during training. What were the red flags? When did anger, in Matt's words, cross the line? "The big thing we looked for was discipline. I don't mean stupid Army discipline, like a crisp hand salute," Reynie explained. "I mean the important stuff." As an officer, he believed strongly in the importance of combatives, or training in hand-to-hand combat—what I heard soldiers refer to more colloquially as gutter fighting. Getting his soldiers in "the pit" was revealing. "What we'd look for is: did they stop when the other guy tapped? Or did they punch one more time? Did they keep twisting his arm? Or did they stop? Or we might say, 'No punches to the face,' and one kid punches their opponent in the face. Little indicators." Same with live-fire exercises. "Fire discipline, right? If I tell my base of fire, 'Lift fire!,' which means cease fire—basically, to stop shooting. Did he stop shooting or did he squeeze off a few more rounds?" One of the soldiers they ended up leaving behind when it was time to deploy had failed these tests, Reynie told me. "Just little things like that. Little things that I trusted the experiences of my NCOs to notice, and what I saw as right or wrong."

An attunement to the "little things" gave Reynie a way to bring into focus some aspect of the otherwise hazy future of a soldier's performance in deployment. When they look for the prohibited punch or the extra rounds squeezed off, leaders like Reynie seek what the field of military psychiatry has long aspired to do: forecast who will hold together in war, and who is likely to fall apart. But even for the experts, making determinations about soldier stability demands clinical acumen, procedural dexterity, and not a little bit of learned intuition. For some, determining soldier stability can seem an exercise in divination, akin to reading tea leaves.

DIVINING STABILITY

> [Service] members should demonstrate behavioral stability and minimal potential for deterioration or recurrence of symptoms in a deployed environment, *to the extent this can be predicted*. . . . This should be evaluated considering potential environmental demands and individual vulnerabilities.
>
> Department of Defense Policy Guidance for Deployment-Limiting Psychiatric Conditions and Medications, November 7, 2006 (emphasis added)

> We're not mind readers, but I think overall, providers get to know their patients pretty well. And could within reason,

> predict how that person's going to be able to manage stressors and cope.
>
> Major Rivera, Army Psychiatric Nurse Practitioner

As suggested by these nods to the limits of prediction, determining who is likely to destabilize in deployment is a craft of divination not a science of forecasting. This craft becomes additionally complex when it involves the clinical and administrative management of mental health and medication used for its treatment. Accountable to the needs of military command and by their roles as both care providers and managers of risk, military health providers are tasked with making assessments about the deployability of soldiers with documented mental and behavioral health needs. They do so through official clinical and administrative concepts of stability as outlined in official policy like the 2006 guidance quoted above. They also rely on their own intuited sense, honed through years if not decades of experience, of what it takes for soldiers to perform effectively once in a deployed environment. As one medic told me of this intuition more generally, "I had a good sense for it, but nothing was ever certain. There were always a few that I thought were just going to break and surprised me, and then there were some really strong ones that did break." Once deployed, military care providers of all stripes must also do the continual work of assessing who has "decompensated" far enough that they should be sent home and whom they might take a chance on and keep deployed.

How providers define and assess "stability" is complex; they do so in ways that blend clinical, administrative, and operational factors. To be deployable in the wars in Iraq and Afghanistan, a soldier with a mental health diagnosis on medications had to be documented as "clinically stable" on the dosage of their medication over the 90 days before deployment. Some soldiers had to additionally apply for medical waivers depending on their mental health diagnosis and the medications used for treatment.[41] DoD guidelines defined "clinical stability" regarding mental and behavioral health in the following terms: "no significant recent deterioration in clinical condition"; "no significant impairment in work or interpersonal functioning"; "no significant risk of sudden incapacitation should condition relapse or recur"; and "no morbid, suicidal, or homicidal ideation, intent or plan."[42] What constitutes "significant risk" and "significant impairment" must be ascertained by the provider, who must "get to know their patients pretty well," as Major Rivera says, and anticipate the kinds of missions and environments any given soldier would likely face. Individuals with psychiatric illnesses treated with psychotropic medications could deploy if they met criteria outlined in DoD and theater policies. Deploying on a psychopharmaceutical typically required a waiver requested by the individual's commander, a process intended to demonstrate to the theater commander that the soldier had been medically examined, was aware of the specific risks of deployment for people with their condition, and that the unit was prepared to provide necessary support.[43]

Divining stability thus demanded projection through time and space—namely, the ability to predict, "to the extent possible," "minimal potential for deterioration or recurrence of symptoms" in a deployed environment. This prediction was based on behavioral stability observed and documented in garrison and in field conditions that could be far different from those the soldier ultimately encountered while deployed.[44] In the act of divining stability, providers had to know something of the specific demands of the soldier's military job, or military occupational specialty (MOS). They had to anticipate the kinds of operational and infrastructural environments the soldier was deploying to and try to project, based on knowledge of a soldier's "positive strengths, skills, training, and previous operational experience," whether that soldier would remain behaviorally stable.[45] (They also did this, fully knowing that a soldier's official MOS often had little to do with the actual work they might be doing once deployed.) They had to consider factors like the "austerity" of the deployment location and mission demands, including the potential effects of sleep deprivation, rotating schedules, fatigue from extended working hours, and environmental stressors such as heat stress, on a given mental health condition.[46] It also meant determining whether the soldier would have access to a reliable supply of medication and what might happen if they ran out. Sometimes, providers had to make these predictions without having deployed themselves.

Military mental health professionals emphasize the multidimensional nature of stability. Army psychologist and Behavioral Health Officer Captain Simpson told me that stability encapsulates "occupational, interpersonal, social, and cross-health domains of function." Providers like

Captain Simpson also emphasize functionality in determining stability. "If there are symptoms and there is impairment, then we have not achieved the stability that we are looking for," Captain Simpson explained. "But a person can still have depressive symptoms and be stable, not having interpersonal or occupational impairment," he went on. "They can still do the job, and there is no harm or risk of further damage to the individual by engaging them in their normal duties. To me, that is stability." This is the functional imperative of operational psychology, evident in the distinction Captain Simpson draws between being symptomatic and being able to do your job. In the wars in Iraq and Afghanistan, soldiers had to evidence stability for at least 90 days before deployment. If a soldier could do that, Captain Simpson says, "awesome, cool. We recognize that it can obviously change, but at least prognosis-wise, 'Hey you're good.'" Of such cases he said, "Whatever coping skills or whatever processing you've done through therapy or meds, whatever it is, is working, and we can *reasonably project* that, barring severe circumstances in which anybody would react, you're going to be all right" (my emphasis).

As Lochlann Jain has written of prognosis in cancer, "the statistical prognosis poses both a stunningly specific (one has x percent chance of being alive in five years) and bloodlessly vague (you, yourself, will either be dead or alive) fact about the future."[47] Providers like Captain Simpson likewise work at the intersection of the specific and the vague, reading what they might know or predict about the specific soldier and their future deployment alongside the sheer indeterminacy of what *could* happen and how that soldier will respond. Prognosis offers "a meager tease toward knowledge" in circumstances where there may be little else.[48]

In the realm of soldier mental and behavioral health, prognosis and "reasonable projection" were all one could expect of a provider; the rest—the possibility for the "severe circumstances in which anybody would react"—was out of their hands. Thus, I met providers like Captain Moore who described honing over the years a kind of "gestalt" regarding soldier stability. The evening light was giving way on his side of our Zoom call as he spoke with me from a picnic table outside the barracks. The contours of his face were fading; soon, I'd be talking to a box of shadows. I had been asking the Army PA about whether, as a provider, he could predict how a soldier would perform on deployment. With seven tours to Iraq and

Afghanistan as an infantryman and two as a PA, Captain Moore brought seasoned insights from across the enlisted-officer divide to the question of who will break and who will not. There's predictive power in "holistic observation," he told me. That's why he paid attention to everyday things like soldiers' interpersonal skills and their handling of conflict. "As a provider, you can tell who is going to have problems," he asserted. But many of these same soldiers, Captain Moore said, are also the most proactive: they tend to seek help from their provider, which enables the provider to work with the soldier well in advance of the deployment to start them on medication and "get them stable on that medication." Reflecting a comfort expressed by some providers I interviewed, the PA told me that the soldiers on SSRIs for depression or PTSD "didn't really pose as much of a concern." "If someone comes into my clinic who I see is on a psych med, if it's for PTSD, we don't even think twice about it," Captain Moore reflected. "It's a normal, day-to-day occurrence. It's benign for us—so ubiquitous. It's not a big deal." I ask him if he considers SSRIs safe in deployment. "Extremely safe," he instinctively replies. "I tell people it's looked more highly upon to take meds if you have an issue than not to be taking meds and having an issue."

Captain Moore also has good trust in the Army's screening process to determine which soldiers are clinically stable, and thus, deployable. The Army prepares soldiers to deploy through a multistage process known as soldier readiness processing, or SRP, a sequence of procedural and documentary activities by which soldiers are evaluated and qualified for deployment. While military medical standards for enlistment and commission are meant to screen individuals entering the military for disqualifying behavioral and mental health conditions, military personnel with psychiatric illnesses treated with psychotropic medications can deploy if they meet criteria outlined in DoD and theater policies. Captain Moore told me that soldiers "are pretty well screened by the time they show up" to the SRP site. When he discusses new medication use with soldiers considering future deployment, he advises them on potential effects and the 90-day policy. He continued, "By that, you can be totally good to go. After those 90 days, you can go anywhere in the world and fight with your team."

Captain Moore had faith in the SRP process to do what it was meant to do, even if it didn't always do it perfectly: it adequately screened for those likely to remain behaviorally stable ("to the extent this can be predicted," as qualified in the DoD guidance) and weeded out those who were likely not to. Captain Moore told me that being documented as clinically stable on medications was itself proof of concept. Soldiers who wanted to deploy badly enough that they committed themself to the personal, clinical, and administrative work of getting diagnosed and medicated were likely to make it through deployment. The stable ones often turned out to be the ones who "fought to be there," the "folks who have screened multiple times and were on meds because they wanted to deploy." "It's the people they don't screen, the people who weren't on meds, that would be the problem," he told me. They deploy but end up having to be flown out because of a mental health emergency—those are "the ones without the coping mechanisms that you want to be concerned about." By Captain Moore's assessment, doing the work to be deemed stable was itself evidence of stability.[49]

Major O'Neill was less rosy about SRP's ability to work as intended. The 40-year-old PA with a nearly two-decade career in the military described the SRP as a process meant to "catch" red flags—a process that was hardly failproof. "SRP only has ten minutes per soldier to quickly scan their medical record to try to catch anything," she said of the process. Details can slip through the cracks. She recalls one soldier who began cutting herself during their deployment to Afghanistan in 2014. "I wanted to evacuate her," Major O'Neill told me, but the commander overruled the recommendation. So, the PA took it upon herself to dig further into the soldier's electronic medical records—not a particularly easy task given their unreliable internet connection. With some persistence, she came to learn about a reported suicide attempt in the soldier's basic training record. "That's one case where I wish we would've caught it at SRP," she laments to me. "Someone who has had a suicide attempt and now is a cutter? I just felt like there were so many red flags and that this person needed to not be in this environment." With this new evidence brought to military command, the soldier was medically evacuated.

For Major O'Neill, predicting in/stability is "detective work," and sometimes the clues only begin to appear once the soldier has deployed, at which point it becomes clear that they need to be sent home. "If I was to look at everyone who is medically evacuated out of Afghanistan in my unit and I went through their whole medical record," she told me, "I would see that they've had things sprinkled in there, right? Like, it wasn't just that being once in Afghanistan was the trigger. They've had a history of childhood trauma, and some problems in basic [training], but they made it through." These people had "enough space" in their medical record and career of proven resilience that "SRP didn't see anything and I didn't see anything. And then on deployment they got triggered, either being away from family, no sleep, or their supervisor's on their ass. So, it triggered something."

Major O'Neill told me that the challenge for her as a provider was that "stability," which she placed in air quotes with her fingers, had no real objective value in the case of mental and behavioral health. "How do you measure that? You can only do an interview or a follow-up appointment with someone to ask, 'How are you feeling? Do you feel better? Do you feel as tired? What's your energy level like?'" By comparison, she explained, if you had to stabilize a patient on blood pressure medication or vitamin D, "it's just some number; you're basing clinical stability on a lab value. At one moment, they're in their normal range according to the lab value, but if they're entering somewhere in the winter with less daylight, their vitamin D might drop or if their stress increases their blood pressure rises." Adjustments to medication could then be made. But there were no lab values to fall back on with mental and behavioral health. "So, you're basing it off of what someone's telling you," she said with a shake of her head, "and they can tell you anything."

Pressure from above can also influence risk management and the work of prediction around soldier in/stability. As a provider helping to prepare her soldiers for their deployment to Afghanistan, Major O'Neill recalls being told by her colonel, "I want as many people as possible." Needing to make the numbers, in a handful of cases in which things could have gone in either direction, the PA worked closely with the SRP site providers to convince them that "this guy's going to be mentally ready. I think he's good. I'll monitor his medications." With the deployment several years behind her, she now questions that reassurance. "Now looking back on it, I think I had people that probably shouldn't have deployed. And probably three of those people that I worked with at the SRP site to get deployed I had to send back because they just couldn't handle it." Staffing pressures could thus influence how fine a filter was used in SRP. Sometimes, the work of divining stability had to be done on a wing and a prayer.

Pressure could also come from soldiers themselves. Psychologist Captain Simpson told me soldiers may underreport symptoms so that they can deploy. "They'll say, 'Ah no, I'm totally good. Nothing's going on. I'm good, Sir. I'm here to fight. Let me go. Let me go kill the bad guys.'" Some among them were "savvy to the regs and requirements," Captain Simpson said, and if they were on a nondeployable medication, they would think, "Okay, I have to show stability, so I'm gonna go in, stop all treatment and say, 'I'm good, I'm great, a miracle happened and I woke up and I was healed.'" At 91 days before deployment, the soldier goes through SRP: "All right, you're all good to go, you're stable, okay. Deploy." But once deployed, they quickly decompensate under the strain of new stressors. "Most of the time, we're able to kind of work with them, to catch them and get down to the truth of the matter," said Captain Simpson of the months before deployment. "But sometimes, stability—reported stability—is not always stability."

PANDORA'S BOX

Divining stability is part of a broader effort by military care providers to predict and manage risk and performance across the time-space of US empire. Medical paperwork, whose trail may extend years prior to deployment, quotidian observations of behavior and performance in training, and the gut intuition of senior NCOs and care providers, alongside the testimony of soldiers themselves, yield the signs from which the future of a soldier's stability might be forecasted. Once deployed, care providers' work does not cease; they must continue to evaluate the ongoing stability of soldiers in relation to dynamic mission demands and infrastructural and occupational factors. Critically, they must also take care that their own interventions do not cause soldiers to destabilize or decompensate.

Continuing soldiers on medications for which they had documented stability prior to deployment posed relatively few major administrative, operational, or clinical concerns to most clinicians I interviewed. But starting soldiers on new medication in deployment could be a different matter altogether. Providers expressed concerns for the unknown potential for impacts on functionality and performance when starting a deployed soldier on new medication, as well as for the uncertainties of medication supply when a prescription was newly initiated. Former field artillery officer and now PA, Major Stuart told me she was hesitant to prescribe new medications for mental health in deployment, emphasizing the instability of the deployed environment itself. This also required the provider to track and document the stability of the soldier on the new medication; if stabilization couldn't be achieved, the soldier was technically required to be sent home.[50] Especially for high OPTEMPO missions, she said, operational demands could constantly shift, making it additionally difficult to decipher how medication affected the soldier's functioning. There were also risks to side effects that were potentially enhanced in a deployed setting, where weapons were in easy reach. All these factors made instances of prescribing new psychiatric medications in deployment far from ideal. "High pucker factor" moments are what Major Stuart and her colleagues would call them, a memorable description of the clenching response that such clinical moments could provoke in the provider.

Initiating therapy in deployment likewise posed its own risks. While psychoeducational counseling and supportive therapy, and even brief cognitive behavioral therapy, are standard parts of the toolkit for mental health providers in deployment, psychologists and social workers told me that they explicitly avoided the "deep dive." At some level, this was due to practical constraints: mental health professionals in the wars in Iraq and Afghanistan were typically responsible for thousands of soldiers, so the ability to have standing therapy sessions with any one soldier was a luxury that the clinician could not afford.

But avoiding the deep dive was also more than a matter of one's hands being tied. "Yeah, I'm pretty hesitant to do that," Captain Simpson told me. "Specifically with trauma work, I was pretty hesitant to do that even though we had some folks that were there who'd had six deployments and had gone through a lot of compounded trauma, who had complex PTSD." These were folks who, prior to deployment, may have been undergoing therapy alongside medication treatment. While their medications were permitted to travel with them, trauma therapy had no place in theater. Captain Simpson gives me the example of prolonged exposure therapy, or PET, an evidence-based therapy for the treatment of PTSD, which involves addressing the trauma through imaginal exposure. With PET, the

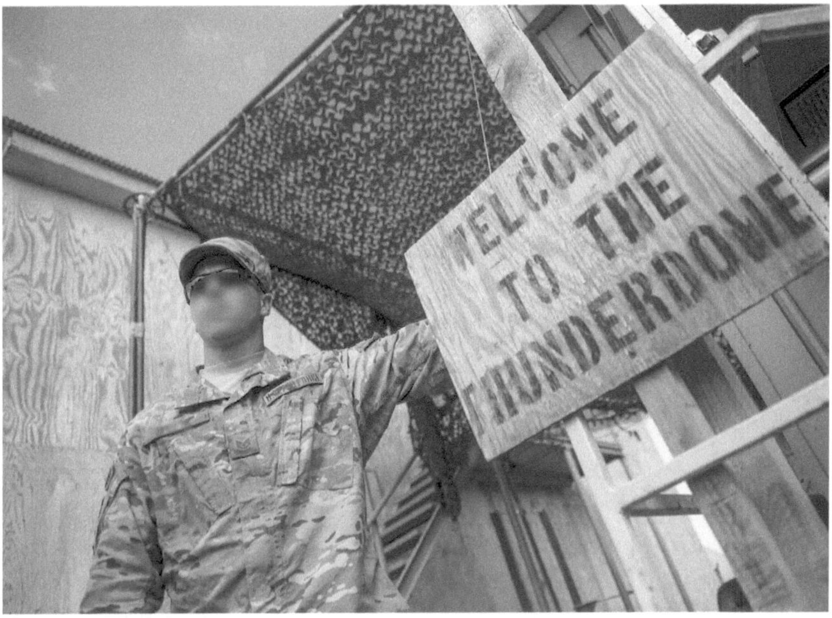

Figure 11. A sign referring to the gladiator arena from the 1985 film *Mad Max Beyond Thunderdome* hangs at Jalalabad Airfield in Afghanistan. Photograph by SSG Justyn Freeman, via DVIDS.

therapist works with the client to change thoughts and feelings surrounding the trauma through in vivo exposure wherein the client is guided to recall events and situations, with the understanding that such exposure allows the client to work through painful memories in an ostensibly safe environment. But deployment is an "environment that is fundamentally unsafe," Captain Simpson tells me. Just imagine that you're sitting with a soldier and guiding them through their imaginal rehearsal and "all of a sudden we're getting rocket attacked and their apex trauma was getting blasted by a rocket." Best not to "crack that open" in that environment.[51]

While medications were leveraged to regain or maintain the stability of soldiers on the battlefield, trauma therapy had no such place. Providers understood deployed settings in the war on terror to be, in Captain Simpson's words, "fundamentally unsafe" (while implying the fundamental safety, by contrast, of the homefront). Cautioning against therapy in deployment, one clinician described for me a hypothetical situation. A soldier might be opening up to a provider during a therapy session on a FOB, she said, only to be vulnerable to a mortar attack in the middle of recounting a story of childhood trauma. This risk was why soldiers should not be brought to an unstable psychological state in a place that was itself unstable. Therapy required safety, both in the sense of a trusted therapeutic relationship and safety from physical and emotional harm, and even the most hardened of military infrastructure could not guarantee the latter. The logic of therapy and safety located the threat outside the military and the walls of the FOB, envisioning the place and occupied people as the sole source of harm. They are not only trauma-inducing; they are hostile to the healing of soldiers' psyches.

Major Rivera, a psychiatric nurse practitioner, likewise told me that there were "boxes you didn't open" in deployment. She told me that therapies like Eye Movement Desensitization and Reprocessing (EMDR) and PET—both of which she characterized as "psychologically more invasive"—weren't things they did in-country.[52] "I think, you know, with anything, you have a risk of destabilizing someone further, right?" she commented about therapy interventions more generally. But additionally, she explained, "some things are not even particularly relevant to what that mission is and what you're doing in country." She gave me the example of a soldier's childhood trauma, something soldiers would want to address with a therapist or counselor at some point "if it's impacting them." But deployment was likely not that time, since "it's not really relevant to the soldier's role. And if they're able to maintain their overall functioning, then it's not something that we would address." Why open that box when it risks destabilizing the soldier in that environment? "Overall, you want people to focus on their mission and to be able to cope well with what they're doing," Major Rivera emphasized. "When you start peeling off the Band Aid, so to speak, you make them more vulnerable."

Soldiers shared similar ideas about compartmentalizing when deployed. Lots of things could need boxing up: an email that your girlfriend was breaking up with you, problems with the kids at school, bills piling up at home, or things seen and done that day on patrol. If you didn't, those things could eat away at you until you couldn't do your job anymore, you couldn't be in game mode. One soldier explained compartmentalizing the death of a friend during his deployment, saying, "I wanted to be alive more than understand what was going on with me." Soldiers described events and their emotions through metaphors of enclosure, invoking fortification and hardening reminiscent of the FOBs they returned to each day. Others talked about "filing things away" or "dumping them" into boxes, lids shut tight, as if they could be stored in the attic of the mind, like the journal into which one medic told me she purged the things she saw each day and pledged not to reread while deployed. These were things that needed to be quite literally contained against the chance of everything coming loose. Yet, not unlike the box in the attic, its presence remained; a reminder that it was there to be "unpacked" later, as needed—perhaps when you were home and away from this place, when you could think again. Or not. But tucking into those things in deployment was not only impractical, since no one could truly help you through all of what you unleashed if you did; it could also take you, as one soldier put it, right to "the edge." Opening boxes could be destabilizing, setting you down a road no one needed you to go.

. . . . .

This chapter has explored efforts to keep stable those who are tasked with the work of stabilization. As a key concept of military and political governance and counterinsurgency strategy that experienced a revival during the wars in Iraq and Afghanistan, stability has also been a central organizing concept in the embodied practice of soldiers and in the governance of mental health among military care providers. Tracing the many inroads into stability takes us into diverse concepts and practices of stabilizing fragile states by exercising control. Providers blend clinical, administrative, and intuitive practice in their efforts to predict and maintain soldier stability, an exercise in prognosis and risk management balancing medication use, operational demands, and the pressures of military command. Soldiers, meanwhile, attune to in/stability by blending ethical reasoning, technical practice, and affective judgment. Where stability is understood to be a behavioral potential that can be chemically modified and medically treated, psychopharmaceuticals and psychopharmaceutical action provide a logic and a definitive means by which providers and soldiers alike seek to control relationships to violence. In the process, they produce moral definitions that distinguish "excess" violence while legitimating the "normal" use of force in counterinsurgency warfare as appropriate, measured, and good.

In the pursuit to stabilize on the battlefield, psychopharmaceuticals were mainstreamed during the war on terror as both quick fix and chronic salve. But how did these pills and tablets come into the hands of soldiers? As we will see in the following chapter, maintaining soldier stability through pharmaceuticals required a pragmatic commitment to supply and logistics: namely, the provisioning of medication to where and when it was needed over the long term. Supplying empire is a vital part of this story of war medicine.

4 Supply

> Logistics is traditionally an unglamorous and underappreciated activity. To generalize, when the battle is going well, the strategist and tactician are lionized; it is only when the tanks run out of gas that people go headhunting for the logisticians.
>
> Lt. General William G. Pagonis, *Moving Mountains,* p. x

While little about Corporal Bey's deployment to Iraq followed a set routine, one thing occurred with unfailing regularity. Nearly every day for five months—close to half his tour—Bey made a point to drop in at the aid station on base. In the beginning, he tried to play it casual. He just happened to be passing by, he would tell the medic on shift, so he thought he'd check in. Had anyone managed to get their hands on some since yesterday? It took a week before these visits became the running joke in the aid station, but Bey didn't mind. The unit had good working relationships with all the medics and their supervising PA, and if anyone could get what he needed, it would be them. So, as predictably as the sun rose and set each day over the concertina wire-laced blast walls surrounding their base, Bey showed up to say hi or, occasionally, to drop off a little something—a few smokes or a pack of gum. A cordial but persistent reminder that he was waiting and in need.

Just days into his deployment, Bey had run out of medication. With dread, he had been counting down his pills, knowing it was only a matter of time. The 25-year-old had been called up to deploy so quickly that there hadn't been enough lead time to arrange to bring with him a bulk supply of medication through his Army provider. So, when it was time to go, Bey kissed his wife and newborn goodbye and left for Iraq with the nine pills he had on hand. The day his bottle of propranolol no longer made its telltale rattle, Bey panicked but knew nothing could be done. A common betablocker, one Bey had been prescribed to reduce physical symptoms of anxiety, the propranolol would have been an easy refill at home.[1] But at the time, Bey was located at a small combat outpost where it was clear he stood little to no chance of getting a refill, so he didn't even try.

Mind and body quickly rebelled. Within days of his medication running out, Bey was waking up in the morning imagining worst-case scenarios of IED blasts and his wife and son left on their own. Those early days without medication were a haze of what he described as "constant catastrophizing" and an ambient feeling of "impending doom." Riding in convoys would cause his heart to race "off the charts," a deeply unsettling sensation for Bey, who had had heart surgery a few years prior. At times, it felt as if his chest would break open. As a calvary scout who traveled regularly on mounted missions, those moments now seemed to string the days together.

When his unit was later moved to a larger installation with an aid station, which would become his regular haunt, Bey saw his chance. The aid station didn't stock propranolol, though, so there was none on hand. The PA put in an order to receive a supply through the military mail pharmacy. In the meantime, personal relationships became key, and the young corporal took to showing his face at the aid station to cultivate them. Aware that the medics regularly traveled out to other installations, Bey eventually got friendly enough with a few of them to ask if they would try to snag some propranolol for him from the aid stations there, enough to tide him over until the full refill came through the mail. "By seeing my face each day," Bey told me, "they were going to be more likely to help me because not everyone is bringing their problems to them every day. So, if something did come up or there was a chance to grab some medication, they would. My thing was just keeping it fresh in their mind." Even then, on the days his symptoms were unbearable, the affected casualness of his visits to the aid station would give way to angry rants on the phone with his wife: how could the world's most advanced military, capable of moving billions of dollars of equipment around the world at a moment's notice, fall so woefully short in delivering him a few pills?

Despite Bey's diligent efforts to cultivate relations and ease flows, the pipeline stayed dry. Bey wouldn't come into any more propranolol until his prescription arrived through the mail. By then, over five months had passed, and Bey had just two weeks left before returning home. The irony of it all was that the medication arrived in true Army bulk-supply style: in the biggest bottle of pills that Bey had ever laid eyes on. In an apt culmination of his many months of dedicated visits and to the genuine applause of all in the aid station, the medics ceremoniously handed off the propranolol to Bey in the oversized manufacturer's bottle—without the usual prescription label indicating his name and dosage, and full of hundreds of pills that ended up lasting him until well after his return home, details he recounted to me with disturbed wonder. From scarcity to utter surfeit. The irony doesn't escape either of us as Bey recounts this mistimed windfall.

Bey's experience is telling, both as a tale of lack and of eventual, albeit belated, surplus. It highlights the efforts and challenges of militaries to get what they need, when and where they need it. As a tale more specifically about the provision of military care, Bey's account also points to contradictions and tensions in the cultural transformation of mental health treatment in the time-space of chronic global war. The arrival of a factory-issued bottle at the tail end of Bey's tour was not only poorly timed; its bulk response misrecognized the tailored and individualized needs of mental health care. Unlike mass vaccinations, the use of psychopharmaceuticals typically requires customization, titration, and maintenance in ways that can sit uneasily alongside the standard-issue approach that the Army does so well. Misalignments between mental health and medical supply and logistics are typically absorbed by military medical and mental health care providers, who must work in the gap between what they have and what they need, and by soldiers like Bey, who must sometimes wait and withdraw.

At the same time, providers and soldiers also share, improvise, hack, and tinker in the space of limitation and possibility that emerges in episodic shortage and bounty. For Bey, that meant a lot more smoking to manage symptoms without the propranolol. It also meant finding passive acceptance, both in the moments when his heart would race and in the long, frustrating wait for his refill. He reconnected with techniques for slowing and focusing his breath. "If there was a task I had to tackle,

I would know how to deal with it," Bey explained. "I also knew my body. I knew I wasn't going to die from it. I knew, eventually, it would be fine." Riding the lightning, is how he put it.

. . . . .

In the wars in Iraq and Afghanistan, psychopharmaceuticals were crucial to the effort to stabilize empire. In practical terms, this required getting the right pills to the right places, in the right amounts, at the right times. The light mobility of medications appears to be an obvious solution to the push for forward care. Yet Bey's long wait and mistimed bounty suggests that this mobility isn't always as simple or as "light" as it might promise.

The mobility of psychopharmaceuticals on the battlefield recalls the ambition of medicine in war more broadly. Battlefield medicine aims to bring care as far forward as possible to meet the injured at the point of wounding. In the wars in Iraq and Afghanistan, improvements in methods used to control bleeding, replace blood, and reduce time to treatment during the so-called golden hour—the 60 minutes following a battlefield injury when proper medical treatment can be crucial to survival—contributed to the highest survival rates for any war in US military history.[2] That meant getting ever-evolving techniques and technologies like self-applied tourniquets, plasma kits, and forward surgical procedures ever closer to the moment and place of severe injury.

But unlike an IED blast or a bullet wound, which demand prompt treatment and evacuation, the chronic and episodic nature of depression and anxiety requires continual maintenance and periodic recalibration in situ. Reflecting the dynamic nature of mental health itself, antidepressants and anxiolytics must also be trialed, titrated, and refilled. Bringing care forward to soldiers with chronic medication needs like Bey thus required an enduring logistical and technical commitment of a different sort than that of combat medicine, one materialized most essentially in the supply and resupply of pills.

This chapter centers the material flows of psychopharmaceuticals and the sustained logistical commitment required to support their chronic use on the battlefield. It asks what these flows reveal about the new role of medication in the in situ management of full-spectrum mental health, and more broadly about chronic war as a project of the carefully timed and unremitting circulation of material things. What is required to get medicine far forward—in this case, the medications of empire that sustain those who sustain *it*? What does it mean in practical terms to keep soldiers in place using chronic medications that must reach them at the right time and in the right place and over the long term of war and occupation? What happens when they fail to come through? Tracing the supply of psychopharmaceuticals enables us to see what is materially required to sustain US military power as force projection. It also reveals the interruptions in pharmaceutical flows and the ways soldiers improvise and get by in the gaps. While the provisioning of antidepressants, antianxiety medications, and sleep aids is important to the story of psychopharmaceuticals in the war on terror, the breaks in supply, lost pills, and empty bottles are equally, if not more, revealing.

Central to this story are the dynamics of logistics and supply, terms I use to identify a broad domain of formal and informal economies and practices by which the material things that sustain military empire get to where they are needed. My use of these terms encapsulates their more conventional meanings describing how US military and private-sector industries synergize and synchronize to procure, warehouse, distribute, maintain, and move supplies, services, and materials—from planes and tanks to toilet paper and medication—across an expansive global US military basing system. But I also use "logistics" and "supply" to recognize the smaller scale workarounds by which military personnel learn to access and get things to one another, particularly when official supply chains fail. These workarounds constitute material and social processes that can deliver but often require cultivated contacts, improvisation, and institutional and localized know-how. Like the friendly visits and occasional packs of gum and cigarettes meant to ingratiate Bey to the medics who were the lifeline to his medication, informal economies and social relations of circulation, exchange, and sharing flourish among military personnel in deployment, and pharmaceuticals are no exception. They sustain soldiers like Bey. Even in times of lack, the prospect of resupply can impart value to relations and keep soldiers in place, awaiting the next delivery.

TOOTH AND TAIL

Armies are built on mobile fighting forces (what the military calls its "tooth"). But they also require extensive support services (their "tail"). They need ammunition, trucks, planes, and tanks; they also need food, linens, paper clips, and caffeinated drinks—and in large quantities, particularly the latter. Collectively termed "materiel," the things of military empire are managed by the US Army Materiel Command. Its task, in its own words, is to "deliver logistics, sustainment and materiel readiness from the installation to the forward tactical edge to ensure globally dominant land force capabilities."[3] The bulk of what the Army needs is procured, contracted, warehoused, supplied, transported, and distributed courtesy of a vast global military and commercial logistics network. A much smaller but personally significant portion travels through the mail to individual soldiers in care packages, and increasingly through online shopping giants like Amazon, whose planetary research extends to overseas military addresses. Most of these items are standard, like the candy, energy drinks, beef jerky, and extra socks ubiquitous to school and church group–assembled care packages. Others are more furtive, like the mouthwash bottles refilled with vodka colored with green food dye, nestled quietly among the candy and energy drinks.

During the war on terror, psychopharmaceuticals likewise moved into overseas deployed settings via routes both official and unofficial, and with varying degrees of documentation. Medications are Class VIII in the Army supply classification system, a class that includes a wide range of medical supplies and equipment, from bandages and medications to blood products and surgical instruments. In the wars in Iraq and Afghanistan, military treatment facilities in theater received bulk shipments of medication through routine logistical channels. Medications would also travel more modestly, carried in the rucksacks of individual soldiers authorized to bring their own supply with them in bulk. Those same soldiers could later refill them through the military mail-order pharmacy system, their aid station, or—if they were lucky to have access to one—through a military pharmacy in-country.[4] In some cases, deployed behavioral health units maintained their own medication supply, taking particular care with controlled substances like benzodiazepines and stimulants. In the rarer case, when a soldier had prescriptions filled by civilian providers outside of (and unknown to) the military, they could arrive, hidden, in the care packages sent by family. In circumstances of desperation, they were sourced locally. Once in the hands of soldiers, they would be tucked away for personal use; sometimes, they would be shared or exchanged.

But unlike packs of gum, tube socks, or even vaccines, psychopharmaceuticals introduce specific supply challenges for the temporalities by which they are prescribed and used. When used as chronic medications, they require continuous supply, yet refills through the mail-order pharmacy could take weeks to months to reach overseas military personnel. A soldier might arrive in theater with a bulk supply of an SSRI they had been taking for years only to have a reoccurrence or worsening of symptoms that required a dosage change or new prescription, a common presentation for soldiers deployed with medication.[5] Or they may not have reported their medication use as required by the Army before they left the station and deployed on an antidepressant different from the first- and second-line antidepressants stocked in the limited deployment formulary, only to run out while in theater.

While the quantity and variety of medications available for prescription in a deployed formulary are generally reduced, in the war on terror this was especially true for psychiatric medications. Even after the push for an expanded formulary by the military mental health community, there was no guarantee that deployed formularies would include providers' preferred medications or the medications their patients were already on. Of those that were stocked, there were often limited amounts, leading to frugal dispensation tactics. Typically, a provider had enough supply to begin the soldier on a certain medication and tide them over until a mail-order pharmacy prescription could be initiated. Medications were flown in or were transported on convoys, the latter of which were susceptible to attacks and didn't always reach their destination.

When it came to the drugs on hand, flexibility and economy were essential. Based on their experiences deployed to Iraq, three military psychiatrists proposed a psychotropic medication formulary in 2007 that recommended 24 medications under the categories of antidepressants/antianxiety medications, benzodiazepines, antipsychotics/antimanics, sleep medications, adrenergic agents, and ADHD medications.[6] Included

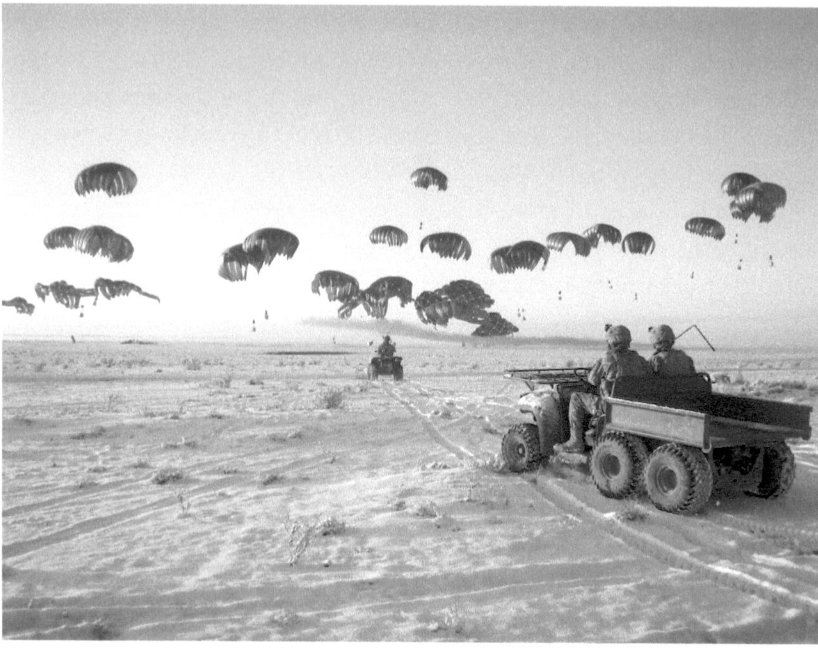

Figure 12. Soldiers wait to retrieve bundles of fuel and supply dropped into their landing zone in Paktika Province, Afghanistan. Photograph by US Army, 101st Division Sustainment Brigade Public Affairs, via DVIDS.

among them are several SSRIs as well as at least two non-SSRI antidepressants. The psychiatrists advised their deploying colleagues to "consider for largest-quantity selection an SSRI that is also indicated for new-onset anxiety disorders"—namely Zoloft (sertraline) and Celexa (citalopram), both of which they described as usually well tolerated for both depression and anxiety symptoms.[7] Bupropion and venlafaxine are good options, they argued, because they have different mechanisms of action than SSRIs and because they can be used in the treatment of other conditions beyond depression: bupropion for ADHD and smoking cessation and venlafaxine for generalized anxiety disorder. Remeron is another advisable choice, "because insomnia is nearly ubiquitous during deployments."[8]

The expansion of the supply and provisioning of psychopharmaceuticals went hand and hand with the evolution of the treatment of combat operational stress casualties, as discussed in chapter 1. Mature infrastructure, to use the military term, was critical to the shift from forward psychiatry predicated on triage and nonpharmacologic treatment to full-spectrum mental and behavioral health care more consistent with outpatient psychiatric practices. Being able to stock and supply psychopharmaceuticals was both enabled by and a sign of the broader transformation of mental health care provision in theater and the enduring nature of war and occupation itself.

Having deployed at the outset of the war in Iraq, Shawn would see nothing of these transformations. In the face of medication scarcity, he would have to improvise his own supply. The field artillery fire-finder radar operator had been among the 130,000 US troops involved in the US-led invasion that began in March 2003. He fell into a bad spot during his deployment, at a time when, in the Army and in the war, "there was no such thing as mental health," as he put it. Shawn's job was to detect combatant forces and alert Army units using a highly specialized mobile radar system that scans for incoming rockets, artillery, and mortar fire. "There was no FOB or nothing," he told me one rainy afternoon in the carpeted quiet of the local public library in his town. He wore a blue pullover, the hood still damp from his sprint from the bus stop. "A lot of people say, 'Well, I was in Iraq at this base.' I'd never seen that. It was just moving from Kuwait all the way to Tikrit, just straight going through, blowing up everything." Shawn was leaving Kuwait to return home as President Bush was declaring major combat operations over in Iraq, the infamous "mission accomplished" banner sailing overhead on the aircraft carrier USS Abraham Lincoln.

Weeks into his deployment, Shawn had reached his limit. Unable to sleep "'cause of the anxiety," his focus grew fuzzy, and his body dragged. His exhaustion made him worry for his own safety and the safety of his team, but he saw few options for help. He explained that the medic, the only provider he had access to, "wasn't there for that kind of psychiatric part." He continued, "'cause, you know, we were supposed to be okay psychiatrically at that point. Our medic wasn't prepared for that." Still, Shawn did have one resource in his favor. Diagnosed with ADHD as a child, he had taken Adderall and Xanax for years prior to enlisting in the Army. This, Shawn told me, together with having mother who is a nurse, made him reasonably well versed in types of psychotropic medication.[9] Desperate for something to help him get some sleep, he and a fellow corporal decided to source their own medication. When their platoon was going through an Iraqi air force base that had been taken over by coalition forces, they saw their opportunity: they raided the pharmacy on base.

Shawn quickly realized that others had had the same idea. They were unable to find the Xanax they were hoping for, likely due to the special mission unit their platoon had followed. "The labels were written in English and Arabic on the shelves," Shawn recalled. "And the whole Xanax line of jars of medications was missing. Someone had gotten there before we did." What they did find were sample packs of the antipsychotic Thorazine. "I didn't know that it had antipsychotic properties, but I had heard from people that they use it in hospitals for psych patients, so I knew it calmed people down," Shawn explained. "So that's what we were carrying out with."

At their limit with no foreseeable options at hand, Shawn and his buddy found a workaround in the ruins of empire. In what was left behind in a ransacked Iraqi military pharmacy, they found enough pills, used sparingly and strategically, to help them get through the remainder of their deployment. Even then, discretion was key. Use of a medication without prescription is technically subject to the Uniform Code of Military Justice. More immediately, they worried about being labeled weak by their command. They also knew they had to be exceedingly careful with a chemical unknown to them, so they broke up the pills to take in small, measured doses at first, alternating their schedules so that one could sleep with the other keeping watch: "in case, you know, combat kicked off, we could at least protect the other guy, make sure they're in their foxhole." By staying awake and alert in the event the other needed protection, the two entered a pact of mutual reliance and secrecy around medication use at a time when supply was otherwise not coming.

THE THINGS THEY CARRIED

In the years after Shawn returned home, battlefield mental health care would see the expansion of deployment formularies, enhanced tracking of prescription requirements, and improved supply chains.[10] Even then, medication stocks were often less robust or regular than deployed providers expected, wished, or were accustomed to given how they practiced in garrison settings. These issues were particularly significant at operationally remote locations occupied by subordinate, smaller units. As one PA put it to me, "If my soldier runs out of medication and they're in the middle of nowhere, it's not like they can just run down to Walmart and fill that prescription." While mail-order pharmacy was an option often preferable to the normal medical supply chain in these locations, mail could lag, depending on helicopter flight availability and mail sort operations at larger FOBs. Soldiers, often, were also on the move. Getting medication refills to them at the right time and place could thus require multiple levels of coordination, proactive planning, premonitory timing, and not a bit of luck. The prospects of unreliable medication supply meant that many PAs I spoke with made a concerted effort to get their patients the maximum allowable amount of medication to carry with them before they left to deploy. "All the other problems fall away when the soldier has his entire duration of deployment in his pocket," one told me. "That was my goal."

But having a deployment in their pocket presumes that soldiers won't need their prescription or dosage adjusted or that they won't lose their medication or get it wet while neck-deep in water. It also presumes that soldiers won't need a prescription for a new diagnosis while deployed. The challenges of initiating a soldier on medication are complex, but of the multiple factors that military providers must consider, questions of supply are front and center. Providers must be able to support follow-up for soldiers started on medication; they must also make sure resupply is available. They need to consider the implications if the soldier runs out or must otherwise abruptly stop their medication, including possible withdrawal effects, impacts on behavior and performance, and risks to others.[11]

Soldiers, too, need to think about how to store and carry their medication, particularly when they are on the move. Medication should preferably be in capsule and not pill form, since the sealed hard gelatin of capsules offers protection from deterioration and makes them easier to swallow without water. With all the other gear soldiers are required to carry, medication bottles only add unwanted bulk, so medication is best stored in plastic zip-top baggies that are lightweight and (relatively) waterproof.

They also allow free movement when soldiers go prone, as they do when taking fire to minimize their profile and stabilize their weapon. Unlike command-ordered medication like malarial prophylaxis, which was typically administered as directly observed therapy, or DOT, wherein a chain-of-command authority distributed the medication to lines of soldiers and watched to ensure they swallowed their dose, antidepressants and antianxiety medications were the personal responsibility of the soldier. The soldier had to maintain and administer their own prescribed supply.

However, even when motivated to do so, adherence to chronic psychotropic treatment was often hindered by practical constraints. Soldiers had to ensure they brought enough medication if they traveled off base, a detail easily overshadowed by other priorities when preparing for missions, or made moot when missions were drawn out longer than planned. In those cases, a soldier's medic—the enlisted medical technician they had easiest access to—would not have what they needed on hand. A soldier's medic would be guaranteed to carry on them small amounts of what are called "sick-call meds," the common over-the-counter medications like the Motrin that soldiers affectionately call "Vitamin M" because of how freely it is given for aches and pains. They would not have on hand the specific SSRI or antianxiety medication prescribed to the soldier by their PA, nurse, or psychiatrist.

These were the kinds of practical concerns that occupied Barb during her deployment to Afghanistan in 2011. A senior combat medic, Barb kept careful track of the inventory in her medic bag: the tourniquets, ACE wraps, chest seals, NSAIDs, morphine, antibiotics, and assorted bandages and dressings, among other medical materiel needed to keep her soldiers alive and healthy. She also kept careful track of her own personal medication. Barb spent much of that deployment giving medical coverage along supply and reconnaissance convoy routes, which amounted to traveling 10,000 miles in nine months, or so she tallied after she got home. The SSRI Lexapro was among the things she carried across those thousands of miles.

Barb had deployed to Iraq several years prior while on Lexapro, having received a waiver that permitted her to deploy after she evidenced clinical stability on a set dosage for three months prior to her departure. While deployed, she began cutting herself. "The cutting started downrange because there was a lot going on, and I wasn't effectively using coping strategies," she shared one afternoon at her dining table. Barb had been going through a divorce at the time, and her then-husband was withholding her children. About four months before she left for Iraq, he assaulted her and sent her to the hospital with a broken jaw. "I don't know, cutting seemed like an . . ." intoned Barb, floating off for a second. "I could control that and the pain in one location," she continued, "and then let it be there, and I didn't have to think about the rest." When a peer reported on Barb, her dosage was upped by a provider at the hospital on the large installation where she was located. She would continue to stay on Lexapro through her second deployment to Afghanistan.

While in Afghanistan, running supply routes as a combat medic gave Barb practical awareness of the networked nature of supply. If soldiers aren't out running supply convoys because they've themselves run out of medication, other supplies run dry. "You have to stay on a certain schedule to make sure ammo, food, water and other life supplies would go to different bases when they would run low. It would come from bigger bases, go out to the smaller," Barb explained. "Like, FOB Lightning is a little base of US soldiers and joint forces in the middle of an Afghan base," she tells me. "So, if FOB Lightning requires us to do resupply for them and if we don't make our route times, then they're going without food, without water, without supplies. And even though Afghan forces in that area are our allies, if they don't have the resupplies, that could shift." Doing the math in her head, Barb told me that if you have a couple of soldiers in a unit who can't do their mission because they're having medication withdrawal effects, "you can't really run the mission at that point. You don't have security trucks, and that pushes you back a week." When medications run empty, so, too, do the lifelines of empire.

The "vital mobility" of humanitarian medicine, writes Peter Redfield, requires a "delicate web of support systems" that must work reliably and seamlessly to deliver technical solutions in places the public health field describes as "resource-poor settings."[12] Like the delivery of humanitarian aid that comes to a halt when the Land Cruiser carrying it punctures a tire, the vital importance of motion in military medicine becomes most visible at points of rupture: when resupply deliveries don't make it or are held up.[13]

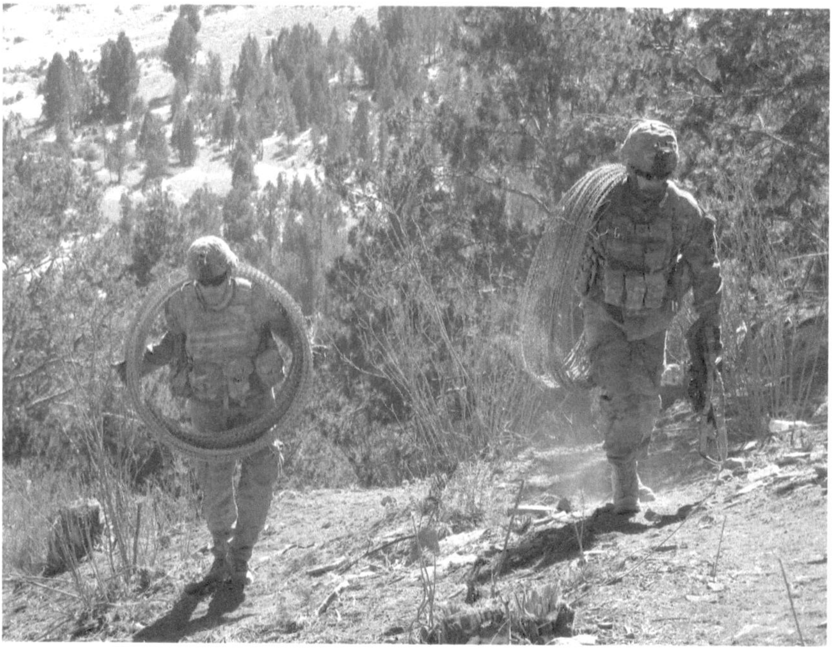

Figure 13. Carrying concertina wire up to an observation post in East Paktika Province, Afghanistan. Photograph by SSG Brandon Rickert, via DVIDS.

Barb herself worried about running out of Lexapro while on the road. "You just gotta make sure you know where your meds are when you're on the road that much. And you can't forget them," she cautioned. "If I was gone for three weeks and I didn't take my medication with me, that was a big problem." If that happened, she would have to hope their unit ended up at a decent-sized base along the way, where she might be able to find a provider to pull her up in AHLTA, the global electronic health-record system used by the DoD. But that was a gamble. To help insure against running out, Barb would keep backup kits in her gear—small zip-top baggies with a few pills that stayed in her go bag and leg bag—in case she forgot to bring her primary bottle.

For soldiers like Barb, the experience of taking chronic medication in the time-space of forward care can often be the experience of running out, or at least the fear of it. To manage that risk, they find small but important ways to take care of the meds that take care of them, tucking them away in small caches on their body and storing them in little plastic baggies. They may count on the timing of supply convoys, the arrival of mail, or a stop at a large installation with robust supplies as they count down their remaining pills and hope to come across a refill at the right place and time. Sometimes, they must manage running out.

EMPTY

For David, running out meant running on empty. A surgical nurse, David deployed early in the Iraq War to a large combat support hospital where, for 12 months, he managed nighttime operations. With two windows adjacent to his cot and a view that looked out onto the entrance to the morgue, space blankets and duct tape could only do so much to make for restful sleeping conditions during the day. Ambien helped.[14] "We'd get off in the morning," David told me, describing his daily routine. "We'd go decompress a little bit, go have chow in the morning together and then we'd all split up and I'd go downstairs and take my Ambien," he said, snapping his fingers, "and wake up when I woke up." The Ambien worked well, almost too well. "I never had an alarm wake me up and I felt like I got sleep. But I couldn't sleep without it," he recalled. "My problem was I was never tired, but I knew I needed to sleep and the only way I got many hours of sleep was the Ambien. So, that's what I did. But when I came home, I never touched it again."

David told me he took Ambien every day during that deployment, or at least, nearly every day. It depended on supply. "I mean, if I didn't have it, I would get nervous," he admitted, though he's quick to tell me he never had any problems while taking it. Referencing strange and unnerving media accounts of people sleepwalking, sleep driving, sleep eating, and unknowingly committing crimes while on the hypnotic, he told me it was hard to believe all the hype since he never experienced or witnessed any problems on Ambien while deployed.[15] This was also early in the war, he reminds me, when there were fewer restrictions around its use—before, as David put it, the Army caught on. Ambien would flow less freely as the war continued. But at least for the time David was at that large CSH in the first years of the war, it seemed his entire medical team was on it.

"I know, just because of the way we joked about it, that everyone was taking it," he recounted. This fact became clearest when they would run out. "When there was a shortage of it, you would hear about it," David says, laughing lightly. "'Hey, they didn't get their supply this week.' That would be what everybody was talking about. Enlisted officers would be talking about it, saying, 'There's no Ambien.'" During times of dearth, members of the team working the nightshift would pool their remaining pills until the next supply came in. Running out entirely made for difficult days of sleep and even more difficult nights on shift. Personal and collective medication use became evident in times of scarcity, when inquiries, grumblings, commiseration, and shared resources pulled people together while waiting for resupply.

Running out posed different kinds of problems for providers trying to treat and ensure adequate supplies for patients, problems that provoked their own kinds of workarounds. Captain Simpson, an Army psychologist, explained to me how he would work with prescribing PAs to consult on patients and strategize medication inventory. This was particularly true at small outposts where the PA might be the only medical professional and had to maintain a lockbox of medication. While Captain Simpson could not prescribe pharmaceuticals to his patients as a psychologist, the PAs often relied on him to provide unofficial counsel, especially when they lacked experience or confidence in prescribing psychopharmaceuticals.[16]

"I would work very closely with the PAs and docs," Captain Simpson told me, particularly in cases in which a soldier might need to be initiated on a new drug, have their dosage increased, or a medication switched. If he diagnosed a soldier with anxiety, for example, he would sit down with the PA and describe the soldier's symptoms. "Then I'd work with them to say, 'Okay, well what do you have?' And a lot of PAs would say, 'Well, let's go look.'" At a smaller outpost, that could involve inventorying a "two-by-two cabinet of just, random stuff." Based on the initial assessment, the PA and the psychologist might arrive at getting the soldier started on a trial of Wellbutrin (bupropion), one of the more common psychopharmaceuticals in standard deployment formularies since it does double duty as a smoking cessation drug. "The doc would go into the back and count how many pills they had and say, 'Okay, I've got 40 pills for my entire outpost. Hope we don't run out.'" Captain Simpson chuckles, recalling the calculated frugality of counting pills.

Providers, too, worried about running out. In situations in which they confronted the limited supplies stored in a footlocker and the like, they had to consider the collective when they prescribed medication to the individual. Patching together supplies sometimes meant putting in a call to a larger installation nearby, or what Captain Simpson called the larger "super-FOBs, the bases that have more supply." "We'd essentially round robin when we were in theater, like, 'Hey, who's got plenty of or an excess of this?' So, you coordinate your different sources." The goal, he explained, was to get the soldier started with what was on hand while getting them connected with a larger supply, ideally, through mail-order pharmacy. But all that required the links in the chain to hold.

For those outside the flow of things, *finding* the chain could itself be challenging. Often, it was a matter of who you knew. In fact, I was told on several separate occasions and always with a gravity intended to impress that deployment is like prison: you can get anything you need so long as you know who to ask and are willing to pay for it. Luis, who deployed to Iraq from 2008 to 2009, boasted about the "steady flow" of Adderall that he was regularly supplied by a sergeant in his unit. This sergeant had been on Adderall for years to treat his ADHD and was able to keep his authorized prescription regularly refilled during his deployment since the smaller base was restocked by weekly convoys to the sprawling Balad Air Base nearby. Luis was a gunner on a gun truck, which meant that he sat up in the turret of an armored vehicle and operated a 50-caliber machine gun—what he lovingly referred to as "my baby, my bread and butter." Luis talked about his time in Iraq as "easy work" in the sense that it was clear what was expected of him: "providing security for the convoy at all costs." At the same time, he talked about the challenges of irregular sleep and an exhausting schedule of 18-hour shifts during which he went out on patrol for multiple days at a time. To remain focused and vigilant on long convoys, he was "hitting up" the sergeant every few days for an Adderall because it "kept my ass awake and alive." The packs of cigarettes he occasionally gave in exchange were nothing, Luis told me, because this sergeant was "saving my life with these drugs."

While the use of stimulants to keep soldiers awake on patrols is hardly a new phenomenon, what is new is how these medications are transformed in their travels and uptake. The way in which Luis's weekly Adderall evaded military regulatory mechanisms and its transformation in war parallels the diversion of high-dose buprenorphine from treatment contexts to informal networks, described by Anne Lovell in France.[17] Two global addiction markets—one in which buprenorphine is valued as a pharmaceutical tool for the treatment of addiction and the other an illicit drug economy—merge through the process of what Lovell calls "pharmaceutical leakage." In this process, "the pharmaceutical object transforms itself from one type of commodity into another one of a radically different rationality and symbolic nature."[18] Having entered theater as a prescribed therapy for one sergeant's ADHD, in the context of Luis's deployment—of daily patrols outside Baghdad at the tail end of the so-called surge of troop build-up in Iraq—Adderall became the "lifesaving" drug that enabled him to remain alert, alive, and attuned in the application of violence.[19] In this way, the Adderall that drifts into the space of theater through the mechanism of medical waivers can, in turn, be potently hacked by soldiers like Luis, who, after a few weeks of irregular sleep and endless patrols, quickly learn to optimize available chemicals.[20]

Sarah learned this, too, during her first deployment to Iraq shortly after the US-led invasion. From within a secure facility called a SCIF in Baghdad's Green Zone, the former administrative center of the Ba'ath Party and the heavily fortified zone that was taken over by US military forces in April 2003, the cryptologic linguist spent her eight-hour shifts continuously monitoring and translating intercepted communications. It was work that she loved doing and, she told me with some pride, was very good at. But her performance came at the cost of sleep, for she found it difficult to wind down at the end of the workday, or rather work night, since Sarah worked the night shift for the entirety of that 15-month deployment.

Occasionally, Sarah would come upon some chemical help. She hadn't wanted to take any medication on a regular basis, she told me. Not that she was a naturopath, she qualified somewhat defensively, but she did worry about the long-term cumulative effects of medication. Something to help her get some sleep every now and then was all she was looking for. Most importantly, Sarah emphasized, it couldn't be anything that might go on her official record and compromise her security clearance. She opted to go a less formal route. Twice a day, members of Sarah's team would travel from the camp to a larger FOB about a 20-minute drive away. There, they would run errands, collect their mail, and pick up food from the chow hall,

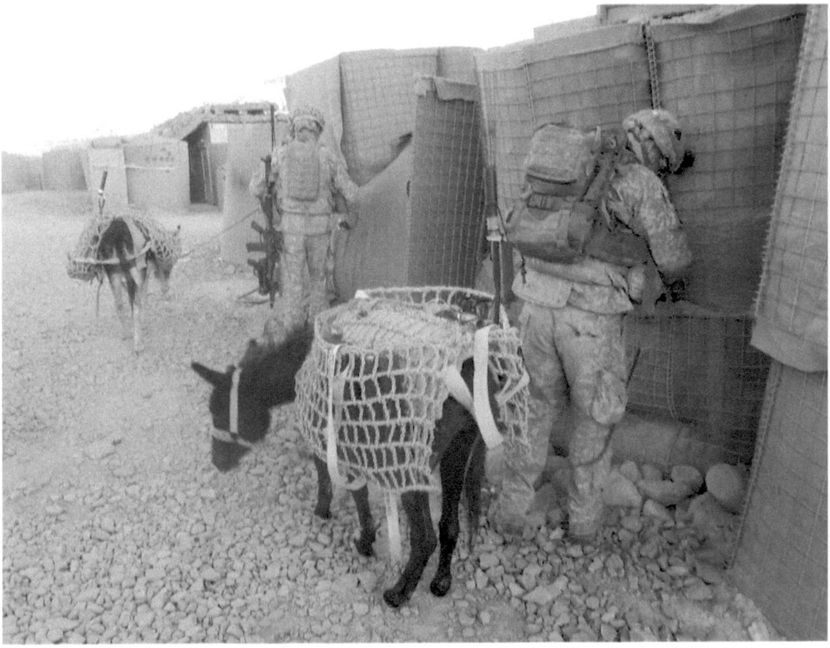

Figure 14. Soldiers untie donkeys carrying counter-radio-controlled improvised explosive device jammers, mortars, MREs, and water for a long-range patrol in East Paktika Province, Afghanistan. Photograph by PFC Brandon Rickert, via DVIDS.

since food runs, however inconvenient, were preferable to eating packaged food rations, known as MREs, day in and day out.

Sarah was able to get other supplies while there, too. It depended on whether she could catch the medic during those short visits on base. If she did, she would explain the situation in a drive-by consult. "You'd just be like, 'Hey, I'm only here for 15 minutes, I don't really have time to go to sick call. This is what I'm having trouble with. Can you help me out?'" The medics were typically obliging, she said, knowing as they did that Sarah's unit didn't have a medic located with them at their camp. Plus, the medics carried small amounts of medication in the pockets of their ACUs. "They would just be like, 'Oh yeah, no, it's totally fine.'" She described the ease of it all. The medics would "just pull stuff out of their shoulder pocket, put it into a little bag, and then they would give it to you and tell you, 'Take one of these at bedtime.'" There was never much—a few pills of trazodone in a small zipper-top plastic baggie with her name, the name of the medication, and minimal instructions written at the top. But it was enough to get by for a time. These spontaneous exchanges—off the cuff, so to speak—were never formally documented in Sarah's record.

Sarah would do that a handful of times before she began to worry that she was asking too frequently and raising eyebrows. She eventually learned to tap into a less direct but more steady supply chain. Sarah's signal intelligence team came to be friendly with the human intelligence folks on base, known colloquially as HUMINTers, "because we're all linguists, right?" One of her HUMINTer friends was able to get "pretty much anything" she needed from her medic, which meant Sarah was able to get the trazodone she wanted through her friend. "I don't know this for sure," Sarah tells me, "but the story is that HUMINTers occasionally traffic in small things to get favors from their sources." This might include things like painkillers, antibiotics, and, apparently, sedatives. Sarah figured the HUMINTers could ask medics for whatever they needed and receive it, presumably for the sake of the intelligence mission. Sarah never formally corroborated this open secret with her friend, but the medication her friend often had on her—in the same little baggies Sarah had received from the medic—was enough to clue Sarah in to where it was coming from. Once Sarah tapped that pipeline, it was as simple as seeking out her friend when she was in need and asking, "'Hey, do you have anything?' And she'd be like, 'I do, hang on.'" Sarah looks a bit sheepish as she recounts these favors, assuring me that she has never been into "recreational drug use or anything." She needed it, Sarah tells me, to do her job. And anyway, she adds, in the end it still came from the medic.

. . . . .

Supply is the lifeblood of military empire, delivering material vitality and force projected over time and distance. Getting things when and where they are needed is fundamental to the control of time and space that is at the core of global US military power in its contemporary expeditionary form. When supply chains deliver antidepressants, sleep aids, and anti-anxiety medications, they sustain the soldiers who fight and hold territory. The lifeblood of empire, followed through the supply and provisioning of psychopharmaceuticals, binds the macro to the molecular, tying the global circulation of medicine to the chemical capacities that enable soldiers to wage war without end.

But supply chains are not always seamless or reliable, even with the maturation of infrastructure and accumulation of experience that come with enduring war. War and occupation also have their pockets of shifting tempo and foci: a military base is razed to solidify the presence and infrastructure at another; troops surge and withdraw. In those ebbs and flows, supply can swell and recede. Even when war winds down, someone must be there to watch the lifelines of empire dry out.

Beyond questions of supply, the mobility of psychopharmaceuticals raises questions about what it means for empire's problems of time and space to be made into issues of supply and logistics: where the deployability of soldiers is a function of arranging bulk medication supply and where surviving exhaustion and sleeplessness are matters of continual refill. Furthermore, what it means for supply to "work" with respect to mental health and the extraction of military labor remains unsettled in contexts in which therapeutic alternatives may not be advisable and medications leave soldiers waiting in place, hoping for a timely refill. The supply and resupply of medication is one narrowly technical solution to enduring war, one which, even when materially achieved, offers no easy victory.

Medicines are meant to be a solution in places where there is no care.[21] Yet much is needed materially to get psychotropic medications into the hands of soldiers and to maintain continuous resupply. Contracts, planes, and trucks to deliver them across the topography of empire are all required, as are military providers to prescribe, monitor, and help titrate the medications, ideally over the long-term. In the far-forward reaches of war and occupation, care and creative resourcefulness are needed by soldiers themselves to ensure they have their medications on them wherever they go and to devise impromptu opportunities for resupply if they run out. Psychopharmaceutical supply in the war on terror was made possible by the infrastructure and time of enduring war and occupation. Yet its flows and breaks also chart the instability of empire at its limits: where human breakdowns meet the breakdowns of supply chains, and at the expeditionary reach of global counterinsurgency, where soldiers on convoy lose their pills, get them wet beyond repair, or forget them entirely.

5 Reaction

Seth asks if I mind if he puts in a chew while we are talking. He's discreet, almost delicate about it, covering his mouth with one hand as he wedges a wad of tobacco into his cheek with the other. The Army Reserve veteran, who first deployed to Iraq as an infantryman during the initial invasion in 2003, is convinced that antidepressants have no place in war. While SSRIs "take the edge off" in a way that's great if you're binge-watching Netflix on your couch on a Sunday afternoon, Seth says that this "dulling down" is entirely maladaptive in a firefight. "You have to be alert at all times, your adrenaline ready to pump at all times. And you have to stay in that mind frame to survive," Seth reflects. "So, SSRIs don't work." Put differently, "When they work, they can get you killed."

Two deployments to Iraq, together with heavy medication use since leaving the Army—what Seth calls being "fed pills" by the VA—have hardened this conviction. At one point in the years after separating from the military, Seth was taking 26 pills a day, including sleep aids and medications for anxiety and depression. He tries to imagine being in that kind of chemical haze on the battlefield. "In a firefight, you have to flank, you have to move in. Chances are, somebody's going to get shot up. That's the chance you take to move forward," he tells me. "So, you have to be, quote, unquote, crazy, *really crazy,* to overpower every instinct you have in order to run into something like that, to do something that puts yourself out there. Dull that down with drugs, and you're going to make a mistake."

I ask Seth to say more about what that dulling would mean for an infantryman like himself. "You need to be rash and unpredictable in combat," Seth continues, running his fingers through his beard as he thinks about how to explain things for me. "Psychopharm takes that away. It balances you out, makes you more human. That's not conducive in that environment." Seth recalls a few soldiers who lost the trust of the team for this reason. "If we don't trust you anymore, we literally keep you away from us, because you could get us hurt or killed by accident or do something stupid. So, we'll send you out: 'Hey, go stand over there, we'll be over here.' That person is literally left out in the cold." They become the shitbag, he says.

Militaries have long sought to keep technology and the environment apart. Examples abound in the history of military logistics and supply. For instance, techniques of "tropicalization" devised by radio engineers and biologists during World War II sought to render the US military's portable radio equipment impervious to the threat of fecund tropical air in the Pacific.[1] The "kit" ubiquitous to contemporary humanitarianism—that familiar "repository of potentially useful implements"—has its own deep history in military equipment and logistics, its techniques of mobility and standardization "the exact opposite of local knowledge in the traditional sense of geographic and cultural specificity of place."[2] Embracing such qualities as miniaturization, portability, and climate proofing, military techniques of equipment design are invested in environmental imaginaries wherein technologies travel as hermetically sealed, "immutable mobiles."[3]

Medications, too, appear encapsulated—in form and in action. Biomedical psychiatry tends to view medications as static objects that carry and produce distinct pharmacologic effects. Taken to be discrete objects, pharmaceuticals common in US civilian life may appear routine and familiar wherever they go, including the battlefield. This separation of chemistry and environment is embedded in military medical bureaucratic and supply practices. Consider the quasi-predictive goal of SRP—the procedural and documentary methods for establishing soldier stability on medication before deployment—and the bulk medication supplies then permitted to follow soldiers into theater.[4] This separation of chemistry and environment is further supported by reductionist-materialist ideas of drugs voiced by some military providers that first-line SSRIs are relatively benign medications, or what one PA I interviewed called "cupcake meds" and another, "baby Tylenol."

However, pharmaceuticals are not stable materials, nor can they be reduced solely to their chemical structure. Pharmaceutical action occurs not only through the medication itself but is potentiated through social and material conditions. In the words of Anita Hardon and Emilia Sanabria, drugs are fluid, "made and remade," and "constantly evolving in relation to their context."[5] Seth reminds us that the meaning of the risk of pharmaceutical use and the embodiment of that risk on the battlefield are actively and dynamically produced. They are also relational, carried by and negotiated among teammates wary of those who lose the trust of the collective. Even seemingly routine medications like SSRIs, Seth suggests, can become uncanny substances in war—familiar yet strange. Or as he put it, they are substances that make you more human, but in doing so, they can get you killed.

This chapter traces the emergent nature of pharmaceutical effects in counterinsurgency warfare, where pharmaceutical action is newly actualized and continually renegotiated in dynamic contexts of risk, violence, and vulnerability, as well as through the corporate structures of military life. It builds on ethnographic observations of military psychopharmaceutical use from previous chapters, where we have seen medication circulate in ways that escape formal regulation, and where SSRIs, mood stabilizers, and stimulants are leveraged for a wide array of purposes beyond the relief of symptoms: to control out-of-control teammates or to power through nightshifts, for example. It also builds on observations in previous chapters about the models of mental health and military performance that soldiers hold in relationship to violence and control. In doing so, this chapter shows how psychopharmaceuticals bring people, infrastructure, technology, weapons, and tactics into uncertain and often volatile arrangements that may work but only for the provisional time-being.

It is useful to think about these unstable formations through the multivalent concept of *reaction*, with its overlapping chemical and militarized meanings. On one level, *reaction* foregrounds the instrumental and performance-oriented ways psychopharmaceutical effects mattered to soldiers, their officers, and military health care providers. As a means of increasing return-to-duty (RTD) rates, psychopharmaceutical use was governed by imperatives to sustain the fighting force under conditions of perpetual war. Yet these drugs were expected to do more than simply keep soldiers in the fight; they were meant to keep them fighting effectively. Liberal humanitarian sentiments of appeasing mental suffering featured minimally in these decisions. Rather, the guiding priority was to maintain mission readiness—or, as Seth put it, to stay in the firefight without becoming the shitbag.

At another level, *reaction* draws attention to the intersubjective and relational aspects of pharmaceutical use, which are arguably intensified in military lifeworlds governed by shared projects of performance and survival. Teammates, for example, attuned to a soldier's medication use to the extent that it impacted collective performance. Prescribing clinicians likewise had to continually evaluate drug effects in relation to changing occupational and operational conditions, including a soldier's job and day-to-day tasks, as well as location and operational tempo.

But concern for psychopharmaceutical use is not just about the extraction of military labor; it is also about risk management. A 2011 report by the Defense Health Board's Psychotropic Medication Work Group found that approximately 23 percent of military personnel were taking "high-risk" medications. The report identifies these medications as those with the potential for significant therapeutic failure when not provided or which, when taken in combination with other drugs, "may increase the *risk of a Service member* in theater (emphasis added)."[6] The concern that psychopharmaceuticals can make the soldier a risk in theater is important to how military providers, command, and soldiers themselves think about medication in deployment. Most soldiers understand psychotropic medication use as a double-edged sword, learning of drug benefits and hazards through personal experience, observation, research, and rumor. Soldiers advise one another on the positives and negatives of specific medications in light of their day-to-day duties and through a risk calculus informed by occupational hazards. Might a sleep aid create danger for the team if a gunner is woken up at two in the morning for an unscheduled night patrol? Do these questions matter for someone in human resources who sits behind a desk all day in a FOB, never leaving the wire? When soldiers talk about medications and concerns about their effects, they give us insight into the capacities they deem necessary to "good" soldiering in counterinsurgency war. In the war on terror, these capacities rested on normative disciplinary, technical, and biopolitical relationships to violence: the ability to pull your weight for the team, to maintain and work your weapons, to discern friend from enemy, and to deploy violence with both efficacy and discriminating moderation.

Risk management around medication use also maintains the illusion that the destructiveness of preemptive war can be controlled and local civilians can be protected from harm, provided soldiers are clearheaded, performing optimally, and not compromised by their medications. This illusion is apparent in the ways providers and soldiers imagine and assess the balance between risk and benefit in medication use. Consider Seth's cautionary tale against antidepressants in which he identified the need for soldiers to be able to run, adrenaline pumping, into a firefight. While foregrounding the requirement for soldiers to be "crazy," the scene Seth painted for us also quietly erased the endangerment of civilians—indeed, the entirety of people and place—as a precondition for unfettered military performance. Crucially, the intensive labor of risk management undertaken by providers, command, and soldiers, which I ethnographically trace in this chapter, was not primarily concerned with the risk to Iraqi and Afghan lives as such or even to soldiers' well-being. Rather, it was ultimately oriented toward securing the strategic success of counterinsurgency objectives, often by implicitly transferring the risk of harm and coercion associated with soldier medication use onto the very people and places under occupation.[7] This chapter thus interrogates risk as an ethnographic object structured by a politics of life and death that assigns unequal value to lives in war.[8]

Attending to the risk and performance-based dimensions of medication reaction also requires recognizing the reactivity of chemicals themselves. Psychopharmaceuticals are one part of a broad ecology of substances used, shared, and experimented with in deployment.[9] A wide range of authorized and unauthorized psychoactive substances that are used for therapy, performance, entertainment, or simply to alter the mood or felt quality of the present moment course through deployed life. These substances can range from prescription medications to the Rip Its and Wild

Tiger energy drinks consumed as fuel to the Benadryl taken before bed as a syrupy nightcap to any number of substances including alcohol and illicit drugs that are obtained through the mail or, with the right contacts, through what soldiers referred to as "the local economy." And then there are the chemical harms of war to which human and ecological life have been willfully exposed, including warfare agents, toxic pollutants, burn pits, and other environmental hazards.[10] Chemicals intermix to produce effects that may enhance, muddle, displace onto, and refract one another, as in a hall of mirrors.

MANAGING RISK

Psychopharmaceuticals are one tool in the kit to keep the deployed soldier deployed. As such, their use in deployment is assessed in terms of the risk posed by potential impairment or changes to the medicated soldier's behavior and performance. But it is also informed by the obverse risk of the soldier's evacuation—namely, the loss of labor and the hazards that loss might pose to the team and unit. As the concern of multiple invested parties, risk management around psychopharmaceutical use ran up the chain of command and reverberated across the lateral relations of deployed military life.

A soldier can come to the attention of command long before being placed on medication, such as when a commander or supervisor directs the soldier to undergo a mental health consultation. In such circumstances, the commander or section sergeant will already have that soldier in their view. If the provider has concerns about the soldier's ability to perform their job or concerns about the risk they pose to themselves or others, the provider will consult with and make a recommendation to military command, including whether to keep the soldier deployed or send them home. If medication is involved, the provider will also consult on the potential risks of medication use given the soldier's day-to-day responsibilities. Though there are many stakeholders invested in the outcome of these discussions and any psychological evaluations that may be performed, consultations between military providers and the chain of command are typically conducted on a "needs to know" basis. As one PA told me, "I won't dive into, like, their sexual trauma as a child or the history of their relationship with their father. It's more, 'This soldier is having depression or anger issues. This is the treatment plan I have for him to see if it can help. I'm recommending we also do this.' And then the commander will say, yes, no, I agree." Those considered "needs to know" may include the soldier's first sergeant, the highest-ranking NCO who likely has direct knowledge of and contact with the soldier.

Command consults involve risk assessments of what typically involve several moving parts. Major Rivera, a psychiatric nurse practitioner, described the command consult as a Venn diagram with overlapping but distinct components involving the patient, the provider, and the chain of command. "The command consultation is super important to me because they can provide me with more context than I could presume," she explained. "They know that soldier. They know that unit. They know the dynamics that are at play. They probably know some information about the family and how deployment has been overall. They also know what their mission is and what they can expect in the near term." As a provider, she would then take all this information and "try to create the most accurate picture of what that person's risk is going to look like in order to make my recommendations." When Major Rivera relies on the command consultation to better understand the personal factors and operational demands at play, risk is implicitly taken to be the risk to the soldier, the unit, and to mission readiness.

Captain Simpson, a psychologist, described the language he uses to connect with command. "The magic words always work," he told me. "Here is the risk to you, here is the risk to the soldier. I want to help you mitigate risk." Given that, if something were to go wrong, responsibility for the soldier would legally fall on command, Captain Simpson taps into that reality when he speaks explicitly of risk during a command consult. "'I want to help you keep your career, and I want to help you take care of your soldier,'" he will say. "So, it was kind of a, 'Hey, you know me, I know you. You know I'll push soldiers as long as they can do it. But when they can't, both you and I know that we need to send them home.' So, when I say, 'We need to pull them off,' you know we need to pull them off. We've done our due diligence. This is not a good situation." In our conversation, Captain Simpson explicitly identified the professional risks that would fall on the shoulders of command should there be a bad outcome; and while the precise nature of the risk to the soldier wasn't made clear by the psychologist, he asserted wanting to avoid what is "not a good situation."

Even while spoken in a language meaningful to command, risk management could feel like it was riding the edge. Commanders could be highly variable in their willingness to take on the liability of soldiers of concern. "Some were very cavalier about it and then others were really risk averse," an NCO told me. Command could be highly engaged with medical providers in the context of the consult; in the experiences of other providers, command minimally heeded provider recommendations, prioritizing the need to keep bodies in place at seemingly "high risk."[11]

Eyes-On

In cases in which a soldier of concern was permitted to stay, that stay was conditional upon the soldier evidencing stability in-country.[12] Keeping a soldier might necessitate modification of their day-to-day duties while it was determined whether they would stabilize on new medication. Upon consulting with the provider and their team, command might decide, for example, to remove the soldier from their platoon doing patrols; but it could also mean rearranging occupational duties to place soldiers in social arrangements in which they might be better observed, encounter fewer stressors, and generally be "out of the way." Among some providers, the possible increase in suicidality with initiation of SSRI therapy was of significant concern. Sometimes, the soldier's ammunition, the firing pin on their weapon, or the weapon itself—even their belt or boot laces, in the event of concern for suicide—might be confiscated.[13] Their access to classified information might also be removed.

Military health care providers were inclined to see this integrated involvement up and down the chain of command as what Major Rivera called an "infrastructure of safety and support" or a kind of "wraparound" care. Consultations with command were also described as critical to the accountability mechanisms by which medical information that might have been held private in the past could now be shared with the chain of command to improve readiness. But where care is tied up with return-to-duty rates and mission readiness, for soldiers of concern this infrastructure could quickly tip into surveillance, monitoring, and infantilizing supervision, or what several NCOs and soldiers pejoratively referred to as "babysitting." NCOs and medics may be deputized to keep an eye on the soldier of concern; they may be told about the medication the soldier is taking and made to watch for behavioral changes. Despite being packaged in a softened, congenial language of "checking in" and "following up," sitting at the center of the Venn diagram necessarily involved being surveilled by others who were waiting for signs of destabilization.

Being removed from your platoon to push paperwork or being otherwise treated like you can't be trusted to do your job—what the Army calls getting "pulled off the line"—could be temporary if a soldier stabilized within a given time frame. While intended to keep the soldier integrated with the unit (a practice grounded in the principles of forward psychiatry), it could also mark them as profoundly apart. Even if, as one NCO put it, the chain of command and medical provider might be discreet about the soldier of concern, speaking only on a "needs to know" basis, everyone tacitly *knew*. As one NCO put it, "Everybody's going to see that one dude handing out basketballs at the gym and know what he's doing there." Despite the relative discretion of pill taking and despite efforts to keep the soldier integrated with the unit, risk management prompted forms of symbolic and physical separation that branded the soldier as not-quite-soldier—or, in the litany of terms soldiers shared to describe the peer who gets pulled off the line for mental health, as the shitbag, problem child, or damaged goods.

Sometimes, they are the snake in the grass.

. . . . .

Risk management can *feel* risky, perhaps most especially to the unit that reabsorbs the soldier of concern. Jonathan, for example, remembers how unsettling it was for his unit to learn that his sergeant had been given medication after an attempted suicide during their deployment to Iraq. As Jonathan described it, "They sent her back for an eval for two weeks and she had to be on observation and stuff. And then they loaded her up with meds and gave her three days to stabilize and then sent her back (to their FOB)." When I asked him how he and others first came to suspect that their sergeant had been put on medication, he told me he knew that she was "on the hardcore stuff," specifically "some of the crazy sleeping meds, like Ambien."[14] "I remember the Ambien because she would have sleepwalking episodes," he told me, shaking his head. "Oh man, like one time? Well, she was a band geek. She brought her flute to Iraq and one time she got found walking around the base in Iraq playing the flute as if she were in marching band. It comes out that she was on Ambien and antidepressants and doing this."

Alongside the threat of sleepwalking on a base replete with weapons, dangerousness materialized in other ways. Given the unpredictable nature of her day-to-day movements on and outside the base, Jonathan's sergeant was ordered to always keep her medications on her. Because of the distinctive rattle the bottle of pills made in her pocket as she walked—a sound that would announce her approach—he and others in the battalion took to calling her "Rattlesnake." As an aural signal of their sergeant's presence and vulnerability, the rattling sound of tablets offers a powerful metaphor for the ways drugs communicate and position the consumer vis-à-vis others when dispensed in theater. The use of psychopharmaceuticals occupies a highly ambivalent position, serving both as warning to others ("she is a potential hazard") and as a symbol of the individual's fulfillment of duty ("she is following orders"). In their medication use, returned military personnel like Rattlesnake simultaneously enacted both the durability and tenuousness of their obligation to the unit and to the mission. Especially when used by the individual to treat symptoms associated with psychiatric disorder, psychopharmaceuticals could ride the cusp between order and volatility, linking together the mission readiness and endangerment of self and whole.

But more than generating concern for safety on the FOB alone, witnessing psychotropic drug treatment attuned Jonathan to profound contradictions at the nexus of medicine and war. Thinking about his sergeant's medicated return to duty, he explained feeling troubled by the ways medication served to maintain mission readiness over and against his sergeant's well-being. "It's pretty underhanded," he said, pausing. "I mean, the lady tried to kill herself. She was 26. And then they send her back less than a month later, back to the same job, same people, same exact situation," he reflected. "Because you know, it can't be that the mission is wrong. The unit itself can't be messed up. Because it's the Army: 'Of course we're always right,' you know?"

Military medicine and military psychiatry medicalize and optimize. They stretch soldiers' limits to keep them in the fight: to withstand more and for longer. In a time of chronic war and a deepening recruitment crisis, medicine was tasked with keeping the empire running. But medicine, too, has its limits—limits that can become turning points. For some soldiers, when the chemical push comes to shove, psychopharmaceuticals foment resistance to the biopolitical and coercive potentials of military medicine, to the war machine that has worn them down, and to the wars themselves. A soldier's medication use—or more commonly, seeing their friends and peers medicated—flips a switch. This, too, can be a reaction to psychopharmaceuticals in war.[15]

POTENTIATING WAR

Psychopharmaceuticals, particularly when used in the treatment of mental health, can evoke both possibility and threat in deployment. Their use draws providers and the military chain of command into the complicated labor of prognostication in dynamic settings, blending the clinical, personal, operational, and tactical with the proverbial wait and see. Concerns on the part of military command, team leaders, and peers to monitor soldiers on new medication center on questions of risk and mission readiness. But these concerns are also about the specific ways that pharmaceutical action can potentiate in settings designed for war and occupation.

The risk that military command and military providers aim to mitigate, after all, is not just the risk of grogginess or fatigue from an SSRI; it's the risk of grogginess and fatigue if you're the 50-cal gunner in a Humvee. The ways soldiers and providers alike evoked different military jobs to talk about risk differentials on the battlefield was profoundly telling of their concepts of mental health in relation to normative distinctions of martial violence. For instance, I often heard soldiers and providers make medication-risk stratifications based on the job and whether that job required regularly leaving the wire. One infantry officer told me, "The people that stay on the FOB all the time, the people who work supply or

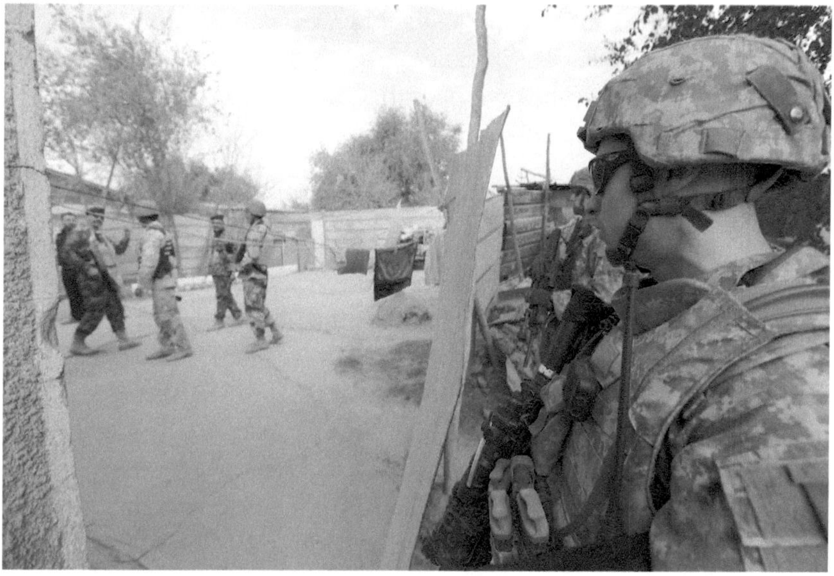

Figure 15. Conducting a "cordon and knock" operation in the village of Kew, Iraq. Photograph by SGT Jacob H. Smith, via DVIDS.

work in the offices? I really wouldn't care if they are impaired. If the office supply person is popping Xanax all day, I could not care less because it wouldn't affect anybody's life." Likewise, an antidepressant dulling the reaction time or situational awareness of a cook located at a built-up FOB may not be a major concern. On the other hand, the infantry soldier leaving the FOB every day is another thing, he said (though he conceded jokingly, a cook zonked on their medications could lead to many more pissed off soldiers).[16] Such risk assessments often revealed implicit hierarchies within the military that prioritize intimacy with combat violence as the only "real" experience of war and by extension see soldiers who regularly leave the wire as shouldering the greatest risk in medication use.[17]

For others, it was the FOB itself—the heavily armed, sealed-off installation that would become the cornerstone of counterinsurgency strategy in the war on terror—that amplified the dangers of undisciplined violence and made psychopharmaceutical use especially risky. In the potent convergence of encapsulated military infrastructure and psychopharmaceuticals, soldiers imagined injuries compounded by weapons and drugs on an almost unspeakable scale. For instance, for Corporal Bey, the problem with medications with psychotropic potential of any kind was that soldiers slept with weapons on FOBs saturated with more weapons. Bey was one of many I spoke with who alerted me to side effects they experienced on mandated antimalarial chemoprophylaxis. Some of these reported side effects were mild and somewhat common: nausea, dyspepsia, and diarrhea. Other reported side effects, though rare, were severe and worrisome: thoughts of suicide, psychosis, and hallucination, among them. Across these accounts, what soldiers like Bey were most eager to talk about were the vivid dreams they experienced on antimalarials, dreams that ranged from diverting fantasy to absurd hallucination to blazing night terrors that jolted you awake in a sweat.

Bey experienced this for himself the first time he deployed to Iraq. It took him just a few weeks to decide that continuing to take his chemoprophylaxis just wasn't worth the risk. Depending on your job, he says, it wasn't uncommon to have live grenades in your room while you slept. "Whatever weapon systems are yours," the cavalry scout told me, "those stay with you the entire time you sleep. You always have a 30-round magazine in your weapon. I could see where things could go bad." You also had to remain ever ready to respond to mortar attacks, including those that could wake you up in the dead of night. Put those threats together with the night terrors and you created the potential for grave mistakes in an already deadly situation, so Bey decided to stop taking his medication. He shared with me his para-epidemiological risk calculus, commenting, "Maybe it's stupid, but I've never even known anybody who had malaria. I figured if malaria kills me in Iraq, then that's natural selection." With a nonchalant shrug, Bey added, "With everything else going on, I wasn't worried about malaria."

Bey's comments suggest that the dangerousness of medication for soldiers emerges not as a discrete effect inherent to the medication itself, but rather in dynamic relation to war making. For Bey, the harm of antimalarials is not the harm of nightmares alone, so much as the problem of their potent convergence with weapons on encapsulated FOBs. These are the harms that potentiate when live grenades and medication come together in the housing containers where deployed soldiers sleep fitfully, awaiting mortar attacks. Psychopharmaceutical risk thus emerges in relation to the ways soldiers routinely incur, enact, and are exposed to harm. It can also implicate the military institutions that prescribe and sometimes mandate these medications. Bey's practical, if grim, calculus of what is more likely to kill him in Iraq underscores how these myriad damages comingle. Harm caused by mortar shells and military doctors, by mosquitos and medicine, by the enemy other and the Army itself, dissolve categorical distinctions: between friend and foe, cure and poison, and life-giving medicine and death-dealing war.

Bey's concern for medicated soldiers sleeping with weapons is also built on ideas of control as a basis for the morality of war violence. Accidental, uncontrolled violence against other military personnel—"friendly fire," as the military calls it—implies the legitimacy of its presumed opposite: the carefully calibrated threat to the enemy other. The problem that psychopharmaceutical use raises in these risk discourses is decidedly not a political one but one that defines uncontrolled violence as a medication side effect and, by extension, the ostensibly controlled use of force as purposeful, restrained, and good. In this way, medicine's "side" effects—here in the form of unbridled and senseless violence, enacted under the haze of sleep—work to define the moral margins of war, "implicitly conferring moral legitimacy on war's core actors and practices themselves" in the process.[18]

Behavioral Potentials

Concern for the risk of military psychopharmaceutical use in deployment typically centered the problem of soldier violence against one's own, as Bey envisioned on the FOB. But medications could also potentiate what some described as the worst elements of human nature in a legal, ethical, and operational context that demanded soldier restraint. Even as these concerns recognized possible "excessive" harm to local civilians as a risk of medication use, the significance of this risk was typically narrowed to the strategic question of how violations in the use of force might undermine the campaign to win hearts and minds. In the normative terms of risk management, the threat to occupied populations mattered to the extent that it threatened the mission.

It was for precisely this reason that Adrian felt strongly that benzodiazepines and stimulants had no place in counterinsurgency warfare. Adrian meets me at the top of a spiral staircase in the lobby of the multistoried steel and glass building where his research lab is located. He's in a checkered button-down shirt, tie, slacks, and a pristine white lab coat, looking very much the part of a physician-researcher. The former officer has been out of the Army for several years now, but despite the career and sartorial change, he retains the posture, stride, and gait that belie his military service. After quick introductions, he turns and walks at a rapid clip to an empty office at the end of a hallway where we sit down to talk. Thoughtful and articulate, Adrian looks back at his Army time and his two deployments to Iraq through layered lenses: as a former infantry officer, but now, too, as a physician.

Adrian works each one of my questions from multiple angles, which I appreciate. He strikes me as the type who talks to think, particularly when it comes to questions of clinical treatment. As we get deeper into the topic of medication use in war, Adrian works assiduously through risk stratifications, talking me through categories of medication and their potential problems in deployment. "Side effects from an SSRI are dizziness, headache, weight gain," he lists, as if reading the side panel of a medication box. "If you're an accountant, that's probably okay," he says with a light laugh. "But if you're out in a combat arms job at a small outpost? SSRIs—maybe everything else—I don't want you on it if I'm your leader." "Things that I care about are: Are you alert? Are you aware of the environment? Can you think clearly? Can you restrain the worst elements of yourself?" Adrian enumerates. "So, in that sense, benzos, absolutely not," he says resolutely. "And antipsychotics?" he continues, "I've never taken one, I have no idea what it feels like. But if you need one, I'm worried that you have a rifle."

"As for stimulants," Adrian continues, "stimulants bother me." He went on to describe why:

> People who have truly practiced counterinsurgency in the way that it's supposed to work—and I don't know ultimately if it does work—but the idea of being among the population and protecting the population, you essentially have to be a community policeman. You have to be able to establish trust. You have to be able to show that you're not a bully. You are an occupying force, but you are not there to take the land, take the oil or whatever. You're

> there to protect them, to make it safe for them to dissociate themselves from the insurgency, right?
>
> Every time that a bullet is fired and kills a civilian, or you know, we arrest the wrong person or knock down somebody's house, you've failed. So, if you're on stimulants, and you're hopped up? We can't afford to shoot the wrong people. So much of counterinsurgency is not shooting when it's easy to.

"Though," Adrian adds, "there is a time when you need to be hopped up, don't get me wrong." "When you know you're going into a battle situation where not all of you are going to walk out of it, you'd better find some false motivation to get yourself through that door," he says, eyebrows raised. Adrian mentions what US accounts would come to call the Second Battle of Fallujah in November and December of 2004, when US and coalition forces led an assault on the city. "Like Fallujah, where all the civilians were gone, we were using tanks to blow holes in buildings, putting hand grenades everywhere, dropping JDAMs [Joint Direct Attack Munitions], yeah." "But for most of the day-to-day stuff," he concludes, "I don't want people on stimulants. Maybe a stimulant is good for like, combat, true, true. But for counterinsurgency, I think it's probably not good."

From Adrian's point of view as a former infantry officer, the risks of the wrong medication are not most immediately about the loss of life or the moral and legal repercussions of civilian harm so much as their strategic and political costs: we can't *afford* to shoot the wrong people. By his risk stratification—versions of which I heard from other officers and military care providers—while SSRIs and benzos may pose supply and performance challenges, stimulants risk the strategic defeat of killing civilians and thus alienating the local population. The concern for being "hopped up" on stimulants marks the threat of uncontrolled violence that is understood to undermine the population-based project of winning hearts and minds.

Stimulants and pharmaceutical action thus provide new chemical terms to articulate the moral authority and legitimacy of "restrained" violence, as justified by liberal concepts of humane warfare. Stimulants may have a place in blowing holes in buildings and dropping JDAMs in combat but not in shooting the (wrong) people. Pharmaceutical use doesn't simply reveal definitions of legitimate violence; it *produces* those definitions through ideas of risk and control. In the ways they potentiate both

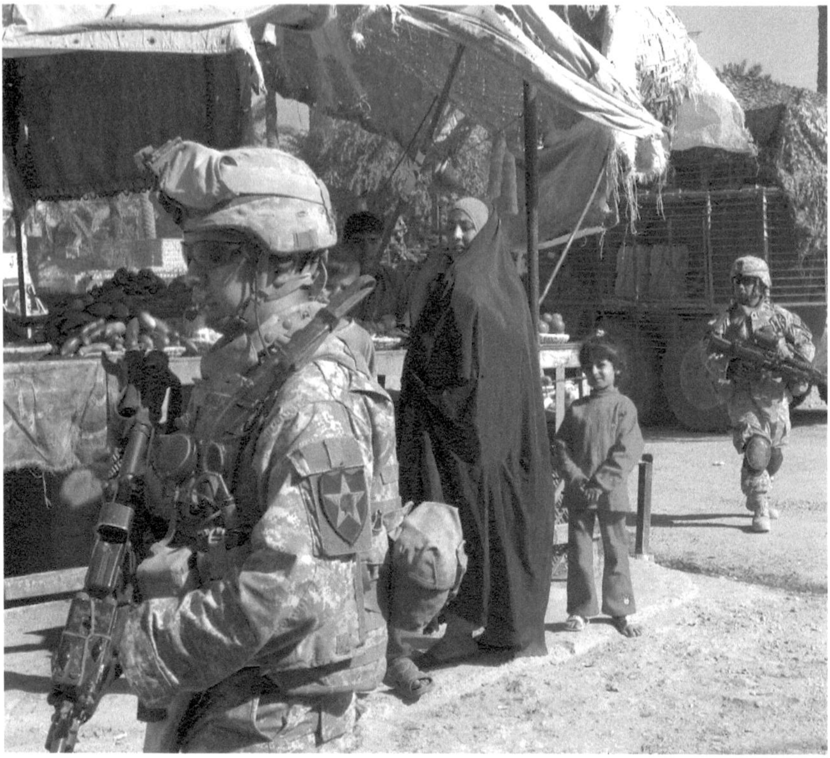

Figure 16. Patrolling a market in Baqubah, Iraq. Photograph by CPT Richard Ybarra, via DVIDS.

the harm of the war machine and, in Adrian's phrase, the "worst elements" of ourselves, psychopharmaceuticals have played an important role in how US military personnel articulate and reinforce the strategic costs as *the* most important consequences of civilian harm and death.

There is a certain "spectacle" of the soldier as autonomous agent in these risk stratifications and the distinctions between more and less legitimate violence that they produce.[19] These scenes seize upon the individual soldier—as a controlled or out-of-control actor, enacting the right or wrong kinds of violence—as the primary site upon which the success of counterinsurgency is imagined to rest. Bracketing off the broader politics of war and occupation and the war-making apparatus that empowers the use of force, such risk stratifications turn the problem of violence into a problem of the mismatch between medication potential and war strategy.[20] At work here are empire's fantasies of control. In this fantasy, a single soldier can win or lose the war and the tens of thousands of local civilians who in fact remained in Fallujah at the time of the siege can be categorically disappeared, as in Adrian's claim that "all civilians were gone," figuratively and literally clearing the grounds for stimulant-driven, "hopped up," unrestrained battle.[21]

It was not uncommon for officers and clinicians to categorize medications in the way Adrian did for me that afternoon. But when it came to the need to keep bodies in place, these theoretical risk stratifications could fall away—not for any singular act of negligence or oversight per se, though those do happen, but out of bureaucratic inertia, the pressure for mission readiness, and a healthy serving of silent conviction. Soldiers, too, came into these medications through any number of formal and informal routes, in moments of desperation, and not uncommonly, as we've already seen, via shared use. Particularly with closely integrated teams, medication use by one soldier could sometimes mean medication use by many. In that collective use, it could become easier to risk riding the edge than to refuse and effortless for magical thinking to take over.

Officers and soldiers assessed performance in different ways in relation to pharmaceutical action and ideas of risk and gain, depending on factors like their day-to-day responsibilities and mission demands. While Adrian said benzos were off the table for his unit, they were more acceptable to Elijah and his team. Elijah, who worked as what the military refers to as a human intelligence collector, was sent on his second deployment in 2011 to Afghanistan. During this deployment, the 23-year-old was tasked with interrogations and debriefings of what he described as "high-valued targets."

While Elijah told me he never took any psychiatric medications himself, he was very familiar with those taken by his teammates. "I mean, you know the people that you deploy with. We're around each other all the time. We sleep in the same room," he said. "There are a lot of forged friendships in deployment. Soldiers would open up and talk about the different types of medication they were taking. 'Oh yeah, I'm taking some sort of antidepressant,' or 'Yeah, I'm taking anxiety medication to help me get

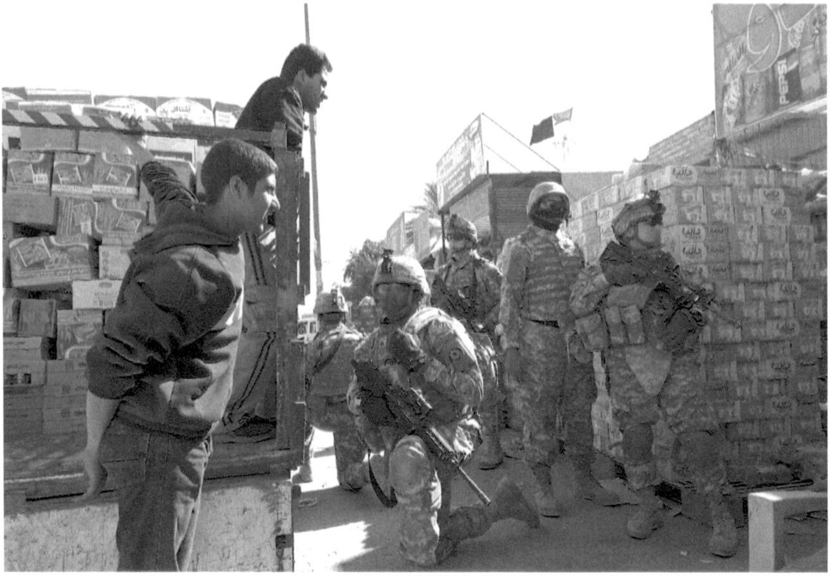

Figure 17. Attracting onlookers at a warehouse in Sadr City, Iraq. Photograph by SSG Michael Pryor, via DVIDS.

by,' and things like that." Knowledge about medications—and not uncommonly, medications themselves—was freely shared.

Elijah said his teammates took medication because of the "emotional and mental toll" of their work. "When it comes to doing interrogations, obviously we're talking to terrorists and insurgents who have killed people. They've affected whole regions," Elijah said. "So, when we're talking to them, as an interrogator, we have to run through different approach strategies to get into their heads and build rapport to get them to open up to us to provide us information." The work was trying. "When you're doing that for hours on end, it can really take a toll on you as a person and in your emotions. And it's really draining, especially for your brain," he recounted. "Having to interrogate somebody for seven hours and you're just playing this game of mental chess with them. You're writing everything down, and you're hearing all this different information about all the violent activities that they've done."

In pointing to the harm of bearing witness to the violence "collected" by human collectors, Elijah evokes what Nadia Abu El-Haj has described as the trauma imaginary of the American soldier as a suffering subject. Elijah's focus on the injurious nature of the work of interrogation for the interrogator and the toll it takes on "you as a person and in your emotions" resonates with the discourse of moral injury. Moral injury frames the consequences of violence "as moral destruction, as damage to the soul," which arises from the virtue of character.[22] As Kenneth MacLeish writes, "tragedies of moral injury arguably contain and miniaturize power asymmetries and complex events within the moral act of a single individual," reframing potentially political questions in terms of transgressions against the soldier's humanity.[23] Medicine works in lockstep with this miniaturization, legitimating psychopharmaceuticals as psychic salve.[24] When you're emotionally drained, Elijah says, you should be able to get the chemical help you need.

Medication could also regulate behavioral potentials in ways that reinforced ethical, legal, and strategic norms of control and restraint that characterize liberal forms of war making. Elijah said several friends accessed antianxiety medications while they were deployed to "calm their nerves." He said that friends would take medication "to kind of take the edge off when they knew they were going to talk to a certain person and knew they were going to need a bit of extra help." I asked him what he meant by that. "As an interrogator, obviously we're not allowed to touch a detainee at all unless it's part of an approach strategy and we're trying to comfort them," Elijah explained. He stated that it's against the law to "physically handle any detainees"—hence, the ostensible reason for the presence of military police during interrogations. Several friends began taking antianxiety medications "because when you start talking to these people, start to get into a groove of collecting information, you witness how somebody is as a person, and you really get into these heated conversations." "I mean, it takes a lot to not reach over a table and knock somebody out," Elijah told me. "It takes a lot of willpower to make sure that you don't do anything that you're not supposed to do." While benzos bring infantry soldiers down in a way that Adrian saw as dangerous for self and team, their action could restrain where willpower failed in the interrogation room.

Adrian and Elijah share one important element in their takes on psychopharmaceuticals: both suggest that behaviors and emotions can be modulated with chemicals. They propose a model of the self that resonates with what Natasha Dow Schüll describes in her study of the entertainment infrastructure in Las Vegas, where the gambling industry is overlaid with an addiction therapeutics industry. While one encourages gambling and the other stops it, Schull observes that both "gear their interventions around a model of the self as an ever-changing configuration of behavioral potentials responsive to external modulation."[25] Likewise, psychopharmaceuticals appear an external means to modulate the behavioral and performance potentials of soldiers, though here the goal is explicitly instrumental—to make soldiers maintain, gain, or reclaim a performance edge. But that edge, as Adrian and Elijah suggest, can take multiple forms.

"SIDE" EFFECTS

Elijah's knowledge of his teammates' medication use is hardly unusual. This kind of knowledge was partly a function of the material conditions of deployment. Within the intimate conditions in which deployed military personnel worked and lived, soldiers learned to read for signs of psychopharmaceutical use by others. They could become accountable to those on medication in new ways as a result, serving as an informal arm of the military-medical risk-management machine.[26] The use of medications by a peer also mattered because it could be exploitable. In convoys and in the barracks, up in the observation post and out in the motor pool, soldiers often saw in their peers' medication use the possibility of a chemical edge for themselves. Prescription medications might be willingly—or less willingly—shared with one's teammates and friends to ease symptoms or improve performance. This meant that pharmaceutical action was often both individually and intersubjectively negotiated, as primary and secondary effects drew soldiers into new ways of relating and performing with one another. But it could also create friction for those on the margins of these forms of shared chemical help. This was the case for Hakeem.

Hakeem enlisted in the Army in 2005 at the age of 20. We met one spring morning at a Barnes and Noble bookstore café, populated mostly by retirees at this weekday hour. Hakeem politely declines my offer to get him a drink, so he waits patiently while I doctor my coffee at the counter. When I rejoin him at the table, he's sitting, baseball cap balled in his hands, looking eager to start. Hakeem begins by telling me that the Army pulled one over him, multiple times. The first time was when a recruiter diverted him toward a more manual, "lower" MOS despite his high Armed Services Vocational Aptitude Battery (ASVAB) score.[27] The recruiter ended up getting Hakeem to enlist as a 63B, a light-wheeled vehicle mechanic. He had hoped to be a military policeman, but he figured being a mechanic would at least keep him relatively safe.[28]

The second time was when he deployed. Hakeem is a telling example of someone who joined the Army to improve his life chances, and he figured that he wouldn't see much combat as a mechanic. But he ended up going off the FOB nearly every day when he was in Iraq in 2006. "I was told all we were going to do was work on cars. The guys who had just come back before us said the worst thing they ever did was go retrieve body parts. They said, 'That's the closest you'll get to combat,' so I thought it was just going to be 12 months of working on cars and watching DVDs." About four months into his deployment, command decided they needed more gun trucks out on the roads, so they came to the mechanic's bay and then and there created three new ones. He ended up operating the 50-caliber machine gun mounted on the roof of their Humvee. "We left the base pretty much every day doing different missions to support the infantry. They kind of just turned us into extra combatants," Hakeem recounts, with a disbelief that hasn't fully attenuated with time.

"At first, it was really scary, because—again—I thought I would never even leave the wire," Hakeem reminds me. "My first time leaving the wire was a ten-minute trip, but I was terrified. My second or third time we got hit. The vehicle in front of me was attacked. It changed my whole perspective on what was really going on," he says. "I thought I would never see war. This brought it home: we're actually at war. So, I grew up pretty fast. Many years in that moment." With time, Hakeem adjusted to the changed circumstances. "Eventually, I got pretty confident with it," he reflects. "I was proud to be the guy protecting all my team."

Adaptability and improvisation were the name of the game. This was the case with medication, too. Hakeem recalls a soldier who was accidentally run over by a Humvee, and when he came back to rejoin the platoon, he was taking several prescription medications. While not permitted to go off the FOB, he was openly sharing his Seroquel, a sleep aid, with his teammates. An atypical second-generation antipsychotic, Seroquel is sometimes prescribed off label in low doses for individuals with sleep problems due to its sedating effects. Hakeem remembers the soldier chopping up tablets to share. At the time, they were working as an on-call team, so their schedule was erratic: they would get called at 2 or 4 a.m. to go pick up a drone or help with some tanks. Sometimes, they didn't sleep for 48 hours straight. So, the team was grateful for the chemical help. To wind down from missions and get to sleep quickly, broken tablets were often supplemented by cough syrup purchased from the PX. The cough syrup, Hakeem said, "was just to get out of here, just to be mentally out of Iraq."

While "it seemed like everybody loved it" and the soldier sharing his supply was hailed a hero of sorts—"like the local drug dealer or something"—Hakeem said it took only one experience on less than half a tablet to scare him away from it completely. Feeling groggy, "messed up," and slow to react when he woke up, Hakeem began to worry about what the Seroquel would mean for the team given the kind of work they were doing. "Especially my job as the crew-serve gunner, I needed to be alert because I was the first line of defense if something were to go wrong," he explained. "To be alert was everything over there. I wanted to get home."

It all came to a head for Hakeem late one day when their team was called up in the middle of the night. The soldier serving as his driver "came to me sweatin' bullets even though it was 20 degrees out." Hakeem explained, "He was zonked out on Seroquel and cough syrup." The soldier told Hakeem that he was messed up and couldn't go out. Hakeem was infuriated and scared. He told the soldier to tell their NCO that he had the flu. "And he went and told him, and our sergeant was like, 'You better get your ass in that truck. We're leaving and we don't have time for that. Be sick later.'" While Hakeem tried to convince the NCO how sick his teammate was, he also didn't want to give him away. "Why not?" I asked. "Because he's been my driver. He's protected me all this time. I love him," Hakeem told me. "But I really hate what he's doing right now."

It turned out to be a bad night. Hakeem said the soldier nearly crashed them into the back of a tank. "He was very inebriated, just zonked out. He wasn't there." Hakeem was visibly agitated as he recounted the near collision. "He got us real close to getting us hurt. I was very angry with him for that. I was angry with the medicines for that. I was angry at the guy giving out the pills. I was angry at the fact that leadership looked away from these guys getting sick off these medicines," Hakeem vented. "So, I grew a disdain for the guys who were abusing these medicines. I thought my friend was going to get me killed that night. Because of them, I almost didn't make it home."

In the corporate setting of deployed military life, care for one another can be pharmaceutical. The physical intimacy of living and working together and an ethos of mutual reliance facilitate knowledge about medication—who is on what and whether the soldier is willing to share. They can also encourage the pooling of chemical resources and collective experimentation. But drugs can produce friction among teammates, particularly when pharmaceutical action proves undisciplined. A drug may make some soldiers groggy while allowing others rest and release. Moreover, its tempo doesn't always align with the tempo of counterinsurgency, as when zonked-out soldiers are woken for an impromptu mission in the middle of the night. Exploiting the power of pills means always riding the edge, never in complete control.

Hakeem's narrative is also telling of the many lateral and longitudinal dimensions along which medication effects potentiate and reverberate outward: between and among soldiers as well as across a lifespan. These, too, are the "side" effects of drugs in war. Medication effects that fateful night were borne by everyone on the team—but they also continue to live on in the ways Hakeem understands his own luck in being able to return home alive. That night was a tipping point in his narrative, marking not only where drugs metabolize into mistakes but also where the junior enlisted meet hard limits in negotiating military hierarchy and the unflinching demands of the mission. For Hakeem, it also marked where love and protection became silence and complicity.

The eagerness (and desperation) of Hakeem's buddies to tap the power of pills, alongside the willful ignorance of leadership about these practices, reveals how deeply routinized the shared use of pharmaceuticals can become, particularly in team-based performance settings. Shared efforts to gain a chemical edge are a distortion of the system itself: on-the-ground practices that uphold the official, instrumental logic of optimizing mission readiness while simultaneously undermining the medical risk-management apparatus meant to regulate medication use. In this sense, the system outpaces itself.

Hakeem was not alone in experiencing the volatility of medication use during deployment, nor was he exceptional in feeling powerless to report problems when things went wrong. How soldiers react to chemical effects and the institutional limits they face in reporting them reveal much about the compounded harms that medicine can produce in settings of war making.

SEEING THINGS

It is an unseasonably warm late-winter morning, the kind that tricks the crocuses into an early bloom. An hour and a half drive out of Chapel Hill has put me on narrow backcountry roads ribboning through small towns and converted farmland. I finally pull into a newish apartment development, one of the generic, could-be-anywhere complexes featuring anodyne tones of blue-gray and part of the commercialized oasis of homes and big-box stores that has forever altered the center of gravity in this small rural town. I walk up the covered flight of stairs to a landing with several pairs of shoes neatly lined up outside the door. Aaliyah has asked that I meet her at her home. She has managed to coordinate our meeting to coincide with her 8-month-old's morning nap. Once asleep in his crib, we sink into her plush living room couch with large mugs of milky coffee, a portable baby monitor providing background white noise to our conversation.

The 33-year-old had left the military the year prior, having enlisted in the Army fresh out of high school. Trained as a chemical biological specialist, or 74D, Aaliyah deployed twice, once to Iraq in 2005 and again to Afghanistan in 2014. While in Iraq, Aaliyah decided to try to quit smoking and was prescribed the antidepressant medication Wellbutrin (bupropion), commonly used to aid smoking cessation.[29] Soon after she began taking it, Aaliyah knew something was wrong. "I was having awful nightmares and cold sweats," she recalled.

When she went back to the prescribing PA, she was told, "Well, do you want to quit smoking? Is that more important or are the nightmares more important? Which one?" Aaliyah walked out of the appointment a bit reassured since the PA didn't seem concerned. Maybe the nightmares were a normal part of adjusting to deployment. She had also heard that antimalarial medication could cause nightmares. Maybe the antimalarials were the problem? She decided to stick it out on the Wellbutrin a bit longer, though she had her doubts. "I wanted to take care of my health and quit smoking, but I also didn't want to feel like I was going crazy." Thinking back on that conversation with the PA, Aaliyah wonders why the PA never offered to switch her to another medication. "There was no, 'Hey, you know, you can try other things,' or 'That's not normal. Those are side effects.'"

Within days, things got worse. She recounted multiple episodes in which she saw things in the pitch black of night, including rats running across the room, that would make her dart out of her trailer. Her roommate reassured her again and again that nothing was there, but Aaliyah couldn't be convinced otherwise. It got to the point that Aaliyah decided to sleep in the command post. She worried that it was the medication; she worried even more that it *wasn't*. "At the time, I wondered if there was something *really* wrong with me, if it wasn't just the medicine. Was I going crazy?" The loss of trust in her own perception of reality and her inability to tell whether these experiences stemmed from the medication or from her own psyche were profoundly unsettling.

If seeing rats in her room was relatively benign, seeing things on the road during Quick Reaction Force night driving was not.[30] "It got really dangerous because I would see stuff on the road—animals, people," Aaliyah explained. "And I would stop in the middle of the road and my truck commander, he would be like, 'Why are you stopping?' I'm like, 'There's something out there.' He's like, 'There's nothing there! I need you to go, you *have* to drive.'" That's when Aaliyah knew she'd become a danger to herself and her team. "Trust is a big issue when you're deployed because you have to be able to trust the person beside you," said Aaliyah. "So, if the person beside me can't trust me, then I'm no good in deployment. I didn't want anybody to feel like they couldn't trust me. But then again, I couldn't trust myself, so I didn't know what to do." At the time, Aaliyah wasn't sure who to turn to. "I didn't want people to think I was crazy and send me home; I also didn't want to be a disappointment to my unit and get sent home. But I also didn't want anybody to really think I was crazy. Then they don't want to be around you."

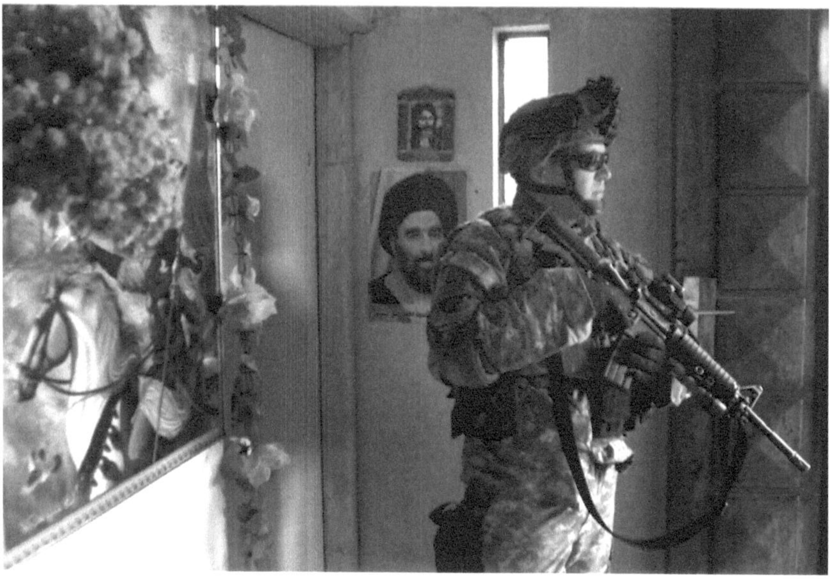

Figure 18. A soldier provides security for his commander in Sadr City, Iraq. Photograph by SSG Russell Klika, via DVIDS.

What psychopharmaceuticals *do* is rarely a straightforward matter, and cause and effect can be all the more challenging to decipher in deployment. Deployment was notoriously disruptive to routines of all kinds; sleep trouble, for example, was common, and dreaming was generally more vivid while deployed. The stress of adapting to a new operational environment and worrying about children and about spouses who were keeping life together at home confounded pharmaceutical action, blurring attempts to identify a singular cause for changes to one's emotional or behavioral state—assuming one even had the mental bandwidth to be attuned to such things. Where psychopharmaceuticals and toxic and environmental harms are common, attributing effects to a specific drug was like boxing smoke.

But attunement itself can also be a risky endeavor, as it was for Aaliyah, since it threatened to reveal that what was wrong had nothing to do with the drugs but rather with *her*. At the time, she could not face the prospect of her own unraveling, nor did she know whom she might tell. Not wanting to disappoint her team or lose their trust, she kept silent and pressed on.

Phenomenological studies of environmental pollution describe how individuals and communities become attentive to contamination through evolving sensory practices and epistemologies; Aaliyah, however, had lost trust in her own sensory and perceptual capacities.[31] If she had what might be generously described as a moment of medication toxicity "discovery," hers came as an act of resignation. A full month lapsed before Aaliyah conceded to her mother, a nurse, what was happening over the phone. Her mother told her to pull herself off the medication, and Aaliyah says her symptoms ceased immediately.[32]

. . . . .

While military proponents have positioned psychotropic medications as important to preserving careers and caring for their own, in the exigencies of deployment, medication mattered almost exclusively in relation to performance, readiness, and risk. Tasked with keeping soldiers soldiering, psychopharmaceuticals in the war on terror have generated possibility and peril. Accounts like Aaliyah's, Elijah's, and Seth's show us how the harms of war are compounded, and are often confounded, by medicine and its unstable role within military institutions at war. Interpretations and experiences of psychopharmaceutical action are shaped by pressures to perform and the desire to protect military others and oneself. How soldiers and care providers evaluate the risks and benefits of medication use also illuminate their models of battlefield mental health and ideas of "good" disciplinary and biopolitical relationships to violence.

Military providers, command, and soldiers work to discipline the uncertainty of medication reaction in war through the stratification of risk. In doing so, they foreground certain forms of violence, elements of war, and subjects of harm while obscuring others, staging both military performance and the impacts of medication in ways that prioritize the strategic outcomes of counterinsurgency and implicitly transfer the risks associated with soldier medication use onto the people and places under occupation. Risk in relation to military medication use thus serves as a key site where definitions of legitimate violence and the politics of life and death in contemporary global liberal war are produced.

Aaliyah's story raises questions about what it means to protect others from oneself in settings of war making. The soldier who becomes a threat to themselves and others is most visible in the concern for suicidal and homicidal behavior. The next chapter considers what happens when psychopharmaceuticals alone fail to contain the risk of the military coming undone from within.

6 Encapsulate

One afternoon toward the final months of his deployment in Afghanistan, Craig was asked by his platoon leader and platoon sergeant to accompany them to headquarters where they needed to take care of an urgent matter. Then a private, the lowest of the enlisted ranks, Craig dutifully followed them to a waiting Humvee. Only after it was apparent that they were headed to the other side of their large FOB did he realize that his senior leaders had made up the story to get him alone. His platoon sergeant explained that they had heard that Craig had been openly talking—perhaps joking?—about harming himself and others in the unit, so they were taking him to see someone, a "buddy of theirs," at the COSC clinic on the FOB. The mental health provider who spoke with Craig that day eventually placed him on a temporary profile, a recommendation made to military command in response to which Craig's duties were restricted, his weapon was confiscated, and he was placed in confinement.

Overnight, Craig went from being out on the roads every day providing armed security to convoys of supply trucks to being confined in a warehouse on base under 24-hour direct supervision by a rotation of soldiers from his unit. During this two-month period, Craig was permitted to leave the warehouse only to go to the latrine, chow hall, and to do laundry, always while accompanied by a peer escort.[1] Expected to continue restricted duties while confined in the warehouse, Craig was tasked with preparing packages of water, food, and ammunition for airdrops. He recalled that time to me as one of confusion and humiliation but also of profound contradiction: "Why am I here? Why am I in a combat zone with no weapon when I'm not allowed to leave this warehouse?" Integrated with his unit yet confined, Craig remained a soldier even though he was no longer trusted not to harm himself or others. His weapon confiscated, he nonetheless remained in and at war.

Throughout this book, I've suggested that as US military policy in the 2000s called for full-spectrum dominance and the US Army became an occupying force in Iraq and Afghanistan, keeping bodies in place became increasingly imperative for a force that was weak in numbers. Psychopharmaceuticals, we've seen, were a key tool in that effort. But the chemical push can reach its limits. Soldiers can, if by competing accounts, become threats to themselves and others. Even then, the imperative remains to maintain the fighting force by stabilizing soldiers like Craig in place in order to return them to duty. This chapter examines a particular but widespread battlefield practice used when pharmaceuticals alone prove insufficient: the formal assignment of soldiers to keep watch over their at-risk peers. It asks what it means in practice to safeguard military life against itself in settings of war.

The unit watch is a widely used tool in the US Army's efforts to address soldiers who present with suicidal or homicidal thoughts.[2] Otherwise referred to as a "command interest profile," and more colloquially as "buddy watch" or "suicide watch," the practice—characterized by continuous direct observation and restrictive measures—is described by military health professionals as a "powerful and controversial method of ensuring safety" for soldiers at risk.[3] As the most common alternative to psychiatric hospitalization in the Army for soldiers who express suicidal ideation, unit watch is said to promote the soldier's rehabilitation and return to duty by avoiding separation from peers, removal from occupational duties, unnecessary evacuation, and the stigma of hospitalization.[4] Unit watch aims to keep soldiers like Craig participating as fully as possible in workday activities and integrated with their unit, while simultaneously providing monitoring by unit peers in situ.

Drawing on the Army concept of the battle buddy—the partnering of fellow soldiers who support each other in and out of combat—the buddy watch is simultaneously conceived as a means of treatment, restraint, surveillance, support, mentorship, and "family" care.[5] It pairs constraint with compelled integration to stabilize at-risk soldiers, strategically mobilizing the military's mechanisms of social control and the Army's corporate ethos for the purpose of protecting the soldier of concern and the unit at large. In practice, however, unit watch commonly foments cynicism and resentment toward the watched. Unit watch structures symbolic and physical processes that I explore in this chapter as a form of *encapsulation,* whereby through intensive surveillance and control, the soldier of concern is alienated, isolated, and separated from within. The relationships and affects generated by unit watch reveal, in fact, the destabilizing nature of safeguarding military life in war, whereby the military body turns in upon and begins to cannibalize itself.

This chapter develops an ethnography of being watched and watching others under the sign of suicidal violence in war. I discuss how unit watch functions, why its use has been both widespread and controversial in the wars in Iraq and Afghanistan, and what its practice reveals about institutional and psychiatric interventions as a form of constraint-as-care in settings of global US military power. The accounts to follow underscore the ambivalent and contradictory forms of sociality that unit watch produces, including coerced obligation, tasked friendship, and forced intimacy. The micropolitics of psychiatric and custodial care between soldiers are shaped by the regimes of power to which soldiers are subjected, the material settings of war's production, and the tensions that emerge in preventing military deaths in settings orchestrated for the application of violence. This chapter considers what it means to mobilize intimacies between soldiers in order to stabilize precarious military life under conditions of coercion, control, and the imperative to endure.

BLACK BOX

The military medical literature identifies suicidal and homicidal soldiers as "one of the most frequent and challenging scenarios" faced by deployed mental health providers.[6] One study that reviewed the charts of 425 deployed soldiers seen by the mental health team at FOB Speicher in Tikrit, Iraq, over a period of ten months in 2004 found that nearly 30 percent had considered killing themselves.[7] About 16 percent of them "had considered killing someone else (not the enemy) within the past month."[8] The pairing of suicidal and homicidal soldiers in the literature is based in part on clinical reasoning: military providers have observed that a large proportion of soldiers presenting with suicidal and homicidal ideation are not diagnosed with severe mental health disorders and thus do not qualify for psychiatric hospitalization.[9] For many of these cases, the unit watch has been promoted as an alternative and more appropriate measure. The discourse of military mental health in deployment also pairs suicidal and homicidal soldiers in a distinct construct of risk that sees them as two sides of the same coin: both represent an internal threat to military life and the ultimate negation of the calibrated threat to enemy others.[10] This risk calculus places "first and foremost priority on limiting access to lethal means," particularly access to firearms.[11] Within this ecology of concern, the unit watch aims to stabilize dangerous soldiers in situ through intensive reintegration into the corporate fold.

While unit watch has been practiced in some form in military settings for decades, its significance would be heightened at a time when the Army was facing growing concern over suicide and homicide. In 2009, the Army reported 160 suicides among its active-duty soldiers, making suicide the third leading cause of death among the Army population. As the report phrased it, "If we include accidental death, which frequently is the result of high-risk behavior (drinking and driving, drug overdose, etc.), we find that less young men and women die in combat than die by their own actions. Simply stated, we are often more dangerous to ourselves than the enemy."[12]

As we've seen with soldier psychopharmaceutical use in previous chapters, unit watch, too, is an exercise in risk management, one that can be especially fraught in settings of war making. "Suicidal and homicidal soldiers can be quite common during deployment, and their treatment is challenging," note three military providers. "Each case presents a dilemma to the deployed provider." Recalling that there was an "epidemic" of sleepwalkers after it became known that sleepwalking would disqualify a soldier from duty in Vietnam, these providers situate the management of suicidal and homicidal threats in the context of the ages-old challenge for military health professionals to maintain the fighting force against so-called evacuation syndromes. "Many soldiers have told us that it is common knowledge among their peers that suicidal or homicidal thoughts or behaviors usually result in withdrawal from duty and discharge from the military" and that they may thus "report these symptoms to facilitate their discharge from service."[13] Unit watch, some have argued, can be particularly effective for those employing threats to separate from service, often on the informal advice of peers.[14] Even then, these providers note that "suicides and homicides do occur in the military, underscoring the importance of thorough evaluation and treatment of all such soldiers."[15]

Whether in a garrison or a deployed setting, it is the responsibility of the military clinician to document the suicide or homicide risk assessment and provide a clear rationale for the unit watch over hospitalization or evacuation. The dilemma for the deployed provider, then, is whether to evacuate the soldier or to attempt to rehabilitate them in theater. The decision to pursue a unit watch is never an easy one. As a form of in situ stabilization, unit watch reflects what Nikolas Rose identifies as a shift from *dangerousness* to *risk* within contemporary regimes of psychiatric control.[16] As an organizing framework for administering people deemed problematic, risk management encourages mental health professionals and allied experts to "frame predictions of future violence in probabilistic terms."[17] It is also "through the notion of risk, and the techniques and practices to which it is linked, that care and control have become inextricably linked."[18] Thus, risk is key to the ways constraint and control as treatment remain "a common practice even in our post-asylum era."[19]

In contexts in which medical evacuation appears the easiest option for safeguarding at-risk soldiers and others, the military medical community has openly grappled with the hefty risks of returning these soldiers to their unit and the legal responsibility and blame that military command and medical providers may face for a bad outcome.[20] The risks of unit watch can be especially difficult for medical personnel to effectively mitigate, and while the unit watch is "often a necessity in a deployed environment" due to the limited medical resources available, "this strategy's risks may outweigh its benefits in a garrison environment," where limited resources are less of a concern.[21] The risk calculus of unit watch and its potential failures have been highlighted by events like the so-called Camp Liberty killings in Baghdad in 2009. Five US military personnel were fatally shot at a COSC clinic by an Army sergeant who, after leaving the clinic under the watch of a guard because of suicidal threats, took an unsecured M16 rifle from his escort, drove back to the clinic, and opened fire.

The unit watch's devolution of monitoring to peers shares kinship with mainstream suicide prevention tools. It is analogous in some ways to the practice of sending a patient home with family members who promise to watch them and control access to weapons, drugs, and pills. Suicide watches in prison may also use procedures similar to unit watch.[22] But while there may be parallels between unit watch and these practices in terms of procedural form, the unit watch diverges in important ways from suicide watch in carceral settings and its civilian-world analogies. Promoted within military mental health circles and to military command as a means of increasing return-to-duty rates among soldiers, unit watch shares with psychopharmaceuticals the aim of "conserving the fighting strength." If the unit watch would be important to the humanitarian concern to preserve military life in the war on terror, especially as suicide and homicide prevention within the ranks became growing concerns for the US public and the Army, it was also expressly promoted as a tool for sustaining mission readiness. As with risk management in psychopharmaceutical use discussed in the previous chapter, managing suicide risk in situ is likewise assessed in terms not only of the risk of retaining the volatile individual but also the obverse risk of evacuating them—namely, the loss of labor and the hazards that loss may pose for the individual, team, unit, and mission.

But even proponents of unit watch can find it difficult to absorb the uncertainty and risk to the unit and themselves. Unit watch has been controversial among military commanders who are tasked with the actual implementation of its recommendations. In the war on terror, many commanders reported discomfort with unit watch as a form of treatment due to a lack of necessary knowledge, abilities, and resources to keep the soldier under watch safe.[23] Medical professionals were generally cautious, given the lack of formal study of the efficacy of unit watch as a treatment option and the fact that discussions in the literature have been largely theoretical. Soldiers and officers I interviewed shared ambivalent, if not overtly hostile, feelings toward the duty of having to watch as well as toward the soldiers they were tasked to watch. Destructive outcomes and failures have also surfaced in the media and case accounts, as in one case when two soldiers at Fort Leonard Wood in Missouri committed suicide in 2000 while on unit watch and another in which the tasked soldiers allegedly taunted the soldier on unit watch to the point that he committed suicide.[24] What unit watch is envisioned to be in theory and what it becomes in practice can be quite different things.

WAR(D)

As with psychotropic medication use on the battlefield in the war on terror, the unit watch draws on foundational principles in forward psychiatry to rehabilitate soldiers as far forward as possible. Through "partnership" between the military clinician and the command team, the unit watch aims "to address the soldier's mental health needs in the least restrictive setting" possible.[25] It is thus part and parcel of a deep and continuing tradition in military forward psychiatry which emphasizes *proximity* to the front lines, *immediacy* of the treatment, *expectancy* of return to duty, and *simplicity* of intervention, principles codified in military combat psychiatry's well-known mnemonic PIES. Recalling language that has been used as far back as World War I that prioritizes rebuilding soldiers' own capacities in war through forward interventions, unit watch is said to help soldiers "regain mastery" over impulsive or dangerous behaviors.[26] By avoiding hospitalization and enabling the watched soldier to maintain some level of occupational functioning, unit watch may also "help the soldier preserve a sense of self-worth and belonging."[27]

Although reflective of the principles of forward psychiatry, unit watch is distinct from other forward psychiatric interventions for the way it explicitly devolves the work of monitoring, confining, and watching onto the at-risk soldier's unit. (In the case of homicidal threats, either the soldier or the threatened target may be moved to another section, with both parties ordered to avoid all contact with each other.) Soldiers assigned as unit watchers typically have no formal health care qualifications or training, and the direct labor of unit watch is often placed, whether officially or unofficially, onto the shoulders of junior enlisted soldiers.[28] In the intimate settings in which soldiers live, eat, sleep, and work together while deployed, proximity becomes the unit watch's prized asset, enabling "positive control" over the watched soldier, while also ideally facilitating the soldier's compliance with treatment and follow-up appointments.[29] The soldier watchers, or "escorts," who are tasked with the close observation of the soldier of concern, are also responsible for initiating immediate contact with mental health services for reevaluation should the soldier's behavior deteriorate. As proponents would have it, this is true forward treatment in situ, a kind of "unit-supported pseudo-inpatient psychiatric treatment capability on or near the front lines of combat"—in essence, an inpatient facility where soldiers provide for the custodial care of soldier-patients.[30] This is arguably PIES in its purest form, offered so far forward that unit peers are doing the work of treatment, and the frontlines become the ward itself.

Proponents argue that in addition to providing monitoring, the unit watch may be less stigmatizing than hospitalization, since members of the soldier's unit are able to continue interacting and engaging with the watched soldier during the treatment period. This is envisioned as having benefits in both directions, keeping the soldier socially supported and mentored by peers, while also mitigating speculation in the unit at large about "what may go on 'in the rubber room.'"[31] Yet the fact that peer observers reserve the power to "escort" the watched soldier for hospitalization should their condition deteriorate suggests that the ward is not fully open to observation by the unit but rather retains a hierarchy of coercive recesses.

There are spatial and material realities to this imaginary of the frontlines as ward. The ready access to firearms that is characteristic of military communities and enhanced in deployment is understood to be a serious risk to be managed in the unit watch.[32] In garrison, soldiers are not permitted personal firearms and assigned weapons are generally secured in locked racks in the unit arms room, with access granted in only limited circumstances. By contrast, in deployed settings, to include installations from large FOBs to small COPs in Iraq and Afghanistan, soldiers generally always keep their weapon on them or near at hand, even at chow or when asleep. While limiting access to firearms in deployment as part of unit-watch procedure can therefore be more difficult due to the sheer saturation of weapons, the encapsulated nature of FOBs in the war on terror also enabled, at least theoretically, a greater capacity to control the soldier's environment, movement, and access. In other words, military installations both undermine *and* enable efforts to secure at-risk soldiers against the threat they pose to themselves and others. Treatment and risk become self-referential.

Mental health providers and command assume the legal and professional risk of a unit watch, yet it is often junior soldiers who shoulder the work of the unit watch itself. As unit watch has been almost exclusively recommended for lower-level enlisted soldiers, many of them young and relatively new to the Army, the idea of "peer" support may motivate this delegation of the work of unit watch.[33] Undoubtedly, it is also motivated by the widespread idea that pulling watch is "dirty work" unfit for NCOs with tasks of higher priority.[34] Tasking soldiers to watch over an at-risk peer, as we will see, produces complex and often conflicting dynamics within the unit.

WATCHING

The unit watch has been used since the 1990s when it was implemented in US military operations in Kosovo. The first rationale and set of guidelines for unit watch would not be published by the Army until much later, in 2011, yet the unit watch was widely used both in garrison and in deployment by the Army during the period of the war on terror. Part of the controversy surrounding its use has been the lack of standardization: it is a highly variable practice, and there is no research into treatment effects and safety, with most clinical practice recommendations based in theory and personal experience.[35] This variability stems in part from the unit watch's intended flexibility in responding to situational factors, including a soldier's assessed risk and operational constraints.

Based on recommendations from the supervising military provider, the command team implementing the unit watch negotiates and agrees to interventions intended to "limit the suicidal or homicidal soldier's access to people, places or objects that might increase the soldier's chances of harming self or others."[36] Such interventions may include searching the soldier's belongings and living quarters for items including the soldier's military-issued firearm, shoelaces, and bed sheet and removing them from their possession; prohibiting the soldier's access to alcohol and drugs; and ensuring attendance at clinical appointments and compliance with treatment. As its name implies, monitoring is the cornerstone of the unit watch's logic and "reflects the unit's attempt to help the soldier refrain from impulsive behavior and maintain positive control over his or her whereabouts."[37] Monitoring can range from less to more restrictive: from assigning a soldier a unit escort who stays with them from first formation until lights out to a 24-hour watch or "CQ watch" in which the soldier under watch must sleep in a room where the unit escort is awake at all times.[38]

As a custodial intervention, the unit watch can produce countervailing effects for those who may have already been receiving other forms of treatment. Such was the case for Craig. Even before his NCOs took him to the COSC clinic via that surprise trip in the Humvee, Craig had already been receiving supportive counseling at the clinic every other week for months, having pursued care voluntarily out of his own concern for his thoughts of harming himself and others. Yet, once placed on unit watch, his regularly scheduled appointments ended abruptly; whether that was because his provider had left the base or because the logic of confinement superseded therapy, Craig would never know. Regardless of the reason, his prescribed medications, which included the benzodiazepine Ativan and the antipsychotic Seroquel for help with nightmares, were never refilled once his unit watch guards, ostensibly acting in accordance with protocols meant to protect against overdose, confiscated the last of his supply. What was furthermore intended to be a few days' confinement—as dictated by Army guidelines and expected by Craig's wife, who had been told that her husband would be medically evacuated by flight back to the US—turned out, in fact, to be two months. Due to a hazy mix of reasons at various levels likely having to do with logistics, cost, and simple bureaucratic mismanagement, Craig ended up finishing out his deployment with his unit, albeit from within the warehouse.

Craig's case suggests that as the unit watch unfolds in improvised ways, constraint can take over for other forms of care. Watching soldiers must improvise, too. While broad guidelines for unit watch exist, at the level of practice, soldiers must learn how to watch. Many are tasked with unit watch having received little if any detailed guidance on what to do and how to do it.[39] While general injunctions to "keep watch" over the person might be supplemented with more specific prohibitions regarding access to places and things, the work of unit watch involves intimate and banal encounters that one must learn to navigate in the course of doing. Fuller, a chief warrant officer with over 20 years in the Army, remembers keenly what it was like to be tasked with unit watch during his early deployments to Iraq when he was a junior enlisted soldier. "There was absolutely zero guidance," he told me flatly, "absolutely none. "Talking with our sergeant, it was, 'What do you think? How should we do it?' And I'm like, 'Who am I to say? I'm not the professional," he recounts, shaking his head. "So, it was very much like, 'Well, just make sure they don't hurt themselves.'"

At the most basic and practical level, Fuller wasn't clear on what the "watching" of unit watch should involve. He recounted one case to me during his 2004 Iraq deployment when they were based at a camp, a semi-permanent military facility, where they had to improvise a confinement room. "They moved this person out of their barracks room into an empty room with a bed and a wall locker and that was it. It was almost like a prison cell, honestly," he recalled. "And it was, 'Okay, this person is on suicide watch.' And it was like, 'Okay, is somebody going to be in the room with them?' 'No, they'll stand outside the room.'" He gave me a look, equal parts frustrated and bewildered. "So, they're going to stand outside the room with the door shut? How is that 'watching'? Define 'watching.'"

The nature of attachment to the one being watched can often be multiple and ambiguous, involving competing messaging and institutional demands. The military medical community aims to socialize soldiers "to envision unit watch as analogous to 'helping a family member in distress'" in order to alleviate the burden of the unit watch and the potential stigma attached to the watched soldier.[40] But for those ordered to do this helping work, conducting the unit watch in such terms is hardly straightforward. One veteran who served on suicide watch for a soldier in his unit while in Iraq told me he felt deeply confused over whether to act on his natural inclination to lend an ear. Should he invite the guy to talk about what was bothering him? Was he even trained to do that on a unit watch? "It's incredibly weird. You have somebody here who is obviously at a very, very low point, and it's, 'Do I try and talk to them?'" he recounted. "I could say,

'What's going on?' But do I even try to talk to them? Do they want to talk about it? I don't know. If I talk to them, is it going to make it worse?"

Recommended protocols are vague. One template memorandum for a 24-hour watch procedure states that "continuous monitoring should occur at all times, including accompanying the Soldier to the latrine and during meals" and that the "Soldier should sleep in a room with a unit member who is awake at all times or in a dayroom . . . so that the Soldier is constantly monitored throughout the night."[41] But what should "continuous monitoring" constitute in practice, and how should intimate boundaries between watcher and watched be negotiated? For example, must the watched soldier always be *in sight?* After her first time serving as a unit-watch guard, Sarah found her friends curious and eager to hear about the technicalities of the work. Their questions gave way to conversations both practical and grimly humorous. "Everyone talks about their funny stories, and someone will be like, 'So, do you watch him shit?' I'm like, 'No dude. I stand outside the door.'" Intrigue over such minutiae suggests that learning to do the work of unit watch often centers on the banal bodily dimensions of watching others, underscoring the negotiated intimacies through which watcher and watched relate to one another in arrangements of care and constraint.[42]

Soldiers informally acquire tips and strategies from one another for how to do the work of unit watch. They also draw on what they themselves know. While Fuller felt that unit watch was more properly the domain of experts, when Sarah was placed on unit watch during her first deployment to Iraq, she called on the knowledge she had accumulated from peers as well as the closest equivalent in the range of her experience. "You kind of know how to watch, like with a detainee. So sort of, tangentially, you kind of are like, 'Okay, so this is how you do it.'" Sarah drew on a personal archive of affective and bodily practice in a manner that is revealing. The transference she easily made between watching detainees to watching at-risk soldiers suggests how practices of constraint and objectification can travel across the embodied work of soldiering.

DIRTBAG

If the restriction of individuals' liberty for the protection of society is part of the mandate of treating threatening individuals through constraint, the unit watch bypasses the concern for agency and individual rights that have featured in public debate in the United States concerning inpatient and community psychiatric care.[43] Unit watch centers the military corporate collective as the unit of concern, under which the individual is already subsumed and their agency potentially (further) sacrificed for the larger good. Indeed, the very effectiveness and efficiency of unit watch is said to rest in the dynamic of confinement from *within* the whole as opposed to seclusion outside the whole. The constraint of unit watch is framed less as the restriction of individual liberty than as care through intensive integration.

But contrary to this logic of integration, more often than not, watched soldiers test rather than confirm the cohesiveness of the unit. While some may avoid sitting next to the soldier at mealtime or forgo striking up conversation in the hallways out of a sense of caution or worry about saying the wrong thing, more commonly, watched soldiers become the easy target of frustration, aspersions, and skeptical remarks as to the nature of their suffering. Due to the economy of labor on deployment, a unit watch typically means an increased workload and the potential for increased risk or hazards as the unit provides personnel to monitor the soldier or scrambles to cover the watched soldier's responsibilities. The watched soldier may therefore be seen as selfish and as sacrificing the team, a shameful charge in a corporate context in which everyone is enjoined to "suck it up" and is inculcated into the ethos that one's weakness, deficiencies, and unperformed labor become someone else's burden. The watched soldier's suffering—and its presumed cause, as conjectured or pieced together through the rumor mill—may be minimized and mocked in a setting where there is a clear hierarchical politics to what kind of suffering is most legitimate and where soldier suffering is a selfish distraction from the "true" enemy threat. It's perhaps unsurprising, then, that soldiers shared a handful of terms to describe watched peers: the problem child, pariah, and the dirtbag.[44] While it's true that cases can be seen as differently legitimate, with some garnering more sympathy than others, by virtue of their granted exceptionality and the added labor taken up by the unit, the watched soldier challenges the very cohesiveness that the unit watch claims to mobilize. In this incongruous state of enjoined care and structural exclusion, the unit watch reveals the fluid lines between care and punishment, where the meanings attributed to constraint by unit peers remain multiple and conflicting.

Further testing this ideal of integration is the fact that watched soldiers are symbolically marked as set apart. In an institutional context in which every soldier is trained to read for minor sartorial differences as signs of rank and unit, unit-watch restrictions can advertise the watched soldier in unspoken, yet overt ways: in the boots held together by rubber bands rather than shoelaces or in the absence of a weapon. Other signs are purposefully designed to shame. For instance, a story came out in *The Daily Beast* in 2009 that orange road guard vests were being used at Fort Benning to single out soldiers on unit watch. "You're in an isolated state," one recruit was reported saying. "You've got the reason you're on suicide watch to begin with on top of the fact that you stick out like a sore thumb," he said. "It's like you're walking around in a zoo, and you're the animal."[45]

Powerful in the accounts of unit watch shared with me was one sign taken to represent the ultimate demotion of soldierness in deployment: the absence of a weapon. Sarah recalled for me how visually jarring it was to see someone without a weapon on the FOB. "Everyone has a weapon. So, if you see someone without a weapon, you know they're on suicide watch or they're in a lot of trouble and haven't figured it out yet," she told me. Sarah described in detail how the three-point tactical sling used in her unit, which hangs a weapon across the torso, made its absence glaringly apparent.

The conspicuous absence of a weapon in deployment undermines the presumed relationship between violence, firearms, and what it means to be a soldier at war. Unit watch restricts access to firearms and other military-issued weapons to ensure the safety of the watched soldier and others, yet in doing so deprives the soldier of the capacity that ostensibly legitimates and secures their role as part of an occupying and fighting force. While recommended alterations to policy have sought to minimize identification of the watched soldier—for example, allowing them to maintain possession of an inactivated weapon whose firing pin or bolt has been removed—the soldier effectively remains in the contradictory state of being a soldier deprived of the capacity for violence.

The conspicuous exclusion of watched soldiers is most visible in communal spaces like the DFAC, or dining facility. Several soldiers tasked with watching others while deployed separately referred to the experience of walking into the dining hall, with one describing it as "a parting of the oceans": everyone gives you a wide berth. Sarah spoke of the awkwardness of being an escort with the watched soldier next to her and trying to sit down at a full table, only to feel the radiating discomfort of others. Simply trying to figure out where to sit in the dining hall meant negotiating countervailing forces of integration and exclusion. "Everyone is weird. If you're escorting somebody and they don't have a weapon, but you're walking with them, it's pretty obvious," she recalled. "So, in the DFAC, there's a little, 'Do we try to sit with people? Do we try to sit over here on the edge?' If you do try to sit on the edge, people kind of make room, but they don't really say anything to you. It's just . . . It's a little awkward." When I asked Sarah to explain this phenomenon, she told me, "I don't know if people avoid the person because they think, 'Suicide is contagious,' or if they think, 'You're a problem child and we don't want to think about you.'" In the end, she suspected both fear and disgust were at play.

Suicide contagion has indeed emerged as a concern for the military. Studies in the Army suggest that the risk of suicide attempts among soldiers increases with the number of previous unit suicide attempts, particularly within smaller units.[46] Brandon, a former Army infantry officer who left the military five years ago, spoke from a military leadership perspective when he attributed the use of unit watch to the need to contain "feelings" of suicide in the unit in order to prevent their spread. "We don't want anyone else to get these feelings, right?" he told me. "We push them aside, so it doesn't affect the rest of the unit, and it doesn't affect the mission, which is the right answer. Unfortunately, that is the right answer. I can't let one bad apple spoil the bunch."

Rather than supporting the watched soldier's integration as PIE principles would promote, Brandon, Fuller, and Sarah instead suggest that the unit watch enacts a process of *encapsulation*: of exclusion, isolation, and separation from within. While intended to integrate, in practice the unit watch works to individuate the watched soldier from inside the collective body. Fuller told me that even senior leaders typically alienate the one on suicide watch, making it clear that the soldier is no longer part of the whole. Fuller described this strange state of being both physically among the unit yet set apart as "living in a fishbowl." "It is dehumanizing," he said. "And if you take someone that's already in a frazzled mental state that maybe has lost touch with reality or he's having a psychotic break, or whatever it is,

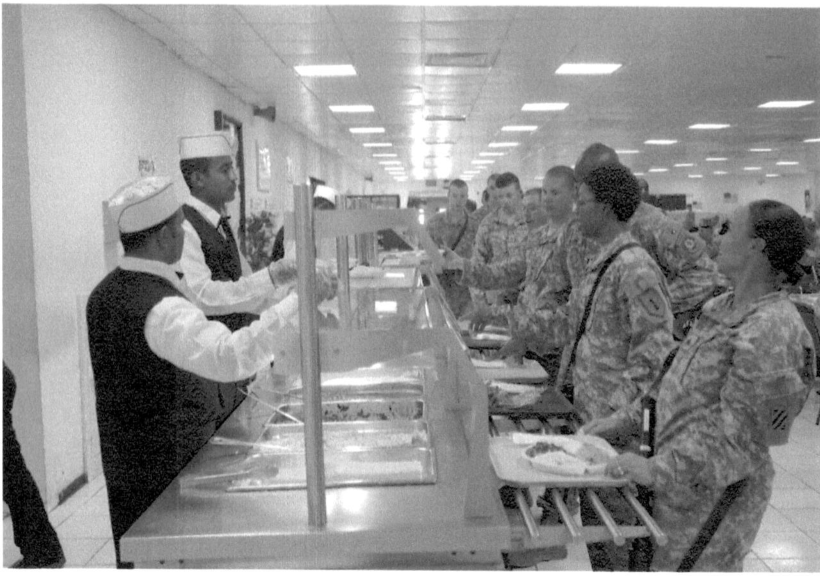

Figure 19. Lining up for lunch at the "Dragon's Lair" dining facility in FOB Falcon in Baghdad, Iraq. Photograph by SSG Nathaniel Smith, via DVIDS.

you take someone that's already mentally weak and you put more stress on them. You point the finger at them even more. Rather than supporting the integration of the soldier, "90 percent of the time, no one talks to the kid," Fuller said. "It's, 'Hey, fuck-o, you're on suicide watch now. Thanks.' And now that's one more rock in that soldier's ruck that he has to carry."

In this intense state of simultaneous scrutiny and disavowal, the watched soldier becomes the lesion around which the system ambivalently folds in on itself. This is expulsion not through extreme spatial separation from the social body as manifest in the asylum but rather through differentiation and confinement from within the corporate whole.[47]

LIFE-GUARDING

Sarah was on her second deployment to Iraq and spending a lot of her downtime playing the multiplayer board game Settlers of Catan with friends in the unit when she was assigned to the unit watch of a fellow specialist named Esposito. A cryptologic linguist, she worked shifts in a SCIF, a secure office limited to authorized personnel located on the top floor of a building on their FOB. Just outside the secure office was a dayroom with a television, a setup that her sergeant determined was ideal for watching Esposito. Given that Esposito had the security clearance to be up in the SCIF and the SCIF required a passcode to enter and exit and had an alarm that would sound when the door opened, their sergeant decided Esposito would be confined in the dayroom while Sarah worked her nightshifts inside the secure office. A mattress was brought in so that Esposito could sleep there at night. Sarah remembered him staying up late most nights, binge watching television series, mostly *Friends* and *Sex and the City*.

Having Esposito in the dayroom turned out to be a good arrangement, Sarah told me, since "it was probably the closest you could get to someone being free." Because she was still responsible for her regular duties during those night shifts while guarding Esposito, she had to periodically step away from her work in the inner office to check on him. "I would have to pop out every hour, so it was a little disruptive to have to go out, but I was also really paranoid," she explained. "But I also didn't want to go out too often and make him feel like I was watching him even though I was watching him. So, it just added this whole extra layer of stress."

Sarah's concern that Esposito not feel watched even as she felt the need to watch him captures the conflict she experienced as both guard and friend. Long before she was tasked with his unit watch, Sarah and Esposito had been game night partners and close buddies. Sarah had also been the one who interrupted Esposito's suicide attempt. It was Sarah who had gone looking for Esposito when he didn't show up for one of their scheduled game nights and who, by some chance of fate, stumbled into the Porta-John where Esposito was sitting with his rifle, butt first on the ground, muzzle pointing upward. It was Sarah who took the rifle from him and escorted him to their sergeant.

The unit watch can set up difficult dynamics, as the unit escort of a watched soldier may be a peer, a teammate, and, not uncommonly, a friend. In fact, Sarah's sergeant deliberately recruited her to be Esposito's primary unit guard precisely because of their friendship. This made striking what

Sarah described as a "balance" in the work of care-as-constraint both complicated and disquieting. How to do the work of watching while still trying to spare her friend's feelings? As the person who saved Esposito's life once, Sarah felt that unit watch tasked her with saving it yet again—and this time in a way that made her overtly responsible for doing so.

As Esposito's friend and his unit guard, Sarah would try to smooth out interactions between him and the rest of the unit by actively resisting the unit watch's tendency to isolate. She described how she would see escorts walking around without talking or interacting with the soldier they were watching. "Sometimes you'll see someone with a weapon and the person without a weapon and the person without a weapon is eating," she said, setting a familiar scene. "The other person's just kind of sitting there. But it all depends on how the individual person handles it, I guess. Like some people feel they're more of a guard." In Esposito's case, "I thought of it like we were friends. I'm sitting with him to make sure he doesn't kill himself, but I'm going to try to make it not awkward."

Going to the dining hall, she would make conversation and eat with him, as if they were "just going to a meal together." But even then, she had to work to facilitate encounters. If someone got up from the table and asked if they could bring something back for anyone, for example, they might ask Sarah if Esposito wanted anything. "I'd be like, 'I don't know, he's a fully grown man right next to me. Ask him.' I would try to make a joke about it. People didn't want to make eye contact with him." It bothered Sarah when other guys from a different part of the battalion, who didn't know Esposito personally, would rotate in as unit guards. When coming off unit guard duty, they referred to Esposito as a thing to be passed along. "The other guys were all just like, very, 'Hey, you got this?' and turn around and go," she recalled. "It's not like they were buddy-buddy, so it was more like they were passing off a radio or something."

Even as Sarah tried to do the work of rebuilding sociality for Esposito, of lending him subjecthood in circumstances where others were inclined to ignore and objectify him, she also noted how the unit watch created odd forms of intimacy. She remembers the time she had to be on watch while Esposito was asleep in his room. Because Esposito's roommate was leaving in the middle of the night for a mission, Sarah was asked to be on watch while they both slept. Sitting on the floor of their sparse, cramped trailer as the two roommates got ready for bed, she resorted to making small talk in a poor attempt to ease the tension:

> He wasn't chatty, so I just was like, "Okay, cool. I guess I'll just stay and wait." They were like, "Yeah, thanks." So, I kind of sat down and just sat there. He was like, "Cool. I'll just sleep." Because he was in his PTs, he's like, "I'll just sleep in my PTs," and I was like, "Cool, thank you. Please don't sleep naked."[48] We made a little joke about that, and he just got in his bed and went to sleep. There was a little conversation but not a lot. He was just trying to go to sleep and then his roommate was also trying to take a nap. I didn't know how long he had until his mission. So, I'm trying not to talk and am just like literally awake in this room full of guys who are sleeping.

This kind of unit-watch duty, where the escort, in effect, watches the soldier sleep, has been described to me as nothing if not deeply and memorably strange. As Sarah put it, "I was just awkwardly sitting in this room watching two dudes sleep." Unit watch can draw soldiers into relationships that can both test and reshape the nature of friendship and collective care. But the injunction to care and the institutional demand for intimacy in unit watch, here experienced as Sarah's closeness to "two sleeping dudes," also reveals, in this particular case, the gendered nature of military embodiment and the gendered forms of protection against death that can emerge in the shadow cast by suicide's possibility.[49] These dynamics recall what Zoë Wool calls "work for life," the "labor and complex attachment" that in the case of veteran and military suicide is always already gendered, implicitly understood to be the domain of girlfriends and wives.[50]

As Esposito's friend and the one who found him that day in the Porta-John, Sarah assumed the duties of his unit watch as a grave and profound responsibility—and with great fear. On their FOB, where weapons were present everywhere and on everyone, Sarah found herself seeing and sensing limitless opportunities for Esposito to hurt himself. "I just felt like a nonspecific tension. I kept remembering what it looked like with him with that rifle," Sarah said. "Because we put our weapons down when we're eating—so, I was always conscious, 'Is he going to suddenly make a grab for a rifle and try to . . . ?'" She recounted how unnerving it was when others in her unit would leave their rifles leaning up against the sofa while in the dayroom, so she would pull them aside and tell them, "Hey, guys, he's going to be up here. He's on suicide watch, so don't leave your guns around."

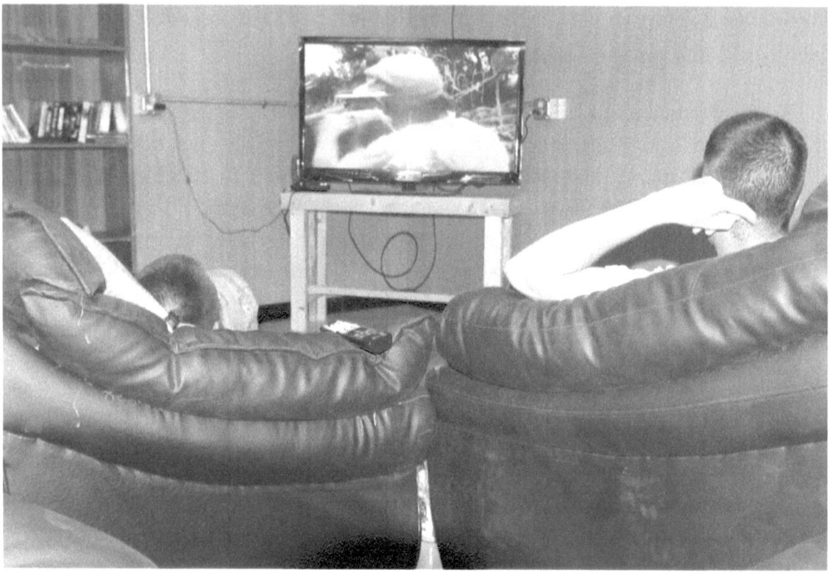

Figure 20. Soldiers stationed at outlying COPs enjoy the amenities and a few days of R&R at FOB Salerno in Afghanistan. Photograph by SPC Tobey White, via DVIDS.

Attuned to the weapons around her as new kind of risk, Sarah found herself constantly scanning their environment for the potential threats it contained. Even mundane objects acquired new meaning. There was a small kitchen on the floor below the SCIF, where they kept an old KA-BAR combat knife they would use to cut food from mermites—insulated food containers typically made of tinned steel—on days they were feeling too lazy to walk down to the dining hall. "We just kept it on the table. But I remember feeling a deep tension that it was there," she recalled. "With my unit, I didn't want to make a big deal of the fact that he was on suicide watch. But there was a big knife there, so I would just go and get a snack and pretend to accidentally take it back into the inner office. Then the guys would come in and be like, 'Hey, where's the knife?' I'd be like, 'Oh, shoot. Sorry, guys. I have it right here.'"

Watchfulness, as Angela Garcia describes of the possibility of suicide in contexts of addiction, can suggest an "ethics of community and a form of care," where "to remain watchful *with* one another—not over or against the others—can offset forms of alienation."[51] For Sarah, watchfulness took shape as an all-consuming vigilance centered on the control of people and objects in a landscape rife with means for violence, all in an institutional and operational context demanding Esposito's eventual and full return to duty. But it also meant sparing Esposito further embarrassment and blame: hiding the need to hide the communal kitchen knife and redirecting peers' questions toward the grown man sitting next to her. Such gestures may be considered radical acts of care in circumstances of objectification and exclusion, of perceived weakness and collective liability. For Sarah, watchfulness against suicide meant recuperating aspects of sociality and selfhood deprived by the dynamics of the unit watch itself.

CATCH AND RELEASE

When Craig returned to the US with his unit after two months in confinement, life went strangely back to normal. As he was going through the processing procedures of returning home from Afghanistan with his unit, as he expected, he "popped like 17 red flags." "I was told, 'Hey, you should visit Mental Health.' So, I did." Craig recalls that a few weeks later, his military care provider told him, "We're really short staffed and you don't seem to be doing that badly, and there's guys from the infantry battalion who are doing really bad, and they need your time slot. Do you really think you need to be here?" After two months of confinement, Craig yielded to the process of return and to the distress of others made visible in that same process. In being discouraged from seeking care once back home, Craig newly realized the profound paradox of his confinement in Afghanistan. Release can reveal the nature of constraint.

At the level of practice, constraint-as-care under the pressure to return soldiers to duty can generate competing responses to distress. In Craig's case, the urgency of his threats resulted in two months of confinement, without access to either his medication or his psychiatrist. Stories like Sarah's reveal that while the unit watch enjoins soldiers to care for their own, it becomes the weighty obligation of tasked watching and felt friendship to restore sociality and personhood against the objectification and isolation that the unit watch produces. Coercive care against suicide in war also confuses expectations about the violence and morality of war itself. As Sarah said with striking clarity of her feeling of sheer ineptitude and lack of preparedness in doing the work of unit watch, "I was not equipped. Keeping someone from killing themselves was literally the opposite of my job there." To prevent death within the very workings of the war machine is, for some, the greatest contradiction of all.

Epilogue

WITHDRAWAL

> Tell me how this ends.
>
> General David Petraeus, 2004

On April 14, 2021, President Joseph Biden announced the full withdrawal of US troops from Afghanistan, beginning May 1 and concluding by September 11 that same year, the twentieth anniversary of the war.[1] The decision, initiated by President Biden and stemming from a formal agreement made by former-President Donald Trump with the Taliban, committed to a troop withdrawal without the involvement of the Afghan government. The war in Afghanistan, Biden said in an address to the nation, was never meant to be multigenerational.

The official end to America's longest war was a chaotic and harrowing final exit, hastened by the speed with which the Taliban regained control of the country once US forces began to pull out. When the Taliban overthrew the US-backed government and captured Kabul on August 15, it forced the US to empty its embassy and frantically accelerate a mass evacuation effort through an airlift executed by the US Air Force, with US ground forces attempting to secure the airfield at Kabul International Airport.

Tens of thousands of Afghans and foreign nationals crowded the runways as they attempted to make their exit before the Taliban completed its takeover of the country. Many had fought the Taliban or had supported Afghan or NATO forces. Desperation drove some to cling to the wings of

US military planes as they took off. Fada Mohammad, a young dentist, fell to his death from a US aircraft. His body was found on a rooftop four miles from the airport.[2] Ten days later, a suicide bombing outside the airport killed 170 Afghans and 13 US military personnel. Three days after that, as one of its last acts in the war in Afghanistan, the US launched a drone strike that killed ten Afghan civilians, seven of them children. The US said it was targeting an Islamic State operative with a car full of explosives intending to target evacuees and military forces at the airport. In fact, the car was that of Zemari Ahmadi, a longtime aid worker for the United States, and nine of his family members.[3]

In this "imperial exit turned spectacle," the world witnessed "empire's flight from the scene of a crime," as Anila Daulatzai and Sahar Ghumkhor have described it. In this flight, the American press expanded its focus beyond US troops to document the devastating realities of "what was unfolding *on the ground*" for Afghans.[4] But in the weeks and months to follow, public attention would return to the suffering of US soldiers and veterans in order to register the failures of the longest-running conflict in US history. Stories in the media and polling surveys reported anger, betrayal, and humiliation over the withdrawal among veterans of the Afghanistan war. As the American public faced the excruciating end to a 20-year war, social media was rife with accounts of military personnel and veterans suffering moral injury as they watched their Afghan "allies," who had worked with the US occupation, abandoned to unknown fates in the hasty withdrawal.[5] Psychologists and psychiatrists warned that framings of the war as a failure and defeat by journalists and foreign policy intellectuals were proving harmful to veteran mental health. "The defeatist narrative dominating even domestic discussions about the US withdrawal from Afghanistan is going to have a tragic impact at home," wrote a reporter for *The Atlanticist*. "The nation has not lost a uniformed service member in Afghanistan since February 8, 2020, but conditions now put service members and veterans at risk for debilitating mental health problems and suicide. *What was it all for? Was it worth it? Why did we bother?* These questions are triggering post-traumatic stress disorder in our men and women who served in Afghanistan."[6]

Local media outlets reported backlogged VA appointments and rising veteran suicide in the immediate wake of the withdrawal, while VA providers encouraged patients to limit news consumption, which could work as traumatic reminders for not just veterans of the war in Afghanistan but also of the Iraq War and the Vietnam War. As one VA psychiatrist who leads an outpatient PTSD clinic at the VA Greater Los Angeles Healthcare System put it, "It's like everything they did—digging wells, helping families build schools, building roads, making areas safe, clearing mines—all these positive things feel like they're erased now. It's very heartbreaking for the soldiers."[7] Policymakers, meanwhile, warned the botched conclusion to the war and the demoralizing speed of the Taliban takeover would discourage young people from joining the military and precipitate an exodus from its ranks, worsening the military's already dire numbers crisis.

In the drift into forever war, medicine was given an impossible task. As US military policy in the 2000s called for full-spectrum dominance and the US Army became an occupying force in Iraq and Afghanistan, psychopharmaceuticals were instrumentalized as a modest but practical tool to keep bodies in place and returning to the same wars. *Stabilizing Empire* has traced the medico-political fantasy of realizing control through chemistry—a fantasy that has proven itself inherently unstable. Military medicine's intensive risk management and soldiers' regulation of their own conduct in relation to the drugs they consume uncannily mirrored the governance and enforced order over occupied territories and populations in the war on terror.

The pursuit of control was also evident in the withdrawal from Afghanistan. In the aftermath of what many described as a devastating failure, efforts to rescript the narrative sought to contain public anger, manage military trauma and moral injury, and shore up the armed forces amid declining numbers. As this book has shown, such efforts to control and stabilize are not simply clinical, ethical, or operational. They are also political. This pursuit continues even after the war's "official" end.

Studying the use of psychopharmaceuticals offers a revealing lens on how soldiers feel, understand themselves and others, and meet the material demands of everyday military life and war making. Psychotropic medications on the battlefield illuminate biomedical and counterinsurgent fantasies of chemical rescue, in which the soldier deemed a threat can be recalibrated and an infantryman on a hilltop hopes that pills will make things better, or at least not any worse. At the same time, psychopharmaceuticals constitute a critical site for the production of the moralities that underwrite contemporary global liberal war.

Psychopharmaceutical use—its embodied effects, military strategic purposes, and the management of its risks—has furnished both the moral vocabulary and practical means through which soldiers have defined what is acceptable and good in these most recent iterations of counterinsurgency war making. The story of psychopharmacy, then, does more than add another chapter to the ages-old tale of soldier drug use. It offers a new angle on this history by showing how battlefield medicine performs critical moral labor, authorizing and condemning particular forms of violence and ways of waging war, "while leaving the war paradigm itself unquestioned."[8]

. . . . .

As the US formally ended the war in Afghanistan, President Biden repeatedly emphasized the need to redirect military assets toward new and evolving threats. While displacement, weakened institutions, and the lasting effects of decades of militarization and conflict continue to structure life in Afghanistan and Iraq, the US military is reconfiguring its global posture, extending its forward presence into new regions.

As this book goes to press, the US has launched a war with Iran—despite ongoing diplomatic talks and without congressional approval. US military policy is also shifting toward China and Russia, as national security strategy and military planners envision threats of the near and distant future. The Department of Defense is predicting that the next major global conflicts will involve what it calls modern LSCOs, or large-scale combat operations. When Russia annexed Crimea in 2014, US military analysts began reimagining the possibility of large-scale conflict between military forces, a concern that has continued to grow with the full-scale invasion of Ukraine in 2022 and the escalation of US-China tension. In October 2022, the Army published field manual 3-0, *Operations*, which asserted the need to focus on, study, and prepare for LSCOs, using the term over one hundred times.[9] The DoD defines LSCOs as high-intensity warfare between nations that are technological peers or near-peers, involving, in its jargon, multi-domain operations, or MDOs—the integration of capabilities across multiple warfighting domains, including air, land, sea, space, and cyberspace. This is compelling the Army to rethink the way it organizes, equips, and fights. After two decades of focusing on brigades rotating in and out of Afghanistan and Iraq, Army leaders are now directing the most significant reorganization of the armed forces since the end of the Cold War, with China setting the pacing challenge.

The troops that the Army envisions needing for the near future of large-scale conflicts is also changing. At a time when nearly half of adolescents in the US have had a mental health disorder at some point in their lives and Congress aims to "turbocharge" recruitment numbers, the Army is having to rethink its policies.[10] In 2024, the Pentagon's expansion of the Medical Access Records Pilot (MARP) eased enlistment for some individuals with an ADHD diagnosis, shortening the time required without treatment and reducing the need for complex waivers under defined conditions. But even as the Army eases eligibility requirements for applicants with ADHD, reforms its waiver process to accelerate recruitment, and mainstreams the language of neurodivergence, the messaging from the White House, by contrast, has been restrictive.[11] In one of his first acts back in office, Trump signed an executive order titled, "Prioritizing Military Excellence and Readiness." While specifically targeting transgender troops, the order also targeted several mental health conditions, "from conditions that require substantial medication or medical treatment to bipolar and related disorders, eating disorders, suicidality, and prior psychiatric hospitalization," deeming them "incompatible" with military service. "The Armed Forces," the order states, "must adhere to high mental and physical health standards to ensure our military can deploy, fight, and win, including in austere conditions and without the benefit of routine medical treatment or special provisions."[12] In this environment—in which the Pentagon is rethinking its paradigm regarding the compatibility of mental health diagnoses and military readiness, while the Commander in Chief of the Armed Forces is officially repolicing the boundaries of the total institution—military psychiatrists are concerned for what this will mean for treatment and stigma in the military. Dr. Stephen Xenakis, a retired Army brigadier general and psychiatrist, warned that the language of the executive order could force soldiers needing treatment to "go underground."[13]

All the while, military medicine is actively preparing for projected warfare. Military medical planners have been looking "back" on the war on terror, as well as on World War II—the last conflict in which the US fought a large-scale war in multiple theaters—in an effort to glean pragmatic lessons for near-future conflict.[14] As military medical planners reimagine large-scale operations of the future, one concern is clear across their predictions: a future conflict with a near-peer adversary will have major implications for access to and mobility of care, including for mental and behavioral health. Contested airspace will likely prevent the establishment of COSC clinics at fixed locations and preclude mental health providers and behavioral health technicians from circulating to forward locations to provide direct support as they did in the wars in Iraq and Afghanistan. Telehealth care may not be able to fully overcome these challenges, as cyber capabilities may also be disrupted. This could mean that soldiers who are the highest priority for acute mental health care—those experiencing suicidal thoughts, emerging psychosis, or acute substance-related problems, for example—may need to be managed in forward environments for longer periods of time. It could mean stabilizing a soldier in place for several days, perhaps weeks, with minimal to no professional supervision or guidance. The military refers to this extended period of care as PFC, or prolonged forward care.[15]

In the setting of prolonged forward care, mental and behavioral health will devolve down the ranks. The military mental health community expects to require additional forward interventions implemented in-place by enlisted providers or by soldiers themselves. Without physical or remote access to mental health professionals, reliance on people and interventions that can work as "service extenders" in forward areas will be increasingly vital. The military mental health community continues to expect that most soldiers requiring mental and behavioral health support will experience COSR, the transient, temporary symptoms that are expected to resolve themselves with supportive intervention.[16] But when options for evacuation or even remote consultation are not immediately available, soldiers will need to rely on themselves and one another to do the work of stabilization.

In the expected absence of providers, the military mental health community is promoting the role of "self-aid" and "buddy aid" for prolonged scenarios of treatment-in-place. This includes mobile applications designed for the self-management of psychological symptoms and to support coping and resilience. For example, the military has shown interest in the Breathe2Relax application, a portable stress management tool that guides users through belly breathing techniques to manage stress and anxiety, and the Virtual Hope Box mobile application, which allows the soldier to set up the app with photos of friends and family, sound bites and videos of loved ones, relaxation exercises, and reminders and reasons for living.

Psychotropic medications have kept soldiers in place in the war on terror, where access to providers was easier than military planners imagine will be the case with large-scale conflict. Particularly when cut loose from diagnoses and normalized for the temporary treatment of symptoms, drugs lend themselves easily to a larger toolkit of "self-aid" therapies. Pharmaceuticals, as we've seen in this book, also shape-shift in what they do and mean in relation to the political-military project of the US empire. This includes the agentive and relational ways that soldiers purposefully hack the power of pills to violent efficacy but also the unpredictable and mercurial effects drugs produce in dynamic settings of war making. No doubt they will shape-shift anew in the time-space of large-scale war.

In the imagined setting of prolonged forward care—a setting that will require agile treatment that can travel separately from the provider and in an institutional environment in which mental health treatment may increasingly go "underground"—psychopharmaceuticals will likely again play a definitive, if ambiguous, role. They will continue to appear as the solution to the time-space dilemmas of military empire, while being deeply unstable in use and effect. With missions increasing in Europe, the Middle East, and the Pacific and the strength of the force a continuing concern, medications that are a routine way of life for many Americans may once again be tapped as the convenient and stealth panacea to the US military empire's challenges of many stripes. As forward care is deputized to soldiers themselves, the heavily seeded ground of psychopharmaceuticals as both civilian and now military medicine will surely foster its continued and expanding use in getting soldiers to get by. For the time being.

Notes

INTRODUCTION

1. All names of interlocutors are pseudonyms. For those no longer in the military at the time of the interview, I use anonymized first names. For those in the military at the time of interview, I use anonymized surnames, sometimes accompanied by rank, to reflect military convention.

2. Military medical care is provided through a continuum of five "echelons" of care. Echelon 1 care is treatment provided by medical assets organic to the unit; echelon 2 care is provided at the brigade and division level; echelon 3 care takes place at forward-deployed combat support hospitals (CSHs); and echelon 4 care occurs in hospitals outside theater. Finally, echelon 5 care is provided at continental-US military and Veterans Affairs (VA) medical centers.

3. The Army does have enlisted medical personnel, known as behavioral health technicians/specialists (BHTs), who work under the supervision of licensed mental health providers (MHPs), such as psychiatrists, social workers, and psychiatric nurses. They are the behavioral health equivalent of the combat medic.

4. Military hierarchy and rank are strictly codified and determine differences including job function, level of responsibility, rules for interpersonal communication, dress, and pay. The two different ways of joining the US military—by commissioning and by enlisting—mark a major division among military personnel: commissioned officers are considered the managers and planners,

responsible for strategizing missions, giving orders, and assigning enlisted soldiers tasks. Among enlisted soldiers, there are 13 Army ranks, which can be broken down into three groups: junior enlisted, noncommissioned officer ranks, and senior noncommissioned officer ranks. In general, climbing the rank structure carries increasing levels of responsibility and demands greater levels of respect and deference.

5. Macroscale analyses that have emerged in the last two decades theorize the US empire in relation to shifts in the forms of imperial practice following the dissolution of the Soviet empire and in light of transformations in capitalist accumulation. See, for example, Michael Hardt and Antonio Negri, 2001, *Empire* (Cambridge, MA: Harvard University Press); David Harvey, 2003, *The New Imperialism* (Oxford: Oxford University Press); Immanuel Wallerstein, 2005, *The Decline of American Power: The US in a Chaotic World* (New York: New Press). My approach follows anthropologists who have called for ethnographic analysis of projects of US empire "in the details." See Catherine Lutz, 2006, "Empire is in the Details," *American Ethnologist* 33(4):593-611.

6. Derek Gregory, "The Everywhere War," *The Geographic Journal* 177(3):238–50. Gregory argues that while commentators emphasized the historical temporality of military violence following the terrorist attacks on the World Trade Center and the Pentagon (e.g., the "post-9/11 wars"), the geographical expanse of the wars conducted by the US also demands analysis. As Stephen Graham notes, this expanding reality is also evident in the shift in US military doctrine from the concept of the battlefield to the multiscalar, multidimensional "battlespace," which "prefigures a boundless and unending process of militarization where everything becomes a site of permanent war." Stephen Graham, 2009, "Cities as Battlespace: The New Military Urbanism," *City* 13(4):383–402, 389.

7. It is essential not to reproduce narratives of post-9/11 rupture and to recognize the long histories of imperial intervention in Afghanistan and Iraq. See Zainab Saleh, 2020, *Return to Ruin: Iraqi Narratives of Exile and Nostalgia* (Stanford: Stanford University Press) on the decades of US imperial interests in Iraq, ranging from the US backing of the 1963 Ba'ath coup to efforts to safeguard American access to Iraqi oil. See Wazhmah Osman and Robert D. Crews, ed., 2025, *Decolonizing Afghanistan: Countering Imperial Knowledge and Power* (Durham, NC: Duke University Press) on the decades of colonial and imperial foreign involvement in Afghanistan from the early twentieth century to the present.

8. Quoted in Maria Ryan, 2019, *Full Spectrum Dominance: Irregular Warfare and the War on Terror* (Stanford: Stanford University Press), 9–10.

9. The term "full-spectrum dominance" appears in the 2004 National Military Strategy of the United States of America, which identifies the need to build a "diverse portfolio of capabilities" able to respond to a spectrum of potential adversaries "including terrorist networks, international criminal organizations and

illegal armed groups that menace stability and security" (4). The 2004 Strategy articulated a goal of "full-spectrum dominance (FSD)—the ability to control any situation or defeat any adversary across the range of military operations" (23). Joint Chiefs of Staff, 2004, *The National Military Strategy of the United States of America: A Strategy for Today; A Vision for Tomorrow* (Washington, DC: Joint Chiefs of Staff).

10. While the Army would increase numbers of mental health personnel during the wars in Iraq and Afghanistan, the ratio of mental health personnel to troops fluctuated and was often significantly lower than the Army's goal of placing one provider per seven hundred troops. United States Army Surgeon General, 2006, *Mental Health Advisory Team (MHAT) IV Operation Iraqi Freedom 05-07 Final Report* (Washington, DC: Army Medical Command), 57. Mental and behavioral health providers in the US Army include psychiatrists, psychologists, licensed clinical social workers, psychiatric nurse practitioners, and BHTs.

11. Peter Redfield, 2008, "Vital Mobility and the Humanitarian Kit," in *Biosecurity Interventions: Global Health and Security in Question,* ed. A. Lakoff and S. Collier (New York: Columbia University Press), 147–72; Peter Redfield, 2013, *Life in Crisis: The Ethical Journey of Doctors without Borders* (Berkeley: University of California Press), 69–97.

12. Military medicine considers the period in the immediate aftermath of traumatic injury, commonly referred to as the "golden hour," to be the most critical for emergency stabilization of a casualty. US troops wounded in the wars in Iraq and Afghanistan had the highest rates of survival of battlefield injuries of any wars in US history. Advancements in acute hemorrhage management, forward surgical support, and rapid air evacuation significantly improved survival rates. Jeffrey T. Howard et al., 2019, "Use of Combat Casualty Care Data to Assess the US Military Trauma System During the Afghanistan and Iraq Conflicts, 2001-2017," *JAMA Surgery* 154(7):600–8. Still, extreme medical interventions on the battlefield can come at extraordinary cost to the health of surviving soldiers. See Emily Mayhew, 2017, *A Heavy Reckoning: War, Medicine and Survival in Afghanistan and Beyond* (London: Profile Books).

13. David Kieran, 2019, *Signature Wounds: The Untold Story of the Military's Mental Health Crisis* (New York: New York University Press), 32.

14. The diagnosis of PTSD was officially added to the American Psychiatric Association's *Diagnostic and Statistical Manual*, or DSM, in 1980. See Allan Young, 1995, *The Harmony of Illusions: Inventing Post-Traumatic Stress Disorder* (Princeton: Princeton University Press) for a groundbreaking historical and ethnographic account of the emergence of PTSD as a cultural product of treatment processes and narratives that shaped Vietnam veterans' experiences.

15. The US Army began using the term "behavioral health" in the 2000s to replace "mental health," on the understanding that "behavioral health" sounded more neutral, clinical, and inclusive of a broader range of issues. The shift in

terminology reflects the Army's broader efforts to lower the barriers for soldiers to seek care and to "destigmatize" mental health during the period of the war on terror, as historian David Kieran has comprehensively documented. Kieran, *Signature Wounds.* I use both terms, with a preference for "mental health," which was the term used most often in interviews with soldiers and veterans.

16. On the political and cultural implications of new military technologies including autonomous weapons and AI warfare, see Roberto González, 2024, *War Virtually: The Quest to Automate Conflict, Militarize Data, and Predict the Future* (Berkeley: University of California Press); Hugh Gusterson, 2017, *Drone: Remote Control Warfare* (Cambridge, MA: MIT Press); Anthony King, 2025, *AI, Automation, and War: The Rise of a Military-Tech Complex* (Princeton: Princeton University Press).

17. For historical surveys of the intersection of psychiatry, the neurosciences, and military interests, see Jonathan D. Moreno, 2006, *Mind Wars: Brain Science and the Military in the 21st Century* (New York: Bellevue Literary Press); Ben Shephard, 2003, *A War of Nerves: Soldiers and Psychiatrists in the Twentieth Century* (Cambridge, MA: Harvard University Press). See also Andrew Bickford, 2020, *Chemical Heroes: Pharmacological Supersoldiers in the US Military* (Durham, NC: Duke University Press) on the biomedical enhancement and protection of soldiers.

18. Nomi Stone, 2022, *Pinelandia: An Anthropology and Field Poetics of War and Empire* (Berkeley: University of California Press), 3.

19. A rich literature in anthropology has examined pharmaceuticals as an instructive lens for inquiry into processes of globalization and localization. While these studies have usefully foregrounded the role of markets, speculative capitalism, and forms of governance in propelling the global mobility of pharmaceuticals, they have yet to detail the role of US militarism and empire as a vector in this mobility. In illuminating this link, I am inspired by the cross-disciplinary scholarship on the chemical histories of capitalism, imperialism, and war. These studies "recognize the multiple levels at which our material entanglements—be they cellular, chemical, or commercial—might be connected to global politics." Vanessa Agard-Jones, 2013, "Bodies in the System," *Small Axe: A Caribbean Journal of Criticism* 17(3):182–92, 192. See, for example, Gabrielle Hecht, 2012, *Being Nuclear: Africans and the Global Uranium Trade* (Cambridge, MA: MIT Press); Timothy Mitchell, 2011, *Carbon Democracy: Political Power in the Age of Oil* (London: Verso); Frank von Hippel, 2020, *The Chemical Age: How Chemists Fought Famine and Disease, Killed Millions, and Changed Our Relationship with the Earth* (Chicago: University of Chicago Press).

20. von Hippel, *The Chemical Age*, 133–240.

21. There is a rich scholarly literature on the ecological, political, and social histories of chemicals in empire building, including historical biographies of specific substances, which is beyond my scope. For an example that also

considers the afterlives of chemical empire, see Townsend Middleton, 2024, *Quinine's Remains: Empire's Medicine and the Life Thereafter* (Berkeley: University of California Press).

22. On alcohol in warfare, see Łukasz Kamieński, 2016b, *Shooting Up: A Short History of Drugs and War* (New York: Oxford University Press), 5–28.

23. On the use of stimulants in World War II and the war on terror, see Kamieński, *Shooting Up,* 104–42 and 263–82. On the multifaceted role of amphetamines in American life, see Nicolas Rasmussen, 2009, *On Speed: From Benzedrine to Adderall* (New York: New York University Press).

24. For an in-depth analysis of the role of pharmaceutical and other technological innovations in the US military's performance enhancement projects from the Cold War era into the twenty-first century, see Bickford, *Chemical Heroes.*

25. On the relationship between globalizing drug production and trade and modern warfare, see Kamieński, *Shooting Up,* 233–42; Paul R. Kan, *Drugs and Contemporary Warfare* (Sterling, VA: Potomac Books).

26. On the role of natural and synthetic drugs in the history of human warfare, see Peter Andreas, 2022, *Killer High: A History of War in Six Drugs* (Oxford: Oxford University Press); Dessa Bergen-Cico, 2012, *War and Drugs: The Role of Military Conflict in the Development of Substance Abuse* (New York: Routledge); Kamieński, *Shooting Up.*

27. David Healy, 2012, *Pharmageddon* (Berkeley: University of California Press).

28. This is a slight decline from 255 million prescriptions in 2018, a dip that researchers attribute to the challenges of accessing and refilling prescriptions at the start of the Covid-19 pandemic. "Top 25 Psychiatric Medications for 2020," PsychCentral, November 2, 2022, https://psychcentral.com/blog/top-25-psychiatric-medications-for-2020#top-25-list.

29. Michael Oldani, 2014, "Deep Pharma: Psychiatry, Anthropology, and Pharmaceutical Detox," *Culture, Medicine and Psychiatry* 38(2):255-78, 257.

30. See Junko Kitanaka, 2014, *Depression in Japan: Psychiatric Cures for a Society in Distress* (Princeton: Princeton University Press); Andrew Lakoff, 2005, *Pharmaceutical Reason: Knowledge and Value in Global Psychiatry* (Cambridge, UK: Cambridge University Press); Adriana Petryna et al., eds., 2006, *Global Pharmaceuticals: Ethics, Markets, Practices* (Durham, NC: Duke University Press).

31. Devised initially for the treatment of shell shock during WWI, forward psychiatric principles would later be used on the battlefield by American and British militaries during WWII to return soldiers back to duty. The principle of treating combat stress close to the frontlines remains an essential doctrine of modern military psychiatry in many nations, yet a wide variety of outcomes have been reported. While published accounts generally suggest they succeed in returning soldiers to duty and that these rates decline the further rear soldiers

are treated, historical rates show considerable variation. Edgar Jones and Simon Wessely, 2003, "'Forward Psychiatry' in the Military: Its Origins and Effectiveness," *Journal of Traumatic Stress* 16(4):411–9 points to a lack of clarity around the effectiveness of these treatments.

32. The more recent BICEPS model expands on its PIES predecessor. It stands for *brevity, immediacy, centrality, expectancy, proximity, and simplicity.*

33. The Vietnam War has been also called the first "pharmacological war" because of the ubiquitous and historically unprecedented use of both prescribed and self-administered psychoactive substances by American military personnel. Kamieński, *Shooting Up*, 188.

34. Sarah Hautzinger and Jean Scandlyn, 2014, *Beyond Post-Traumatic Stress: Homefront Struggles with the Wars on Terror* (New York: Routledge), 6.

35. Nadia Abu El-Haj, 2022, *Combat Trauma: Imaginaries of War and Citizenship in Post-9/11 America* (New York: Verso).

36. The key place given to biomedicine in the moral economy of care for soldiers is not particular to psychopharmaceuticals. See Jennifer Terry, 2017, *Attachments to War: Biomedical Logics and Violence in Twenty-First Century America* (Durham, NC: Duke University Press) on the significance of regenerative and rehabilitation medicine to what is "owed" to soldiers. On the moral economy of exchange between soldiers and civilians, see Zöe Wool, 2015, *After War: The Weight of Life at Walter Reed* (Durham, NC: Duke University Press), 97–129.

37. For example, see Erik Baard, 2003, "The Guilt-Free Soldier," *The Village Voice*, January 21; Lisa Chedekel and Matthew Kaufman, 2006, "Mentally Unfit, Forced to Fight," *Hartford Courant*, May 14; Richard Friedman, 2013, "Wars on Drugs," *New York Times*, April 6; Jennifer Senior, 2011, "The Prozac, Paxil, Zoloft, Wellbutrin, Celexa, Effexor, Valium, Klonopin, Ativan, Restoril, Xanax, Adderall, Ritalin, Haldol, Risperdal, Seroquel, Ambien, Lunesta, Elavil, Trazodone War," *New York Magazine*, February 6; Mark Thompson, 2008, "America's Medicated Army," *Time*, June 5.

38. Senator Barbara Boxer, quoted in Kieran, *Signature Wounds*, 73.

39. Bret A. Moore et al., 2012, "Assessment and Management of Acute Combat Stress on the Battlefield," in *Military Psychology: Clinical and Operational Applications*, ed. C. Kennedy and E. Zilmer, 73–92 (New York: Guilford Press), 87. Historically, the Army had a lower suicide rate than the US at large, but this would begin to shift in 2004, when it began rising from a previously stable rate of fewer than 10 per 100,000 to over 20 per 100,000 by 2008, an 80% increase. Timothy Lineberry and Stephen O'Connor, 2012, "Suicide in the US Army," *Mayo Clinic Proceedings* 87(9):871–8. See also Thomas Howard Suitt III, 2021, "High Suicide Rates among United States Service Members and Veterans of the Post-9/11 Wars," Costs of War Research Series.

40. The use of SSRIs, along with factors such as the use of sleep prescriptions and mental health evaluations, was associated with suicides among active-duty

members between 2005 and 2007. Jeffrey Hyman et al., 2012, "Suicide Incidence and Risk Factors in an Active Duty US Military Population," *American Journal of Public Health* 102(S1):S138–46. The Department of Defense Suicide Event Report (DoDSER) reported in 2010 that psychotropic medications were used in nearly one-third of decedents prior to suicide, most frequently antidepressants (*n*=33, 22.45%) and antianxiety medication (*n*=14, 9.52%). United States Department of Defense, 2011, *Department of Defense Suicide Event Report: Calendar Year 2010*, https://www.dspo.mil/Portals/113/Documents/2010-DoDSER-Annual-Report.pdf, 136.

41. Antina Von Schnitzler, 2013, "Traveling Technologies: Infrastructure, Ethical Regimes, and the Materiality of Politics in South Africa," *Cultural Anthropology* 28(4):670–93, 672.

42. Andrew Barry, 2005, "Pharmaceutical Matters: The Invention of Informed Materials," *Theory, Culture & Society* 22(1):51–69, 57.

43. See, for example, Salih Can Açıksöz, 2019, *Sacrificial Limbs: Masculinity, Disability, and Political Violence in Turkey* (Berkeley: University of California Press); Erin Finley, 2011, *Fields of Combat: Understanding PTSD among Veterans of Iraq and Afghanistan* (Ithaca, NY: Cornell University Press); Grégoire Hervouet-Zeiber, 2026, *War and the Pull of Life: Ex-Combatants in Putin's Russia* (New York: Fordham University Press); Susie Kilshaw, 2009, *Impotent Warriors: Gulf War Syndrome, Vulnerability, and Masculinity* (New York: Berghahn Books); Seth Messinger, 2003, "Incorporating the Prosthetic: Traumatic Limb Loss, Rehabilitation and Refigured Military Bodies," *Disability and Rehabilitation* 31(25):2130–4; Wool, *After War*.

44. Moving beyond the combatant focus of military medicine, important ethnographies have detailed broader relationships between medicine and statecraft in contexts of occupation and conflict. Omar Dewachi, 2020, *Ungovernable Life: Mandatory Medicine and Statecraft in Iraq* (Stanford: Stanford University Press); and Saiba Varma, 2020, *The Occupied Clinic: Militarism and Care in Kashmir* (Durham, NC: Duke University Press) have illuminated how militarization and imperial and colonial modes of governance have shaped medicine and its institutions and professionals in Iraq and Kashmir, India, respectively. See also Sugandh Gupta, 2021, "A Shifting Hospital and Shifting Dependencies in Jammu and Kashmir," *Somatosphere*, https://somatosphere.com/2021/shifting-hospital-dependencies-jammu-kashmir.html/.

45. Kieran, *Signature Injuries*, 7.

46. Medical anthropologists have documented how drugs transform culturally constituted selves; they have also illuminated the complex and contradictory effects of psychotropic medication use more specifically. See, for example, Michael D'Arcy, 2019, "'It Tastes Like Order': Psychotic Evidence for Antipsychotic Efficacy and Medicated Subjectivity," *Ethos* 47(1):89–107; Jerry Floersch, 2004, "The Subjective Experience of Youth Psychotropic Treatment," *Social Work in*

Mental Health 1(4):51–69; Jacinthe Flore et al., 2019, "Unraveling Subjectivity, Embodied Experience and (Taking) Psychotropic Medication," *Social Science & Medicine* 230:66–73; Janis Jenkins, ed., 2011, *Pharmaceutical Self: The Global Shaping of Experience in an Age of Psychopharmacology* (Santa Fe, NM: School for Advanced Research Press); Allison Schlosser and Kristi Ninneman, 2012, "The Anthropology of Psychopharmaceuticals: Cultural and Pharmacological Efficacies in Context," *Culture, Medicine, and Psychiatry* 36(1):2–9.

47. See Roger Cooter, 1993, "War and Modern Medicine," in *Companion Encyclopedia of the History of Medicine, Vol. 2*, ed. W. F. Bynum and R. Porter, 1536–73 (London and New York: Routledge) for a critical analysis of how such narratives have been perpetuated in histories of military medicine.

48. Terry, *Attachments to War*, 12.

49. A SCIF, or Sensitive Compartmented Information Facility, is a secure room for the handling and protection of the most sensitive classified information available to military personnel.

50. Kamieński explains that standard Army instruction for the use of speed during the Vietnam War—20 milligrams of dextroamphetamine for 48 hours of combat readiness—was rarely followed and that amphetamines were given out, as one veteran described it, "like candies." Łukasz Kamieński, 2016a, "The Drugs That Built a Super Soldier," *The Atlantic*, April 8.

51. Compare to Bickford's description of his work as a signals intelligence linguist for the US Army at Field Station Berlin before the fall of the Berlin Wall. While he did not have access to psychotropic medications, "caffeine and sugar would keep me going for hours and help alleviate the stress and exhaustion of sitting with headphones on." Bickford, *Chemical Heroes*, 21.

52. Evidence of sharing, possessing, or using someone else's prescription medications can disqualify a soldier from duty and is punishable under Article 112a of the Uniform Code of Military Justice. Random drug testing is a constant presence in the military. The frequency of these tests can vary, but their unpredictability is intended to promote the military's strict no-drug policy, including the use of nonprescribed medications.

53. On medicine and synchronization in war, see Jocelyn Lim Chua, 2020a, "Bloody War: Menstruation, Soldiering, and the 'Gender-Integrated' United States Military," *Critical Military Studies* 8(2):139–58.

54. Cf. Thomas Gregory, 2020, "The Costs of War: Condolence Payments and the Politics of Killing Civilians," *Review of International Studies* 46(1):156–76.

55. On how war's destruction and medicine's harms coalesce, see Varma, *The Occupied Clinic*. See also Emma Varley and Saiba Varma, 2019, "Medicine's Shadowside: Revisiting Clinical Iatrogenesis," *Anthropology & Medicine* 28(2):141–55 on the political and social dimensions of medical iatrogenesis.

56. Michel Foucault, 1977, *Discipline and Punish: The Birth of the Prison* (New York: Pantheon Books).

57. Medicine is, of course, not the only field mobilized for the protection and enhancement of military life. Bickford has richly documented how military, private, and university-based research into US military performance enhancements track across a wide range of scientific fields including biotechnology, genomics, synthetic biology, neurobiology, metabolic enhancements, and microbiome manipulation. Bickford, *Chemical Heroes.*

58. In 2018, Bales's lawyers asked the US Supreme Court to consider that the antimalarial drug mefloquine may have played a role in Bales's behavior. Mandatory mefloquine prophylaxis was broadly directed in the war in Afghanistan beginning in 2002 and during the initial 2003 invasion of Iraq. After contraindications and enhanced warnings regarding the drug's neuropsychiatric effects were added to its label warnings in 2009, the Army dropped mefloquine as its preferred protection against malaria.

59. I build here on Catherine Lutz and Kathleen Millar's argument that war is a "privileged site of morality production." Catherine Lutz and Kathleen Millar, 2012, "War," in *A Companion to Moral* Anthropology, ed. D. Fassin, 482–99 (Hoboken, NJ: John and Wiley Sons), 482. War, they argue, isn't simply governed by ideas of what is acceptable or wrong on the battlefield; war is in fact central to morality production, as it works to define what is right and wrong not only on the battlefield but in society more broadly.

60. Scholars of bioethics and philosophy have debated the legal and ethical implications of the performance-enhancing and therapeutic use of psychotropic medications by US military personnel. See, for example, Jessica Wolfendale, 2008, "Performance-Enhancing Technologies and Moral Responsibility in the Military," *American Journal of Bioethics* 8(2):28–38. See also Sidney Axinn, 1989, *A Moral Military* (Philadelphia, PA: Temple University Press) for a philosophical study of morality and military action. Whereas these approaches generally draw on normative concepts and values in military ethics, my analysis examines these as cultural and political constructs that confer legitimacy or obscure forms of violence and their effects.

61. Atwood Gaines, 2012, "From DSM-I to III-R; Voices of Self, Mastery and the Other: A Cultural Constructivist Reading of US Psychiatric Classification," *Social Science & Medicine* 35(1):3–24, 13.

62. The scholarly literature on gender and the performance of masculinities is robust and beyond the scope of this book. For a foundational piece, see Catherine Lutz, 1996, "Engendered Emotion: Gender, Power, and the Rhetoric of Emotional Control in American Discourse," in *The Emotions: Social, Cultural, and Biological Dimensions*, ed. R. Harre and W. Gerrod Parrot, 151–70 (Thousand Oaks, CA: Sage) on the role of "emotional control" in both popular and scientific constructions of gender and power in American discourse.

63. Harold Braswell and Howard Kushner, 2012, "Suicide, Social Integration, and Masculinity in the US Military," *Social Science & Medicine* 74(4):530–6, 533.

On emotional control and military masculinity, see Eyal Ben-Ari, 1998, *Mastering Soldiers: Conflict, Emotions, and the Enemy in an Israeli Military Unit* (New York: Berghahn Books); Hillary Schaefer et al., 2021, "The Military Hypermasculine Mystique: Sex, Status, and Emotional Control at the United States Military Academy," *Psychology of Men & Masculinities* 22(4):611–26. On the gendered nature of military embodiment, more broadly, see Chua, "Bloody War"; Kevin McSorley, 2013, *War and the Body* (Oxfordshire, UK: Routledge); Oma Sasson-Levy, 2003, "Feminism and Military Gender Practices: Israeli Women Soldiers in 'Masculine' Roles," *Sociological Inquiry* 73(3): 440–65; Wool, *After War.*

64. Stanley McChrystal, 2009, "Tactical Directive" (Kabul, Afghanistan: International Security Assistance Force).

65. See chapter 3 on the construction of occupied Iraq and Afghanistan as chaotic and the role of the "cultural turn" within the US military in deciphering and weaponizing culture.

66. See Talad Asad, 2007, *On Suicide Bombing* (New York: Columbia University Press) on how the idea of horror as a reaction to suicide bombing alongside the condoning of "necessary violence" by democratic governments is fundamental to contemporary iterations of liberal war.

67. A rich literature in sociology, medical anthropology, science and technology studies, and related fields has theorized risk and its governance. Identified as a hallmark of the modern, risk discourses have more recently been connected to neoliberalism, in which risk avoidance is a critical component in the formation of responsible, self-regulating subjects. Scholars in the social sciences have also illuminated dynamics of inequity that unfold through the uneven distribution of risk. The discourse, calculation, and control of risk is foundational to medicine and psychiatry. For foundational texts in this broad literature, see Ulrich Beck, 1992, *Risk Society: Towards a New Modernity* (Thousand Oaks, CA: Sage); Michel Foucault, 1991, "Governmentality," in *The Foucault Effects: Studies in Governmentality,* ed. G. Burchill et al., 87–104 (London: Hargraves); Sarah Lochlann Jain, 2006, *Injury: The Politics of Product Design and Safety Law in the United States* (Princeton: Princeton University Press); Deborah Lupton, 1999, *Risk* (New York: Routledge); Nikolas Rose, 1998, "Governing Risky Individuals: The Role of Psychiatry in New Regimes of Control," *Psychiatry, Psychology and Law* 5(2):177–95.

68. Derek Gregory, 2008b, "The Rush to the Intimate," *Radical Philosophy* 150(1):8–23, 12.

69. See chapter 3 of this book.

70. Cf. Edward W. Said, 1979, *Orientalism* (New York: Vintage Books). See D. Gregory, "The Rush to the Intimate."

71. An important and growing body of anthropological scholarship has illuminated the effects of war on civilian populations, costs that have been largely invisible compared to the experiences of combatants, and particularly, US soldiers.

These costs include the disproportionate loss of life, public health consequences, and harm to social, infrastructural, and ecological worlds that persist long after conflict's official end. See Hayder Al-Mohammad, 2012, "A Kidnapping in Basra: The Struggles and Precariousness of Life in Postinvasion Iraq," *Cultural Anthropology* 27(4):597–614; Dewachi, *Ungovernable Life;* Omar Dewachi et al., 2014, "Changing Therapeutic Geographies of the Iraqi and Syrian Wars," *The Lancet* 383(9915):449–57; Eleana Kim, 2016, "Toward an Anthropology of Landmines: Rogue Infrastructure and Military Waste in the Korean DMZ," *Cultural Anthropology* 31(2):162–87; Catherine Lutz and Andrea Mazzarino, eds., 2019, *War and Health: The Medical Consequences of the Wars in Iraq and Afghanistan* (New York: New York University Press); Kali Rubaii, 2019, "Tripartheid: How Sectarianism Became Internal to Being in Anbar, Iraq," *PoLAR* 42(1):125–41; Kali Rubaii, 2023, "De-Centering Death: The War on Terror and the Less-Than-Lethal Paradigm," *American Anthropologist* 126(3):497–508. See also Munira Khayyat, 2022, *A Landscape of War: Ecologies of Resistance and Survival in South Lebanon* (Berkeley: University of California Press) on life and creative resistance amidst perennial conflict.

72. Begoña Aretxaga, 2003, "Maddening States," *Annual Review of Anthropology* 32(1):393–410, 402. On the discursive and material force of fantasy in counterterrorism, see Ben Anderson, 2011a, "Facing the Future: US Counterinsurgency Doctrine and the Pre-insurgent," *Theory, Culture & Society* 28(7-8):216–40; Joseba Zulaika, 2014, "Drones and Fantasy in US Counterterrorism," *Journal for Cultural Research* 18(2):171–87; Joseba Zulaika and William Douglas, 2016, *Terror and Taboo: The Follies, Fables, and Faces of Terrorism* (Oxfordshire, UK: Routledge).

73. The "psy" sciences have played a key role in statecraft and international governance in the war on terror. See Alison Howell, 2011, *Madness in International Relations: Psychology, Security, and the Global Governance of Mental Health* (New York: Routledge) on the role of the psy sciences within the international realm in the work of stabilization and global security; and Neil Krishnan Aggarwal, 2015, *Mental Health in the War on Terror: Culture, Science, and Statecraft* (New York: Columbia University Press) on the weaponization of psychiatry in the war on terror. Vanessa Pupavac, 2001, "Therapeutic Governance: Psycho-Social Intervention and Trauma Risk Management," *Disasters* 25(4):358–72 provides a broader analysis of the problematization of psychological dysfunctionalism in contemporary international policy and social-risk management.

74. The figure of the "crazy vet" as both vulnerable and threatening has featured in American film and literature and reveals wider anxieties and conflicts in societal values regarding intimacy with war violence. See Kenneth MacLeish, 2009, "Wounds of War and the Dilemmas of Stereotypes," *Savage Minds,* September 27, https://savageminds.org/2009/09/27/wounds-of-war-and-the-dilemmas-of-stereotype/.

75. Given the limitations of analyses that privilege the US war-making subject as the primary site for registering the consequences of war, anthropologists have written from the lived landscapes and settings in which war is waged, centering precarity, loss, and resilience in the midst of war and serial conflict while denaturalizing the values and paradigms that can structure both military and scholarly paradigms of war and violence. See, for example, Anila Daulatzai and Sahar Ghumkhor, 2023, "Afghanistan, Racial Melancholia, and Loss That Exceeds Loss," *Critical Times* 6(2):202–11; Munira Khayyat, 2023, "War, from the South," *Public Culture* 35(1):113–34; Rubaii, "Decentering Death."

76. Melody Petersen, 2009, "US Military: Heavily Armed and Medicated," *NBCNews*, May 19.

77. British Forces Broadcasting Services, 2024, "British Army Dishing Out Too Many Antidepressants to Treat PTSD, Says Former Soldier," *Forces News*, March 31.

78. Primary care providers have been leveraged as "mental health force multipliers" in the war on terror. Christopher Warner et al., 2007, "The Evolving Role of the Division Psychiatrist," *Military Medicine* 172(9):918–24, 922.

79. Medications were prescribed to 41% of treatment-seeking individuals, and antidepressants were prescribed to 74% of all diagnosed patients with a medication treatment plan. Kimberly Schmitz et al., 2012, "Psychiatric Diagnoses and Treatment of US Military Personnel While Deployed to Iraq," *Military Medicine* 177(4):380–9.

80. Larry Applewhite, Nathan Keller, and Adam Borah, 2012, "Mental Health Care Used by Soldiers During Counterinsurgency Operations," *Military Medicine* 177(5):501–6, 504.

81. National Center for PTSD, 2004, *Iraq War Clinician Guide*, 2nd ed. (White River Junction, VT: National Center for PTSD), 10.

82. Friedman, "Wars on Drugs."

83. Defense Health Board, 2011b, "Defense Health Board Recommendation Memorandum Pertaining to Psychotropic Medication Prescription Practices and Use and Complementary and Alternative Medicine Use 2011-09," September 23, Falls Church, VA, 10.

84. Andrew Tilghman and Brendan McGarry, 2010, "Medicating the Military," *Military Times*, March 17.

85. Keith Brown and Catherine Lutz, 2007, "Grunt Lit: The Participant-Observers of Empire," *American Ethnologist* 34(2):322–8; see also Jocelyn Lim Chua and Lacy Jo Evans, 2018, "Collaborative Research Between Student Veterans and Faculty in Higher Education," *Journal of Veteran Studies* 3(1):122–38, 123.

86. Jocelyn Lim Chua, 2020b, "Medication by Proxy: The Devolution of Psychiatric Power and Shared Accountability to Pharmaceutical Use among Soldiers in America's Post-9/11 Wars," *Culture, Medicine & Psychiatry* 44:565–85.

87. On the production and performance of ignorance claims by military bureaucracy, see Catherine Lutz, 2019, "Bureaucratic Weaponry and the

Production of Ignorance in Military Operations on Guam," *Current Anthropology* 60(S19):S108–21.

88. This aligns with Matt Kenard's observation that "it is in the interest of recruiters to interpret recruiting standards loosely, as a failure to meet their targets means they have to attend a punitive counseling session, and persistent failure hurts their chances for promotion." Matt Kenard, 2012, *Irregular Army: How the US Military Recruited Neo-Nazis, Gang Members, and Criminals to Fight the War on Terror* (London: Verso), 24. These pressures were arguably heightened given the severe recruitment challenges faced by the US military during the war on terror, discussed in chapter 2.

89. Per DoD data from 2023, individuals who self-report as American Indian or Alaska Native, Asian, and Native Hawaiian or other Pacific Islander collectively make up less than 6% of active-duty members of the US military. Asians constitute 3.6%. Military personnel who self-report as White make up the highest percentage of active-duty members, at 68%, while those who self-report as Black or African American represent 17.6%. United States Department of Defense, 2023, "Profile of the Military Community," https://download.militaryonesource.mil/12038/MOS/Reports/2023-demographics-report.pdf.

90. The Human Terrain System, or HTS, was a US Army program launched in 2007 that embedded anthropologists and other social scientists in military teams in Iraq and Afghanistan. The program was highly controversial and generated vociferous debate on the ethics of working with US military, intelligence, and security organizations. On October 31, 2007, the Executive Board of the American Anthropological Association (AAA), the scholarly and professional organization for anthropologists, issued a statement outlining the ways the HTS project violates the AAA Code of Ethics. American Anthropological Association, 2007, "American Anthropological Association Executive Board Statement on the Human Terrain System Project," https://americananthro.org/about/committees-and-task-forces/human-terrain-system-hts-project/. On these debates, see Maximillian Forte, 2011, "The Human Terrain System and Anthropology: A Review of Ongoing Debates," *American Anthropologist* 113(1):149–53; Roberto J. González, 2009, *American Counterinsurgency: Human Science and the Human Terrain* (Chicago: Prickly Paradigm Press); Montgomery McFate, 2005, "Anthropology and Counterinsurgency: The Strange Story of Their Curious Relationship," *Military Review* 85(2):24–37.

91. The entanglement of the social sciences and American power has a long history. See David Price, 2016, *Cold War Anthropology: The CIA, the Pentagon, and the Growth of Dual Use Anthropology* (Durham, NC: Duke University Press) on the strategic use of anthropological research by the Pentagon and CIA during the Cold War.

92. Clara Han, 2020, *Seeing Like a Child: Inheriting the Korean War* (New York: Fordham). Han offers a moving narrative of how familial memories of violence diffuse through everyday domestic life.

93. Collaboration with and the mentoring and training of military-affiliated and student veterans in qualitative research were key components of this project. See Chua and Evans, "Collaborative Research Between Student Veterans and Faculty in Higher Education."

94. The prevalence of reported polypharmacy in 2016 was the highest among the Army (14.5%) and lowest for the Marine Corps (7.4%). Richard Eide and Shauna Stahlman, 2018, "Polypharmacy Involving Opioid, Psychotropic, and Central Nervous System Depressant Medications, Period Prevalence and Association with Suicidal Ideation, Active Component, US Armed Forces, 2016," *Medical Surveillance Monthly Report* 25(6):2–9, 2. In a 2010 report, the Army noted the increased use of prescription antidepressants, antianxiety drugs, and pain medications in its ranks, reporting that 14% of the force was taking an opiate medication, with 95% of these individuals taking oxycodone, often in addition to prescriptions for depression and anxiety. United States Department of the Army, 2010, "Army Health Promotion, Risk Reduction, Suicide Prevention Report 2010" (Washington, DC: United States Department of the Army), 83.

95. Dave Baiocchi, 2013, "Measuring Army Deployments to Iraq and Afghanistan," RAND Corporation.

96. The remaining 14% had begun as enlisted and been promoted to officer.

97. For more aggregate data from the research, see "Enduring War: Psychopharmaceticals and Soldiering in America's Post-9/11 Wars," UNC Dataverse, https://dataverse.unc.edu/dataverse/chua.

CHAPTER 1. BUILDUP

1. Not all aspects of the care infrastructure could follow the movement of pills. Psychopharmaceuticals could reach far-forward settings like this one, but those environments often rendered documentation of treatment encounters rare or irretrievable. The variability of medical documentation practices and limitations to comprehensive medical review could raise clinical challenges, including those related to polypharmacy, such as potential medication contraindication, drug interactions, and overlapping prescriptions.

2. The Korengal Valley and the fighting that took place there were popularized for US audiences by the work of British photographer Tim Hetherington and American journalist and author Sebastian Junger. Junger's 2010 book *War* and his films *Restrepo* and *Korengal* document his experiences embedded with the soldiers manning the Restrepo outpost. Sebastian Junger, 2010, *War* (New York: Twelve Books).

3. See David Vine, 2015, *Base Nation: How US Military Bases Abroad Harm America and the World* (New York: Metropolitan Books) on America's sprawling network of overseas bases and the US national security policy of far-flung

forward presence in the decades after World War II. Vine notes that at the height of the US occupations of Iraq and Afghanistan, "the total number of bases, combat outposts, and checkpoints in these two countries alone topped one thousand" (3). Bickford, *Chemical Heroes,* also refers to the "military-pharmacology complex" that will continue to grow "as the military increases its focus on preparing to dominate the pharmacological battlefield" (15).

4. Military mental and behavioral health care providers were often embedded with or attached to combat units and combat operational stress control (COSC) teams. Given the low density of mental health assets, providers relied heavily on "battlefield circulation," traveling regularly on short, multiday trips to various bases and outposts to provide immediate, forward care, building relationships with unit commanders and observing mental health trends in the process. They were typically responsible for wide geographic areas of treatment coverage. Tim Hoyt, 2025, "Preparing Mental Health Support for Multi-Domain, Large-Scale Combat Operations: Current Progress and Future Directions," *Military Medicine* 190(2):50–6, 51–2. On the mobility of military mental health providers in the provision of care, see Jocelyn Lim Chua, 2022, "Escaping the Clinic: Exposure as Care among Military Medical Professionals at War," *Medicine Anthropology Theory* 9(2):1–25.

5. See chapter 4 on medication supply.

6. Norman Camp, 2011, "US Army Psychiatry Legacies of the Vietnam War," in *Combat and Operational Behavioral Health*, ed. E. Ritchie, 9–42 (Falls Church, VA: Office of the Surgeon General of the United States Army), 11–12.

7. In a survey conducted in 1967, Army physicians used prochlorperazine to treat gastroenteritis in 45% of cases where psychopharmaceuticals were used. William Datel and Arnold Johnson, 1978, *Psychotropic Prescription Medication in Vietnam* (Washington, DC: Walter Reed Army Institute of Research).

8. Camp, "US Army Psychiatry Legacies of the Vietnam War," 28.

9. Datel and Johnson, *Psychotropic Prescription Medication in Vietnam*, 9. Insufficient data exists to assess the impact of the use of these medications on the psychiatric casualty rate during the Vietnam War. See also Peter Bourne, 1970, "Military Psychiatry and the Viet Nam Experience," *American Journal of Psychiatry* 127(4):481–8 which notes that "while these drugs have been effectively used in Viet Nam with certain groups, their overall impact has been relatively slight. Rest, emotional support, the opportunity to ventilate, and time to reintegrate adaptive capacities that are temporarily overwhelmed have proven infinitely more effective than any specific pharmacological agent in enabling the average patient to return to duty" (487).

10. See Michael Perlman, 1975, "Basic Problems of Military Psychiatry: Delayed Reaction in Vietnam Veterans," *International Journal of Offender Therapy and Comparative Criminology* 19(2):129–38; Raymond Scurfield, 1993, "Posttraumatic Stress Disorder in Vietnam Veterans," in *International Handbook*

of Traumatic Stress Syndromes, ed. J. P. Wilson and B. Raphael, 285–96 (New York: Plenum Publication).

11. United States Department of the Army, 1998, *Combat Stress Control in a Theater of Operations Field Manual 8–51* (Washington, DC: United States Department of the Army).

12. United States Department of the Army, *Combat Stress Control in a Theater of Operations Field Manual 8–51*, 8–6.

13. United States Department of the Army, *Combat Stress Control in a Theater of Operations Field Manual 8–51*, 8–5.

14. Frederick Hanson, 1949, *Combat Psychiatry: Experiences in the North African and Mediterranean Theaters of Operation, American Ground Forces, World War II, Vol. 9* (Washington, DC: United States Government Printing Office), 3.

15. Even during the Vietnam War, when psychopharmaceuticals were used liberally, military providers remained concerned for the "fixation of a sickness role suggested by taking medication." Brett Schneider et al., 2011, "Psychiatric Medications in Military Operations," in *Textbook of Combat and Operational Psychiatry*, ed. E. Ritchie, 151–62 (Washington, DC: Office of the Surgeon General of the United States Army), 152.

16. For example, sections 9-8 and 11-1 outline doctrinal changes in the use of medication in treating service members diagnosed with mental disorders while deployed: "Ongoing treatment and/or therapeutic modalities are essential to improving a Soldier's chance to RTD (return to duty) whether in theater or after evacuation. . . . These modalities include medication, individual psychotherapy, group psychotherapy, and appropriate therapeutic occupations." United States Department of the Army, 2006a, *Combat and Operational Stress Control: Field Manual 4-02.51* (Washington, DC: United States Department of the Army), 9.

17. See chapter 3 for a full discussion of how clinical and behavioral stability on a psychopharmaceutical is evaluated before and during deployment.

18. The 2003 MHAT-I study, which was the first comprehensive assessment of the military behavioral health care system in Iraq, found that the rate of return went from 11% in Kuwait down to just 3.6% in Landstuhl, Germany, while forward-deployed behavioral health units reported returning to duty 97% of soldiers seen. United States Army Surgeon General, 2003, *Operation Iraqi Freedom* (OIF) *Mental Health Advisory Team (MHAT) Report (MHAT-I)* (Washington, DC: Army Medical Command), 14.

19. The command team in a US Army company typically consists of officer leadership—namely, the unit commander and executive officer—and senior enlisted leadership. Military clinicians commonly work with the command team to address individual soldier's mental health needs. See chapters 4 and 5 for more on how this relationship works in the management of psychopharmaceutical use and in suicide risk management, respectively.

20. Schneider et al., "Psychiatric Medications in Military Operations," 154.

21. The Division Mental Health (DMH) unit consisted of a psychiatrist, a psychologist, and a social worker and three to five enlisted mental health specialists. Around 2005, the Army would transition the DMH structure to a more modular, decentralized model of Brigade Combat Teams (BCTs). BCTs were designed to be mobile, with multiple BCTs under the control of the division, yielding more providers and allowing for the "projection of resources" to commanders at lower levels, including at the battalion and company levels. Christopher H. Warner et al., 2007, "Division Mental Health in the New Brigade Combat Team Structure: Part I Predeployment and Deployment," *Military Medicine* 172(9):907–11.

22. "Drift" has been used in political circles and in the media to describe the gradual, haphazard, and aimless manner by which the US military and American political strategy have pursued a state of continual war. For example, political commentator Rachel Maddow's 2013 book, *Drift: The Unmooring of American Military Power,* suggests that the power to declare America's wars has been incrementally usurped by the executive branch. Rachel Maddow, 2013, *Drift: The Unmooring of American Military Power* (New York: Crown). A White House statement in the aftermath of the US withdrawal from Afghanistan stated, "At the outset, America's goal was never to nation-build. But, over time, this is what America drifted into doing." White House, 2023, "US Withdrawal from Afghanistan," April 6, https://bidenwhitehouse.archives.gov/wp-content/uploads/2023/04/US-Withdrawal-from-Afghanistan.pdf.

23. Military accession rules—the policies, procedures, and standards established by the DoD that determine eligibility of applicants to enter, or "access," the military—are intended to ensure the physical, medical, and moral fitness of recruits and officers. See United States Department of Defense, 2018, "DoDI 6130.03, Vol. 1: Medical Standards for Military Service: Appointment, Enlistment or Deduction," Washington, DC: Department of Defense, especially 45–7.

24. Civilian providers don't automatically report to the Army, and it is possible to seek care without the Army knowing, especially if the soldier pays out of pocket or doesn't use military insurance, like TRICARE.

25. Robert Burns, 2004, "Pentagon: 40,000 US Troops Being Sent to Iraq for a Year," *Associated Press,* May 3.

26. Lawrence Korb and Sean Duggan, 2007, "Caught Off Guard: The Link Between Our National Security and Our National Guard," Center for American Progress, https://www.americanprogress.org/article/changing-to-meet-new-challenges/.

27. Schneider et al., "Psychiatric Medications in Military Operations," 154.

28. Schneider et al., "Psychiatric Medications for Deployment," 682. This finding is confirmed by the 2003 MHAT-I study, which found that deployed psychiatrists reported inadequate psychotropic medication stocks "to minimize

avoidable evacuations of Soldiers requiring acute/maintenance pharmaceuticals." United States Army Surgeon General, MHAT-I, 35.

29. Murty Savitala and George Dydek, 2004, "US Army Reserve (Medical) Soldier Prescription Challenges during Operation Iraqi Freedom," *Military Medicine* 169(12):937–41, 937. Reports also suggest that DoD-deployed private contractors—typically older than deployed soldiers and subject to less uniform and stringent deployment requirements—also contributed to complex supply needs by pharmacy services in theater. Dave Whaley et al., 2018, "Considerations for Retrograding Deployed Army Pharmacy Operations: What about Department of Defense Civilian Contractors? Lessons from Kosovo," *Military Medicine* 183(1-2):e19–23.

30. Jocelyn Lim Chua, 2020c, "Pharmaceutical Creep: US Military Power and the Global and Transnational Mobility of Psychopharmaceuticals," *Medical Anthropology Quarterly* 34(1):41–58.

31. This would not be the first time that the use of chemical substances by soldiers at war would emerge as a concern of "contamination." See Jeremy Kuzmarov, 2009, *The Myth of the Addicted Army: Vietnam and the Modern War on Drugs* (Amherst, MA: University of Massachusetts Press) on how the image of the "drug-addicted GI" associated with the Vietnam War was promoted by the antiwar movement.

32. Edna Lomsky-Feder et al., 2008, "Reserve Soldiers as Transmigrants: Moving Between the Civilian and Military Worlds," *Armed Forces & Society* 34(4):593–614, 594.

33. See chapter 2 on the US Army's recruitment challenges during the war on terror.

34. The overreliance on undertrained and unprepared National Guard and Reserve soldiers filling the Army's ranks would also fuel critique from opponents of the Iraq War. While in the early 2000s the Army National Guard formally positioned itself for domestic disaster response, by 2004, National Guard soldiers sent to Iraq were one-third more likely to be killed in Iraq than their active-duty counterparts, due in part to the fact that Guard and Reserve troops were frequently assigned to high-risk missions. Dave Moniz, 2004, "Rate of Guard Deaths is Higher," *The Spokesman-Review*, December 13.

35. Kieran, *Signature Wounds*, 33.

36. US Army Surgeon General, MHAT-I, 16.

37. Camp, "US Army Psychiatry Legacies of the Vietnam War," 7.

38. Schneider et al., 2011, "Psychiatric Medications in Military Operations," 153.

39. Ritchie published these proposals after preparing to deploy with a unit providing frontline mental health intervention in Somalia in 1993, only to find minimal guidance on what medications to bring. The proposals recommended emergency medications including the benzodiazepines lorazepam and diazepam and the neuroleptic haloperidol. For maintenance medications, Ritchie advised

antidepressants, anxiolytics, and sedatives, including just one tricycle antidepressant and one SSRI, reflecting clinical practice at the time which suggested that patients could be easily switched from one antidepressant to another without problem. Elspeth Cameron Ritchie, 1994, "Psychiatric Medications for Deployment," *Military Medicine* 159:647–8.

40. Simon H. Pincus and David M. Benedek, 1998, "Operational Stress Control in the Former Yugoslavia: A Joint Endeavor," *Military Medicine* 163(6):358–62, 361.

41. United States Department of Defense, 2006, *Policy Guidance for Deployment-Limiting Psychiatric Conditions and Medications* (Washington, DC: Assistant Secretary of Defense).

42. The lack of empirical data on medication usage in theater during the war on terror itself presented a challenge to the development of evidence-based recommendations, since most data guiding recommendations comes from nonmilitary populations, a challenge that would persist during the wars. The 2006 policy would be continuously updated over the period of the wars, with over a dozen iterations.

43. United States Department of Defense, *Policy Guidance for Deployment-Limiting Psychiatric Conditions and Medications*, 4. Some of these exclusions involve medications that require infrastructural support that cannot be guaranteed in deployment, such as medications like lithium requiring special storage considerations or laboratory monitoring.

44. Kieran, *Signature Wounds*, 75.

45. Vincent F. Capaldi and Hanna Zembrzuska, 2015, "Thrust into the Breach: Psychiatry in a Combat Zone within 1 Year of Residency Completion," *Academic Psychiatry* 39:410–5, 413.

46. The DoD's research investment in epidemiological studies of the health of the military was first established in 2000 with the Millenium Cohort Study, which was originally designed to address health concerns of veterans of the 1990–1991 Gulf War. The largest prospective collection of health data in US military history, this longitudinal cohort study was originally scheduled to run 21 years but was modified to include additional waves of service members every three years during the war on terror to study health outcomes across the life course. It is now scheduled to continue for the lifetime of most participants (until 2068) and has over 260,000 enrolled participants. See Sheila Castañeda et al., 2023, "Cohort Profile Update: The US Millennium Cohort Study—Evaluating the Impact of Military Experiences on Service Members and Veteran Health," *International Journal of Epidemiology* 52(4):e222–31.

47. Emily Yates-Doerr, 2015, *The Weight of Obesity: Hunger and Global Health in Postwar Guatemala* (Berkeley: University of California Press).

48. Marc A. Cooper et al., 2011, "Provision of Mental Health Services in Operation Iraqi Freedom 05-07," in *Textbook of Combat and Operational Psychiatry*,

ed. E. Ritchie, 137-49 (Washington, DC: Office of the Surgeon General of the United States Army), 139.

49. Kieran, *Signature Wounds*, 55–7. For example, while the public and media saw PTSD as a permanent, debilitating disease, Walter Reed researchers and VA officials understood post-traumatic stress as one of several potential reactions to combat and one that could vary in severity, progression, and duration.

50. Leonard Wong, 2006, *CU @ the FOB: How the Forward Operating Base is Changing the Life of Combat Soldiers* (Carlisle Barracks, PA: Strategic Studies Institute), 2. While initiated and developed in the context of military operations in Iraq and Afghanistan, the FOB concept has also been adopted domestically to maintain National Guard troops in support of US Border Patrol along the US-Mexico border. Donna Miles, 2006, "Concept Perfected in Iraq, Afghanistan Used along US Border," American Forces Press Service, December 4.

51. FOBs and COPs were envisioned as key to the US military "surge" strategy when an additional 30,000 troops were sent to Iraq in 2007 to quell insurgent activity. Military proponents argued they helped to establish a more permanent presence of force by enabling patrols, while facilitating relationships with Iraqi locals. FOBs were strategically scattered throughout the most populated areas of the country, and near major crossing routes. See Eugene J. Palka, 2016, "Operation Iraqi Freedom (OIF) and the Use of Forwarding Operating Bases (FOBs)," in *Military Geosciences and Desert Warfare: Past Lessons and Modern Challenges*, ed. E. McDonald and T. Bullard, 205–19 (New York: Springer).

52. Palka, "Operation Iraqi Freedom (OIF) and the Use of Forwarding Operating Bases (FOBs)," 206.

53. Telehealth has been part of the US military health system in deployment settings since the early 1990s. In the wars in Iraq and Afghanistan, its uses included teleconsultations for infectious diseases and behavioral health and telepsychiatry. See Cathaleen Madsen et al., 2023, "Telehealth in the Military System: Impact, Obstacles, and Opportunities," *Military Medicine* 188(1):15–23 for an overview of the history of telehealth in the military health system.

54. Edward Brusher, 2011, "Combat and Operational Stress Control," in *Combat and Operational Behavioral Health*, ed. E. Ritchie, 59–74 (Falls Church, VA: Office of the Surgeon General of the United States Army), 60.

55. Cooper et al., "Provision of Mental Health Services in Operation Iraqi Freedom 05-07, 139.

56. Cooper et al., "Provision of Mental Health Services in Operation Iraqi Freedom 05-07," 138.

57. Cooper et al., "Provision of Mental Health Services in Operation Iraqi Freedom 05-07," 139.

58. United States Department of the Army, *Combat and Operational Stress Control: Field Manual 4-02.51*, 8-6.

59. Maria Morgan et al., 2023, "Adjustment Disorder in US Service Members: Factors Associated with Early Separation," *Military Medicine* 188(7-8):e1501–07.

In the Army, adjustment disorder was diagnosed in 27.6% of soldiers evacuated from Iraq and Afghanistan for psychiatric reasons. James Rundell, 2006, "Demographics of and Diagnoses in Operation Enduring Freedom and Operation Iraqi Freedom Personnel Who Were Psychiatrically Evacuated from the Theater of Operations," *General Hospital Psychiatry* 28(4):352–6. It was diagnosed in 30.8% of psychiatric hospitalizations among soldiers deployed to Iraq and Afghanistan. Barbara E. Wojcik et al., 2009, "Hospital Admissions Related to Mental Disorders in US Army Soldiers in Iraq and Afghanistan," *Military Medicine* 174(10):1010–18. Adjustment disorder rates are generally greater in military populations compared to general civilian populations. See Amber McKenzie et al., 2023, "Adjustment Disorder in the Armed Forces: A Systematic Review," *Journal of Mental Health* 32(5):962–84; Charles H. Van Wijk, 2024, "Prevalence Estimate for Adjustment Disorders in the South African Navy," *Clinical Practice and Epidemiology in Mental Health* (20):e17450179301661. It is more than twice as likely to be diagnosed in women than men in the active-duty population. Jouhayna Bajjani-Gebara et al., 2021, "Adjustment Disorders in US Active Duty Military Women: A Scoping Review for the Years 2000 to 2018," *Women's Health Issues* 31:S33–42. While acute stress reaction is known to be very relevant to military populations, far fewer studies have documented or estimated the prevalence of acute stress reaction in the military, compared to adjustment disorder. One study puts the percentage of self-reported combat-related acute-stress reactions among soldiers at 17.2%. Amy Adler and Ian Guttierez, 2022, "Acute Stress Reaction in Combat: Emerging Evidence and Peer-Based Interventions," *Current Psychiatry Reports* 24:277–84, 280.

60. Acute stress disorder is recognized as a diagnosis within the International Classification of Diseases, or ICD.

61. Liana Matson et al., 2022, "Management of Acute Stress Reactions in the Military: A Stepped Care Approach," *Current Psychiatry Reports* 24:799–808, 800. Medication may be used as part of a strategy to prevent chronic trauma responses, though evidence on this point is mixed.

62. The *Diagnostic and Statistical Manual* (DSM) *V* defines adjustment disorder as a time-limited disorder characterized by excessive emotional or behavioral symptoms in response to a traumatic event or other identifiable life stressor, which interfere with social and occupational functioning. American Psychiatric Association, 2013, *Diagnostic and Statistical Manual of Mental Disorders*, 5th ed. (Washington, DC: American Psychiatric Publishing).

63. On the clinical difficulties of distinguishing acute adaptive responses from psychopathology in military treatment in the war in Iraq, see National Center for PTSD, *Iraq War Clinician Guide*, 11–13.

64. National Center for PTSD, *Iraq War Clinician Guide*, 17.

65. Concepts of psychiatric casualty and combat reactions in military psychiatry have a long and complex history that lies outside the scope of my analysis. For concise historical and contemporary perspectives on concepts of post-combat

reactions and disorders, see Edgar Jones, 2006, "Historical Approaches to Post-Combat Disorders," *Philosophical Transactions of the Royal Society B* 361:533–42; Bret Moore and Gregory Reger, 2007, "Historical and Contemporary Perspectives of Combat Stress and the Army Combat Stress Control Team," in *Combat Stress Injury: Theory, Research, and Management*, ed. C. Figley and W. Nash, 161–81 (New York: Routledge/Taylor & Francis Group); Thomas Mareth and Alan Brooker, 1985, "Combat Stress Reaction: A Concept in Evolution," *Military Medicine* 150(4):186–90. For cultural analyses of how systems of meaning have shaped the repertoire and expression of symptoms of war-related disorders and psychiatric breakdown in combat, see Edgar Jones and Simon Wessely, 2005, *Shell Shock to PTSD: Military Psychiatry from 1900 to the Gulf War* (East Sussex, UK: Psychology Press); Young, *The Harmony of Illusions*; Kilshaw, *Impotent Warriors*; Simon Wessely, 2006, "Twentieth-Century Theories on Combat Motivation and Breakdown," *Journal of Contemporary History* 41(2):268–86. See Hans Pols and Stephanie Oak, 2006, "War and Military Mental Health: The US Psychiatric Response in the 20th Century," *American Journal of Public Health* 97(12):2132–42 for a brief but useful historical overview of US military psychiatry.

66. W. H. R. Rivers, 1919, "Psychiatry and War," *Science* 49(1268):367–9.

67. Mareth and Brooker, "Combat Stress Reaction," 187.

68. Mareth and Brooker, "Combat Stress Reaction," 186.

69. Even before the expansion to COSR, the Army recognized that many soldiers seen for mental health care present with problems that it categorized as occupational and personal in nature. In a 1993 study at an Army mental health community center, the V-codes "Phase of Life" Disorders and "Occupational Problem" constituted 51% of diagnoses, with "very few" medication prescriptions written for the entire clinical population. V-codes denote situations that are not psychiatric disorders themselves but may be of clinical significance. James E. McCarroll et al., 1993, "Clients, Problems, and Diagnoses in a Military Community Mental Health Clinic," *Military Medicine* 158(11):701–5, 702–3.

70. Moore and Reger, "Historical and Contemporary Perspectives of Combat Stress and the Army Combat Stress Control Team," 166.

71. Javier seemed to imply that this was not the case for all providers, and indeed I found that in interviews, some PAs expressed less concern with starting soldiers on new medications in deployment, perceiving medications like SSRIs as relatively "harmless" compared to other categories of psychopharmaceuticals.

72. See chapter 5 on how military providers stratify risk in clinical care and manage potential medication side effects in relation to these considerations.

CHAPTER 2. CHRONIC

1 Kenneth MacLeish, 2020, "Churn: Mobilization-Demobilization and the Fungibility of American Military Life," *Security Dialogue* 51(2-3):194–210.

2. The Clinton administration cut national defense by more than half a million personnel and $50 billion in inflation-adjusted dollars during this period. Jack Spencer, 2000, "The Facts about Military Readiness," The Heritage Foundation, September 15.

3. David McCormick, 1998, *The Downsized Warrior: American's Army in Transition* (New York: New York University Press), 105.

4. By 2007, the number of US-paid private contractors in Iraq exceeded that of American combat troops. More than 180,000 civilians, including American, Iraqi, and foreign contractors, were working in Iraq under US contracts, compared to the 160,000 soldiers stationed in Iraq. T. Christian Miller, 2007, "Contractors Outnumber Troops in Iraq," *Los Angeles Times,* July 4. The US government subcontracted out myriad operational tasks to private military companies like DynCorp and Blackwater, who received billions of dollars in government largesse to carry out the occupation of Iraq. On the privatization of the US military industry, see Jeremy Scahill, 2007, *Blackwater: The Rise of the World's Most Powerful Mercenary Army* (New York: Nation Books); P. W. Singer, 2003, *Corporate Warriors: The Rise of the Privatized Military Industry* (Ithaca, NY: Cornell University Press).

5. Congressional Research Service, 1998, "Military Readiness, Operations Tempo (OPTEMPO) and Personnel Tempo (PERSTEMPO): Are US Forces Doing Too Much?" January 14, 3.

6. Military recruitment concerns could be said to date back to the conception of the all-volunteer force in 1973, when critics cautioned that a military composed entirely of volunteers would not provide sufficient troops for a lengthy ground war. The proliferation of overseas missions has also coincided with rising college attendance and an expanding job market, which have undercut recruitment. The challenges continue: immediately after the apparent end of the war on terror with the final 2021 withdrawal from Afghanistan, the DoD fell far short of its recruiting goals, with the lowest recruiting numbers since 1999. Ethan Brown, 2023 "The Ghost of GWOT Haunting the Military Recruiting Crisis," The Modern War Institute at West Point, https://mwi.westpoint.edu/the-ghost-of-gwot-haunting-the-military-recruiting-crisis/. After historic lows in 2022 and 2023, all major branches of the military met or exceeded recruitment targets in 2025.

7. This is but one illustration of MacLeish's argument that the worthiness of soldiers can shift in accordance with "military prerogatives of mobilization and demobilization—that is, the ability to put people and resources in motion for war-making purposes and then to release or abandon them as needed." MacLeish, "Churn," 195.

8. Nearly a quarter of new military recruits needed some type of waiver in 2006, up from 20% in 2003. Roughly 30,000 moral waivers were approved annually between 2003 and 2006. Associated Press, 2007, "Military Granting More Criminal Waivers," February 14. The military divides moral waivers into six categories: felonies, serious and minor nontraffic offenses, serious and minor traffic

offenses, and drug offenses. Data released in 2008 showed that the Army gave out 511 moral waivers to soldiers with felony convictions in 2007. Recruits accepted into the Army and Marines that year included 87 convicted of assault or maiming, 130 convicted of nonmarijuana drug offenses, seven convicted of making terrorist threats, and two convicted of indecent behavior with a child. Elana Schor, 2008, "US Army Increases Use of Moral Waivers to Meet Demand for Troops," *The Guardian,* April 21.

9. Eric Schmitt, 2004, "US Army Lowers Recruit Standards." *Deseret News,* October 1.

10. Stop loss was initially used in the 1990–91 Gulf War and later in Bosnia and the Kosovo Air campaign. Because of the involuntary nature of this extension, in a campaign speech in 2004, then–presidential candidate John Kerry described stop loss as a "backdoor draft." John F. Kerry, 2004. "Address Accepting the Presidential Nomination at the Democratic National Convention in Boston," https://www.presidency.ucsb.edu/documents/address-accepting-the-presidential-nomination-the-democratic-national-convention-boston.

11. United States Department of the Army, *Army Health Promotion, Risk Reduction, Suicide Prevention Report,* 1.

12. United States Department of the Army, *Army Health Promotion, Risk Reduction, Suicide Prevention Report,* 1.

13. Defense Manpower Data Center, "Profile of Service Members Ever Deployed," cited in Board on the Health of Select Populations, 2010, *Returning Home from Iraq and Afghanistan: Preliminary Assessment of Readjustment Needs of Veterans, Service Members, and Their Families* (Washington, DC: National Academies Press), 25.

14. Kieran, *Signature Wounds,* 142.

15. The stated policy during the wars was one year deployed and one year at home for active-duty soldiers, one year deployed and five years at home for National Guard, and one year deployed and four years at home for Reserve. The Army was not the only branch deploying with shortening deployment-to-dwell ratios. At one point, the Marine Corps was deploying units to Iraq for approximately seven months, with a seven-month dwell time between deployments. Congressional Record, 2007, "Text of Amendments," Congressional Record Vol. 153, No. 139, September 19.

16. Accounts shared with me by Special Forces soldiers and veterans, as well as personal accounts reported on Reddit, generally reflect much higher operational tempo than conventional forces, especially in the early-to-mid years of the war on terror, with some reporting as many as ten months deployed per year with just two months at home, an extreme deployment-to-dwell ratio of roughly 1:0.2.

17. Congressional Record, 2009, "The Current Status of US Ground Forces," Senate Hearing 111–66, April 22.

18. Concerns over the consequences of admitting mental health problems and seeking treatment are especially prevalent among military aviation personnel. Blake Lollis et al., 2009, "Major Depressive Disorder in Military Aviators: A Retrospective Study of Prevalence," *Aviation, Space, and Environmental Medicine* 80(8):734–7; Joseph McKeon et al., 2009, *A Review of the US Army Experience Using Selective Serotonin Reuptake Inhibitors in Aircrew* (Rucker, AL: United States Army Aeromedical Research Laboratory). Aviation personnel who are diagnosed with a mental health problem are often disqualified from flying until it is established that the problem has been treated and symptoms resolve. While "grounded," pilots do not receive flight pay.

19. Paul is referring to soldiers engaged in "ground combat" or "ground warfare," which refers to fighting that typically involves land forces such as infantry, combat vehicles, and artillery. In referring in shorthand to "ground guys," Paul reproduces the privileging of proximity to martial violence as the authoritative basis of war experience. Paul does so through what is referred to in military discourses as the "ground truth," wherein "on-the-ground" experience of combat and violence count as the only "real" military activity and, indeed, as the "real" itself. See Thomas Randrup Pedersen, 2017, "Get Real: Chasing Danish Warrior Dreams in the Afghan 'Sandbox,'" *Critical Military Studies* 3(1)7–26; Thomas Randrup Pedersen, 2019, "Ambivalent Anticipations: On Soldierly Becomings in the Desert of the Real," *Cambridge Journal of Anthropology* 37(1):77–92.

20. On the gendered politics of "ground truth" and military hierarchy, see Katharine Millar and Joanna Tidy, 2017, "Combat as a Moving Target: Masculinities, the Heroic Soldier Myth, and Normative Martial Violence," *Critical Military Studies* 3(2):142; Joanna Tidy, 2016, "The Gender Politics of 'Ground Truth' in the Military Dissent Movement: The Power and Limits of Authenticity Claims Regarding War," *International Political Sociology* 10(2):99–114.

21. For instance, one website providing financial advice to military members states, "If you're on deployment, why not maximize your pay by getting into the action? By volunteering for hazardous duty, a service member can earn up to $225 extra per month. Again, the key to maximizing your current pay is taking advantage of the military pay system." "Making Extra Money, Military-Style," InCharge Debt Solutions, November 30, 2021, https://www.incharge.org/military-money/military-life/making-extra-money-military-style/.

22. Kieran, *Signature Wounds*, 32.

23. Quoted in Kieran, *Signature Wounds*, 32. In an interview with Kieran, Castro went on to say, "clinicians in the military didn't know how to treat people with PTSD . . . [On] 9/11, maybe 10, 15 percent [of clinicians] knew how to do it" (32).

24. Remington Lee Nevin, 2017, "To Squander the Fighting Strength? Personal Experience with Preventive Psychiatry and the Dilemma of Wartime Public Mental Health," in *Psychiatrists in Combat: Mental Health Clinicians'*

Experiences in the War Zone, ed. E. Ritchie, C. Warner, and R. McLay, 145–56 (New York: Springer).

25. Nevin, "To Squander the Fighting Strength?," 150.

26. Elspeth Cameron Ritchie, 2011, "A Mixed Message about Stigma in Military Mental Health Care," *Time*, July 5.

27. Defense Health Board, 2010a, "Defense Health Board Psychotropic Medication Work Group Complementary and Alternative Medicine Work Group Meeting Minutes," Arlington, VA, November 3, 5. Reporting high prescription rates of antidepressants by general medical providers at an outpatient mental health clinic at a US air base in southern Iraq, one study describes prescribing providers as "fairly perceptive of airmen and soldiers suffering from anxiety and depression, even when they presented to the medical clinic primarily with physical complaints and/or were reluctant to discuss their emotional disposition." Military general providers in this study conveyed the "strong desire" to help military personnel who were "suffering emotionally," which may have contributed to high antidepressant medication prescription rates. Wayne Chappelle and Vicki Lumley, 2006, "Outpatient Mental Health Care at a Remote US Air Base in Southern Iraq," *Professional Psychology: Research and Practice* 37(5):523–30, 527.

28. Soldiers likewise talked about speaking to the chaplain as the first resort option over mental and behavioral health. One NCO told me that when he was a junior soldier, one of his warrant officers told him, "Hey, just be careful with that. I understand you have issues. Go see the chaplain. Don't see mental health because now you've got to check that box."

29. Every branch of the military has its own creative monikers for military psychiatrists and psychologists, though one common term across all branches of service is the largely derisive "Wizard," whose military use dates at least as far back as the Vietnam War. The title of Douglas Bey's memoir, *Wizard 6*, for example, refers to his radio call sign while he was the combat psychiatrist for the First Infantry Division in Vietnam. Rumored to be great and powerful, in the story the Wizard of Oz turns out to be nothing more than a charlatan operating from behind a curtain, a further unflattering commentary on the authority of military mental health professionals. Douglas Bey, 2006, *Wizard 6: A Combat Psychiatrist in Vietnam* (College Station, TX: Texas A&M University Press).

30. For more on the value of "stealth" mental health in the Army as a means of widening access to mental health care, see Chua, "Escaping the Clinic," 11–15.

31. Defense Health Board, 2011a, "Defense Health Board Joint Meeting Psychological Health External Advisory Subcommittee Psychotropic Medical Work Group Complementary and Alternative Medicine Work Group," Feb. 24–5, Bethesda, MA, 11.

32. Defense Health Board, 2011b, "Defense Health Board Recommendation Memorandum Pertaining to Psychotropic Medication Prescription Practices

and Use and Complementary and Alternative Medicine Use 2011-09," September 23, Falls Church, VA, 17.

33. The prescribing of psychotropic medications to patients without a psychiatric diagnosis, especially by nonpsychiatric physicians, is also common in civilian medical practice in the US. One study showed that over 60% of adult outpatient visits at which a new psychotropic prescription was initiated showed no psychiatric diagnosis recorded for the visit. Taeho Greg Rhee and Robert A. Rosenheck, 2019, "Initiation of New Psychotropic Prescriptions without a Psychiatric Diagnosis among US Adults: Rates, Correlates, and National Trends from 2006 to 2015," *Health Services Research* 54(1):139–48.

34. "Counterintelligence Agent 35L," US Army, https://www.goarmy.com/careers-and-jobs/signal-intelligence/languages-code/35l-counterintelligence-agent.

35. See, for example, Finley, *Fields of Combat*; Kilshaw, *Impotent Warriors;* Kenneth MacLeish, 2012, "Armor and Anesthesia: Exposure, Feeling, and the Soldier's Body," *Medical Anthropology Quarterly* 26(1):49–69; Messinger, "Incorporating the Prosthetic;" Wool, *After War.*

36. See Chua, "Bloody War," 145–7.

37. In most cases, military service members who accumulate 20 or more years of active service are eligible for sizeable monthly retirement pay at the end of their career, as well as other benefits. The 20-year-mark is therefore significant for careerists, who are typically working toward that mark.

38. On the use of SGB for the treatment of military-related PTSD, see Eugene Lipov and Elspeth Cameron Ritchie, 2015, "A Review of the Use of Stellate Ganglion Block in the Treatment of PTSD," *Current Psychiatry Reports* 17(8):63.

39. At the time of this project, I mostly heard about SGB as a treatment for PTSD from Special Forces soldiers.

40. The term "reset" is often used to describe the purpose of dwell time in both official circles and among soldiers. See MacLeish, "Churn," on the ways terms used by both the military and in scholarly framings analytically compartmentalize war in space and time.

41. Rajiv Chandrasekharan, 2007, *Imperial Life in the Emerald City: Inside Iraq's Green Zone* (New York: Vintage Books).

42. Morten G. Ender, 2012, "Boredom: *Groundhog Day* as Metaphor for Iraq," in *The Oxford Handbook of Military Psychology*, ed. J. Laurence and M. Matthews, 311–24 (New York: Oxford University Press).

43. Thomas L. Friedman, 2004, "'Groundhog Day' in Iraq," *New York Times*, November 12.

44. David Abrams's ironic 2012 novel, *Fobbit,* vividly portrays the stark divide between the strange normality of the air-conditioned, fast-food life on Iraq's FOBs and the brutality of war just yards away, while showing how the two worlds are deeply connected. Other terms and acronyms have been used to capture

the dilemmas of the fobbit and noninfantry soldiers more generally, including REMF (rear echelon mother fucker) first popularized during the Vietnam War, and POG (people other than grunt). David Abrams, 2012, *Fobbit* (New York: Black Cat).

45. Going outside or "crossing" the wire had deep significance in the wars in Iraq and Afghanistan. Understood as a masculinized rite of passage, crossing the wire marks in spatial terms the proximity to violence and combat that confers gendered authority and legitimacy on military personnel, motivates the work of soldiering, and structures military desires for "the real." See Morten Brænder, 2016, "Adrenalin Junkies: Why Soldiers Return from War Wanting More," *Armed Forces & Society* 42(1):3–25. It is also significant to the ways others in positions at the margins of military communities, like embedded journalists and researchers, approach and claim "insider status." On the significance of leaving the wire in relation to the practice of military medicine, see Chua, "Escaping the Clinic."

46. Pedersen, "Get Real."

47. eArmyU is an Army distance education program. Some reenlisting soldiers were eligible to receive a free laptop computer through this program.

48. On boredom and military life, see Victoria Basham, 2015, "Waiting for War: Soldiering, Temporality, and the Gendered Politics of Boredom and Joy in Military Spaces," in *Emotions, Politics and War*, ed. L. Åhäll and T. Gregory, 128–49 (New York: Routledge); Amanda Laugesen, 2016, *"Boredom is the Enemy": The Intellectual and Imaginative Lives of Australian Soldiers in the Great War and Beyond* (Oxfordshire, UK: Routledge); Bård Mæland and Paul Brunstad, 2009, *Enduring Military Boredom: From 1750 to the Present* (New York: Springer).

49. Mæland and Brunstad, *Enduring Military Boredom*, 1.

50. Hydroxycut is a brand of dietary supplement marketed to help with weight loss and to boost energy and mental focus. It was initially withdrawn from the US market in 2004 due to cardiotoxicity associated with its use of ephedra as a primary ingredient.

51. Wong, "CU @ the FOB," 9.

52. Wong, "CU @ the FOB," 10.

53. Wong, "CU @ the FOB," 9–10.

CHAPTER 3. STABILITY

1. The collection of biometrics was part of the Pentagon's broader quest to mine "big data" in the effort to measure and forecast the sociocultural and psychological states of populations and predict insurgent attacks during the war on terror. This included data from newer technologies including biometric databases,

remote sensors, and mobile phones, as well as intelligence gathered from traditional sources such as police and military records and soldiers' accounts. Roberto J. González, 2015, "Seeing into Hearts and Minds: 'Big Data,' Algorithms, and Computation Counterinsurgency," *Anthropology Today* 31(4):13–18.

2. See, for example, Anderson, "Facing the Future"; Ben Anderson, 2011b, "Population and Affective Perception: Biopolitics and Anticipatory Action in US Counterinsurgency Doctrine," *Antipode* 43(2):205–36; Elizabeth Dauphinee and Cristina Masters, eds., 2007, *The Logics of Biopower and the War on Terror* (London: Palgrave MacMillan); Derek Gregory, 2008a, "The Biopolitics of Baghdad: Counterinsurgency and the Counter-City," *Human Geography* 1(1):1–21; D. Gregory, "The Rush to the Intimate"; Julian Reid, 2013, *The Biopolitics of the War on Terror: Life Struggles, Liberal Modernity, and the Defence of Logistical Societies* (Manchester, UK: Manchester University Press). See also Rubaii, "Tripartheid," on how divide-and-rule policies introduced by the US after 2003 in Iraq enacted the political categorization of people by sect, producing differences that "became internal to being" among Sunni communities in Anbar province.

3. Anderson, "Population and Affective Perception," 205.

4. D. Gregory, "The Rush to the Intimate," identified a "cultural turn" in contemporary counterinsurgency comprised of a heterogeneous assemblage of practices and representational regimes, ranging from the recruitment of anthropologists and other social scientists into the Human Terrain System (HTS), the use of computer-based interactive training programs, and simulated Iraqi villages for military training. This cultural turn should not be taken only as a paradigm shift in military affairs but also as an overt attempt to "change public perceptions of the nature of warfare itself," particularly after the leaking of images and US public knowledge of the strategies of abjection and torture used against Muslim men in US custody at Abu Ghraib prison. Derek Gregory, 2010, "Seeing Red: Baghdad and the Event-ful City," *Political Geography* 29(5):266–79, 277.

5. Neta Crawford, 2013, *Accountability for Killing: Moral Responsibility for Collateral Damage in America's Post-9/11 Wars* (Oxford, UK: Oxford University Press).

6. McChrystal, *Tactical Directive.*

7. See T. Gregory, "The Costs of War" for a similar argument about the strategic aims of condolence payments by the US military to Iraqi and Afghan civilians.

8. Roger Mac Ginty, 2012, "Against Stabilization," *Stability: International Journal of Security and Development* 1(1):20–30.

9. Stabilization discourse predates this period, having crept into governance and intervention parlance in the mid-1990s, including in relation to economies undergoing the shock doctrine of rapid liberalization and the withdrawal of state support. See Naomi Klein, 2007, *The Shock Doctrine: The Rise of Disaster Capitalism* (New York: Metropolitan Books).

10. One PA told me: "Some of the most stable folks I had were the ones that previously had been exposed to combat and were diagnosed with PTSD and were on medication." "They knew what to expect," he said. "It doesn't mean that they liked it, but they knew what to expect." PTSD-expert Charles Hoge, who headed the largest US research program on the mental health and neurological effects of the wars in Iraq and Afghanistan at Walter Reed, has likewise suggested that "the reality was that a lot of those guys who had PTSD [and] who had learned to cope with their PTSD symptoms were exactly the guys you wanted on your team down range . . . .They have that emotional control. They have that ability to channel anger. They have that hypervigilance that's necessary for that environment." Kieran, *Signature Wounds*, 67. This is arguably consistent in some ways with classic tenets of military combat psychiatry, which have argued that "the battle-tested soldier is better trained because he is battle trained." Stephen W. Ranson, 1949, "The Normal Battle Reaction: Its Relation to the Pathologic Battle Reaction," *Bulletin of the US Army Medical Department 9*, Supplement:3–11, 7.

11. Contrary to the common claim that the US military's turn to counterinsurgency in the war on terror was a new strategy, in fact these contemporary tactics are part of a long history of "armed social work" put in the service of imperial militaries around the world. See Patricia Owens, 2015, *Economy of Force: Counterinsurgency and the Historical Rise of the Social* (Cambridge, UK: Cambridge University Press).

12. US Department of the Army, 2008, *Stability Operations Field Manual 3-07* (Washington, DC: United States Department of the Army), 5-8.

13. US Department of the Army, *Stability Operations Field Manual 3-07*, 5-8.

14. Anderson, "Facing the Future," 216.

15. It would also involve other kinds of professionals and personnel in the battlespace, including academics, private contractors, NGO workers, and civilian security personnel.

16. While the graphic photos that were published made the abuse at Abu Ghraib into an international scandal, photos taken by Marines in the aftermath of the Haditha killings were never released. In an oral history for the Marine Corps, General Michael Hagee, who was the commandant of the Marine Corps at the time of the killings, bragged about keeping the photos secret, saying, "The press never got them, unlike Abu Ghraib." Madeleine Baran, 2024, "The Haditha Massacre Photos that the Military Didn't Want the World to See," *The New Yorker*, August 27. The Haditha massacre registered minimally with the US public.

17. Results from the MHAT IV indicated that 14% of soldiers and Marines screened positive for depression, 13% screened positive for anxiety, and 31% screened positive for acute stress. United States Army Surgeon General, *MHAT IV*.

18. United States Army Surgeon General, *MHAT IV*.

19. United States Army Surgeon General, 2008, *Mental Health Advisory Team (MHAT) V Operational Iraqi Freedom 06-08* (Washington, DC: Army Medical

Command). See J-R Sébastien Blanc et al., 2018, "Association Between Unethical Battlefield Conduct and Mental Health: Implications for Leaders and Ethical Risk Assessment," *Psychology of Violence* 8(2):250–8, which proposes a "Triad of Ethical Risk" model linking mental health problems including PTSD to unethical battlefield conduct through anger disregulation.

20. By the time of MHAT IV, mental health personnel, programs, and resources in theater had established their basic functions in a combat environment and their roles were expanded into forensic and administrative psychiatry, specialty services not typical of combat psychiatry and not discussed as part of the domain of combat and operational stress control in the COSC field manual. The request for these expanded services by commanders and soldiers reflected an increasing need for sanity boards and command-directed mental health evaluations performed in theater, a development that some link to the rise in moral waivers given to recruits and to the link reported in the MHAT IV between mental health problems and unethical behaviors among soldiers. Cooper et al., "Provision of Mental Health Services in Operation Iraqi Freedom 05-07," 139.

21. Ben Klappe, 2011, "Rules of Engagement," in *International Military Missions and International Law*, ed. M. Odello and R. Piotrowicz (Boston: Martinus Nijhoff Publishers).

22. "US Rules of Engagement for Iraq E–1–6," WikiLeaks, February 4, 2008.

23. Hautzinger and Scandlyn, *Beyond Post-Traumatic Stress*, 6.

24. Kenneth MacLeish, 2022, "Moral Injury and the Psyche of Counterinsurgency," *Theory, Culture & Society* 39(6):63–86, 64.

25. T. Gregory, "The Costs of War," 159.

26. Cf. Said, *Orientalism*. See D. Gregory, "The Rush to the Intimate."

27. Paraphrasing MacLeish, "Moral Injury and the Psyche of Counterinsurgency," 71.

28. Rubaii, "Decentering Death," 498.

29. "US Army Special Operations Recruiting," goarmysof.army.mil, https://www.goarmysof.army.mil/SF/.

30. Laminated pocket cards that distilled RoE were often supplied to soldiers to help keep them apprised of the most recent directives in the "rapidly changing situations that characterize COIN operations." United States Department of the Army, *Counterinsurgency Field Manual* 3-24 (Washington, DC: United States Department of the Army), x.

31. On the role of emotions in soldiers' perceptions of imminent threat, the use of lethal force, and the deadly consequences for local civilians, see Thomas Gregory, 2012, "Dangerous Feelings: Checkpoints and the Perception of Hostile Intent," *Security Dialogue* 50(2):131–47. Gregory analyzes incident reports of Iraqi civilians who were killed or injured at coalition checkpoints, illuminating "perceptual practices or regimes of affect that marked certain bodies as dangerous, hostile or even threatening before they arrive," 132.

32. I build here on MacLeish's argument that the moral injury framework of individual transgression fails to account for the complex affective, embodied, and technical dimensions of military experience. MacLeish, "Moral Injury and the Psyche of Counterinsurgency," especially 73–9.

33. The term "baseline" commonly surfaced in several interviews with both soldiers and military providers. Like "stability," it was used in diverse ways but generally referred to the idea that each soldier has a behavioral reference point from which stability and instability could be ascertained.

34. One infantryman told me that the only reason he was able to go out every day on patrol was because he had given up caring about his own life and was singularly focused on protecting his buddies. He told me that while someone like me "might see that as sick, crazy, or suicidal," it was precisely what made him a good soldier.

35. The Special Forces soldiers I spoke with were candid to share that they had much easier access to psychopharmaceuticals than their conventional Army peers. One discretely intimated the fact that this included illicit drugs when he told me that elite units could essentially source anything they wanted. See Seth Harp, 2025, *The Fort Bragg Cartel: Drug Trafficking and Murder in the Special Forces* (New York: Penguin Books) which connects illicit drug use and drug trafficking in the Special Forces to overdose deaths and unresolved murders at Fort Bragg.

36. Nikolas Rose, 2003. "The Neurochemical Self and its Anomalies," in *Risk and Morality*, ed. R. Ericson and A. Doyle, 407–37 (Toronto: University of Toronto Press), 410–11.

37. Natasha Dow Schüll, 2014, *Addiction by Design: Machine Gambling in Las Vegas* (Princeton: Princeton University Press), 223.

38. Matt's evocation of a civilizational divide in forms of violence recalls liberal constructs "of what is cruel and what is necessary." These constructs condemn the cruel and inhumane atrocities perpetrated by the savage other while justifying or condoning the violence of democratic governments as principled and morally advanced. Asad, *On Suicide Bombing*, 2.

39. See chapter 2 for a discussion of the Army's recruitment challenges and the use of moral waivers during the war on terror.

40. It is commonly assumed and has been argued that the increase in moral waivers was directly responsible for creating adverse morale, discipline, and attrition problems for the military. See, for example, Kenard, *Irregular Army*. Government analyses have suggested somewhat mixed results. In 2006, based on analyses conducted by the Army and the RAND Corporation, a Government Accountability Office report stated that, "while those with conduct waivers tend to perform as well as those without conduct waivers, they are more likely to be separated for adverse reasons, such as behavioral issues." United States Government Accountability Office, 2009, "Military Personnel: Army Needs to Focus on Cost-Effective Use of Financial Incentives and Quality Standards in Managing Force

Growth," GAO Report Number GAO-09-256, 32. Framing its analysis in terms of institutional risk management, one study found that waivered recruits were "not *inherently* risky and are often better performers, with lower attrition risk" than non-waivered recruits but that the "'riskiness' of the waivered population" can vary depending on the number of waiver combinations and type of waiver. Lauren Malone and Neil Carey, 2011, "Waivered Recruits: An Evaluation of Their Performance and Attrition Risk," *CNA Analysis and Solutions*, 2–3.

41. This reflects standards for minimum fitness requirements, known as MOD standards, for personnel deploying to the US Central Command (USCENTCOM) Area of Responsibility, a geographic region that stretches from Northeast Africa across the Middle East to Central and South Asia as defined by the Unified Command Plan. Previous MOD standards required a 60-day timeframe before deployment to determine stability and assess the need for further care for newly diagnosed medical and psychological conditions or newly prescribed medications. Beginning with MOD 13, updated in 2017, the new requirement was a 90-day window with no issues for most conditions.

42. United States Central Command, 2019, *MOD 14 to USCENTCOM Individual Protection and Individual/Unit Deployment Policy (3 Oct), Tab A: Amplification of the Minimal Standards of Fitness for Deployment to the CENTCOM AOR* (Washington, DC: USCENTCOM), 9.

43. The DoD offers broad guidance on medical conditions and deployments, defining medical standards and placing limits for deployment on service members with "acute or unstable illnesses, chronic illnesses requiring frequent visits or monitoring, and illnesses likely to be aggravated by the deployed environment." United States Department of Defense, 2010, *DoD Instruction 6490.07 Deployment Limiting Medical Conditions for Service Members and DoD Civilian Employees,* https://www.esd.whs.mil/Portals/54/Documents/DD/issuances/dodi/649007p.pdf; James C. West, 2016, "Guest Perspective: Deployment, Mental Health Conditions and Psychotropic Medications—Good to Go?" *Center for Deployment Psychology,* April 19, https://deploymentpsych.org/blog/guest-perspective-deployment-mental-health-conditions-and-psychotropic-medictions-good-to-go. Additional guidance specifically pertaining to mental health conditions and medications used to treat them was released with a policy memorandum, with guidance requiring that individuals demonstrate "a minimum of three months stability" on their current treatment. Operational commanders issue additional guidance on medical standards for military personnel deploying to their geographic region. For instance, USCENTCOM, which encompasses Iraq and Afghanistan, issued guidance for deployment to the region that amplified DoD requirements and identified specific limitations on medical conditions and medications.

44. United States Department of Defense, "Policy Guidance for Deployment-Limiting Psychiatric Conditions and Medications," 2.

45. United States Department of Defense, "Policy Guidance for Deployment-Limiting Psychiatric Conditions and Medications," 2–3.

46. United States Department of Defense, "Policy Guidance for Deployment-Limiting Psychiatric Conditions and Medications," 4.

47. Sarah Lochlann Jain, 2007, "Living in Prognosis: Toward an Elegiac Politics," *Representations* 98(1):77–92, 78.

48. Jain, "Living in Prognosis," 78.

49. Another PA similarly told me that if a soldier has established care with a therapist, he is more likely to see that soldier as "stable" because he has the therapeutic relationship and will have resources to make use of when needed. Such soldiers in treatment are "self-aware," which he took as a sign of stability.

50. There are many ways providers work around this when first prescribing psychopharmaceuticals that might require a waiver or evidence of stability in-country. They might, for example, not initiate a profile or document a psychiatric diagnosis. See chapter 2 for more on how these decisions are made on a case-by-case basis and how providers use subclinical and time-limited diagnoses.

51. The history of western military psychiatry reflects shifting attitudes toward repression and abreaction in theater. During WWI, for example, most physicians saw little value in abreaction. The anthropologist and physician W. H. Rivers argued that volunteer soldiers broke down because their lack of experience left them ill-prepared to know how to repress unwanted emotions. Rivers, "Psychiatry and War." This emphasis would change with time and with shifting ideas of soldier mental health and the role of treatment in theater. As Jones and Wessley note, "Changes in culture towards the end of the twentieth century witnessed a greater acceptance of disclosure, ventilation and the expression of feelings. Psychological debriefing became an important element in forward psychiatry. This development reflected the tension between military needs (suppression of fears to return to duty) and an individual's therapeutic goals, which emphasized a cathartic release of tension." Jones and Wessely, "'Forward Psychiatry' in the Military," 417. While forms of counseling and psychological debriefing were mentioned by my interlocutors, they generally agreed that the repression of certain emotions while in theater was necessary for soldiers to continue to perform.

52. EMDR is an evidence-based psychotherapy that has been recommended by the VA and DoD for the treatment of PTSD. It involves having the patient pay attention to a back-and-forth movement or sound while prompted to recall an upsetting memory to shift how that memory is processed.

CHAPTER 4. SUPPLY

1. Propranolol has been a drug of interest to the US military, given its potential role in disrupting the consolidation or reconsolidation of traumatic memories

characteristic of PTSD, though study results have been mixed. See, for example, Elizabeth Hoge et al., 2012, "Effect of Acute Posttrauma Propranolol on PTSD Outcome and Physiological Responses During Script-Driven Imagery," *CNS Neuroscience & Therapeutics* 18:21–7; Roger Pitman et al., 2002, "Pilot Study of Secondary Prevention of Posttraumatic Stress Disorder with Propranolol," *Biological Psychiatry* 51(20):189–92. As part of the Psychological Kevlar Act of 2006, which aimed to implement preventative and early-intervention measures to protect troops against stress-related psychopathologies, the prospect of propranolol administration both in the immediate aftermath of an event and prophylactically has generated significant ethical debate. On military interest in propranolol, see Bickford, *Chemical Heroes*, 202–10. On ethical debates regarding military propranolol use, see Elise Donovan, 2010, "Propranolol Use in the Prevention and Treatment of Posttraumatic Stress Disorder in Military Veterans: Forgetting Therapy Revisited," *Perspectives in Biology and Medicine* 53(1):61–74; Wolfendale, "Performance-Enhancing Technologies and Moral Responsibility in the Military."

2. Howard et al., "Use of Combat Casualty Care Data to Assess the US Military Trauma System During the Afghanistan and Iraq Conflicts, 2001-2017."

3. "AMC—The Army's Materiel Integrator," Army Material Command, https://www.amc.army.mil.

4. In 2006, the Army opened the TRICARE mail order pharmacy program, which enables soldiers to have refills of medication shipped directly to them.

5. Brett Schneider et al., 2007, "Psychiatric Medications for Deployment: An Update," *Military Medicine* 172(7):681–5, 682.

6. Schneider et al., "Psychiatric Medications for Deployment," 683.

7. Schneider et al., "Psychiatric Medications for Deployment," 683.

8. Schneider et al., "Psychiatric Medications for Deployment," 683.

9. During the war on terror, a candidate with ADHD could enlist in the military as long as they met certain criteria or qualified for a medical waiver. Candidates were also required to go without medication treatment for ADHD for at least two years prior to enlistment. United States Department of Defense, "DoDI 6130.03, Vol. 1," 50. In 2024, the DoD eased restrictions for applicants with ADHD by allowing them to enlist without a waiver if they had not received treatment for the condition within the past year.

10. The phrase "the things they carried" comes from the title of the well-known collection of war stories of the same name by American novelist Tim O'Brien about a platoon of soldiers in the Vietnam War. Part memoir, part fiction, the 1990 collection begins with a title story describing what the soldiers must carry with them, both literally and figuratively, as they march: food, flak jackets, grenades, and canteens, as well as secrets, memories, grief, and terror. Tim O'Brien, 1990, *The Things They Carried* (Boston: Mariner Books).

11. On risk stratification and management around medication use, see chapter 5.

12. Redfield, *Life in Crisis*, 71.

13. Redfield, *Life in Crisis*, 69–71.

14. Ambien is a prescription sedative used for the short-term treatment of insomnia. The active ingredient is zolpidem, a sedative-hypnotic, that works by depressing the central nervous system.

15. See Romy Hoque and Andrew Chesson Jr, 2009, "Zolpidem-Induced Sleepwalking, Sleep Related Eating Disorder, and Sleep-Driving: Fluorine-18-Flourodeoxyglucose Positron Emission Tomography Analysis, and a Literature Review of Other Unexpected Clinical Effects of Zolpidem," *Journal of Clinical Sleep Medicine* 5(5):471–6. While David spoke of Ambien as relatively innocuous, compare with Jonathan's story in chapter 5.

16. Military psychologists can go through a two-year, highly competitive fellowship to obtain prescribing privileges, but this is very rare. General providers in the wars in Iraq and Afghanistan have reported lower comfort levels with prescribing psychotropics compared to other medications and less knowledge about common psychological symptoms, complications, and treatments. Defense Health Board, "Defense Health Board Psychotropic Medication Work Group Complementary and Alternative Medicine Work Group Meeting Minutes," 5.

17. Anne Lovell, 2006, "Addiction Markets," in *Global Pharmaceuticals: Ethics, Markets, Practices*, ed. A. Petryna et al., 136–69 (Durham, NC: Duke University Press).

18. Lovell, "Addiction Markets," 138.

19. Importantly, supply doesn't guarantee that the timing of the use of drugs will synchronize with the mission. Luis told me about a handful of times when he took a pill expecting that they would be heading off base, only for things to be delayed or rescheduled. He recalled furiously polishing his weapon to bide the time until the medication effects wore off.

20. Military personnel have also been known to "shop" for multiple providers who can prescribe medications for ADHD to access additional amphetamines. Detecting overlapping prescriptions in theater can be delayed given how the medical records system is designed. Defense Health Board, 2010b, "Defense Health Board Joint Meeting Psychological Health External Advisory Subcommittee Psychotropic Medication Work Group Complementary and Alternative Medicine Work Group," December 2–3, Rockville, MD, 28.

21. Scholars have written about the evolving role of pharmaceuticals in global health practices in which infrastructure may be poor or lacking, evidenced for example by the antiretroviral rollout and the emergence of the category of "essential medicines": a list of drugs defined by the WHO as "basic, indispensable, and necessary for the health of the population." See João Biehl, 2007, "Pharmaceuticalization: AIDS Treatment and Global Health Politics," *Anthropological Quarterly* 80(4):1083–126; Jeremy Greene, 2011, "Making Medicines Essential: The Emergent Centrality of Pharmaceuticals in Global Health," *BioSocieties* 6(1):10–33.

CHAPTER 5. REACTION

1. Boyd Ruamcharoen, 2024, "Tropicalizing the Portable Radio: Electronics and the US Military's Battle against Fungi in the Pacific War," *Technology and Culture* 65(2):497–529.

2. Redfield, "Vital Mobility and the Humanitarian Kit," 161.

3. Bruno Latour, 1987, *Science in Action: How to Follow Scientists and Engineers through Society* (Cambridge, MA: Harvard University Press).

4. See chapter 3 on soldier readiness processing, or SRP.

5. Anita Hardon and Emilia Sanabria, 2017, "Fluid Drugs: Revisiting the Anthropology of Pharmaceuticals," *Annual Review of Anthropology* 46:117–32, 118.

6. Defense Health Board, "Defense Health Board Joint Meeting Psychological Health External Advisory Subcommittee Psychotropic Medication Work Group Complementary and Alternative Medicine Work Group," Dec. 2–3, 21.

7. Cf. T. Gregory, "The Costs of War."

8. Emily Gilbert argues that condolence payments by the US military to civilians in the wars in Iraq and Afghanistan—up to $2,500 for death and $1,500 for injury—suggest both the objectification of and little value placed on not just enemy troops but also civilian populations, especially as compared to the sacred life of American soldiers. Emily Gilbert, 2015, "The Gift of War: Cash, Counterinsurgency, and 'Collateral Damage,'" *Security Dialogue* 46(5):403–21. Didier Fassin has likewise suggested that an important distinction is made between the sacred lives of Western soldiers, whose individual deaths are counted and honored, and the deaths of non-Western civilians, "whose losses are hardly tallied and whose corpses sometimes end up in mass graves." Didier Fassin, 2012, *Humanitarian Reason: A Moral History of the Present* (Berkeley: University of California Press), 24. On the politics of life and death in the war on terror, see Judith Butler, 2016, *Frames of War: When Is Life Grievable?* (London: Verso Books); Thomas Gregory, 2012, "Potential Lives, Impossible Deaths: Afghanistan, Civilian Casualties and the Politics of Intelligibility," *International Feminist Journal of Politics* 14(3):327–47; Kandida Purnell, 2018, "Grieving, Valuing, and Viewing Differently: The Global War on Terror's American Toll," *International Political Sociology* 12(2):156–71. On the limitations of the military and liberal paradigm focused on lethality, see Rubaii, "Decentering Death."

9. Here, I take inspiration from scholarship on the ethnography of chemicals, chemical selves, and chemical life. Recognizing that "chemicals have seeped into the ethnographic imaginary," anthropologists and others have engaged the formation of new subjectivities, socialities, and forms of life that emerge with modern chemistry's pleasures and toxicities in late capitalist contexts. Nicholas Shapiro and Eben Kirksey, 2017, "Chemo-Ethnography: An Introduction," *Cultural Anthropology* 32(4):481–93, 481. See, for example, Kim Fortun, 2012, "Ethnography in Late Industrialism," *Cultural Anthropology* 27(3):446–64; Anita Hardon et al., 2013, "Chemical Sexualities: The Use of Pharmaceutical

and Cosmetic Products by Youth in South Sulawesi, Indonesia," *Reproductive Health Matters* 21(41):214–24; Elizabeth Roberts, 2017, "What Gets Inside: Violent Entanglements and Toxic Boundaries in Mexico City," *Cultural Anthropology* 32(4):592–619.

10. Burn pits are shallow pits in which waste from military bases ranging from plastic water bottles to medical waste is burned. They were the primary model of waste management used by the US military in Iraq and Afghanistan. See Kenneth MacLeish and Zoë Wool, 2022, "Burn Pits: US Military Waste as War Violence," Society for Cultural Anthropology, January 25; Zoë Wool, "All That is Solid Burns into Smoke: US Military Burn Pits, Petrochemical Toxicity, and the Racial Geopolitics of Displacement," *Catalyst* 9(1):1–22. See also Kali Rubaii, 2020, "Birth Defects and the Toxic Legacy of War in Iraq," *Middle East Research and Information Project.*

11. Because uniformed psychologists like other care providers are obligated to "put the mission first" when evaluating or treating a soldier, there can be times when psychologists encounter clear incongruence between the best interests of a soldier and the interests of the military as an institution. The ethics literature refers to this as the "dual loyalty" of military medical professionals.

12. See chapter 4 on the clinical discourse of stability and how variable concepts of stability can be among military providers.

13. On suicide and homicide risk management among military personnel in deployment, see chapter 6.

14. While Ambien was reported by soldiers I interviewed to have been widely used relative to other psychotropic medications in the war on terror (see David's story in chapter 4), Jonathan's description of Ambien as "hardcore" emphasized the fact that Ambien has been associated with potentially dangerous, though uncommon, behaviors like sleepwalking. It's also likely that Ambien was not widely available given the timing and location of his deployment.

15. In Jonathan's case, this experience would become part of his journey into antiwar activism. See Jocelyn Lim Chua, 2018, "Fog of War: Psychopharmaceutical 'Side Effects' and the United States Military," *Medical Anthropology* 37(1):17–31.

16. See Millar and Tidy on the normative imagination of "combat" and its investments in what they call the "heroic soldier myth." Millar and Tidy, "Combat as a Moving Target."

17. Pedersen, "Get Real"; Pedersen, "Ambivalent Anticipations." Interestingly, these models imagine a war machine that runs apart from its machinery. They also conceive the only "true" risk as lying outside the FOB.

18. Lutz and Millar, "War," 486.

19. My argument builds on MacLeish's analysis of the limitations of the concept of moral injury and its construction of the soldier as an autonomous agent, specifically his notion of the "spectacle of moral transgression," for which he

builds on Lauren Berlant's "spectacle of decision." As MacLeish observes, if "the spectacle of decision" is "a rather impoverished model for how people actually inhabit their capacity for action," in Berlant's formulation, "perhaps moral injury's 'spectacle of moral transgression' may be similarly limiting if we recognize that the soldier is not an autonomous actor, but a body subjected to and empowered by the war-making apparatus." Kenneth MacLeish, 2013, "'Our Job is Not to Decide': War-Making and the Limits of Moral Injury," Meeting of the American Ethnological Society, Chicago, IL., 7. Lauren Berlant, 2007, "Slow Death (Sovereignty, Obesity, Lateral Agency)," *Critical Inquiry* 33(4):754–80.

20. Paraphrased from MacLeish, "'Our Job is Not to Decide," 7.

21. In 2004, the densely populated industrial city of Fallujah had an estimated population of 250,000 to 300,000 residents. While many of the city's residents fled before the assault, between 30,000 and 50,000 are believed to have remained during the fighting. Rory McCarthy and Peter Beaumont, 2004, "Civilian Cost of Battle for Fallujah Emerges," *The Guardian*, November 13.

22. El-Haj, *Combat Trauma*, 127–8. El-Haj argues that the ascendance of the figure of the traumatized soldier and its "moralist antipolitics" during the period of the war on terror was built in part on the recognition of their psychological pain and suffering as a victim of violence, thus affirming their inherent humanity.

23. MacLeish, "Moral Injury and the Psyche of Counterinsurgency," 76. Researchers consider moral injury a distinct phenomenon from PTSD; the concept of moral injury recognizes that "some combat and operational experiences can inevitably transgress deeply held beliefs that undergird a service member's humanity." Shira Maguen and Brett Litz, 2012, "Moral Injury in Veterans in War," *PTSD Research* 23(1):1–6, 1. While moral injury has the potential to widen the conversation beyond the biopsychiatric framework of PTSD, El-Haj argues that, in the American political environment in which national conversations excluded political questions about the nature of the wars in its moral obligation to the figure of the traumatized soldier, the concept of moral injury remains "radically severed from questions of the politics and ethics of the post-9/11 wars." El-Haj, *Combat Trauma*, 129. Indeed, MacLeish argues that moral injury fits into a "contemporary incarnation of just and humanitarian warfare in which violence itself is cast as a 'humane' instrument—when wielded by the right (Western) hand—and combatants' feelings about killing become part of the justificatory apparatus of war-making." MacLeish, "Moral Injury and the Psyche of Counterinsurgency," 65.

24. PTSD, particularly its incarnation in the form of combat PTSD in the war on terror, has commanded a similar power to limit political conversations. El-Haj, *Combat Trauma*. On the power of trauma to authenticate the moral and political suffering of victims more generally, see Didier Fassin and Richard Rechtman, 2009, *Empire of Trauma: An Inquiry into the Condition of Victimhood* (Princeton: Princeton University Press).

25. Schüll, *Addiction by Design*, 227.

26. Chua, "Medication by Proxy."

27. The ASVAB is a standardized test typically taken during the recruitment process. Designed to predict academic and professional success in the military, ASVAB scores are used to determine eligibility for military branches, rank, and career fields.

28. Despite constituting the formal mechanism by which states and militaries enroll personnel, the actual process by which militaries persuade young people to join their ranks has been minimally documented. Jessica Lavariega Monforti and Adam McGlynn, 2010, "The Poverty Draft? Exploring the Role of Socioeconomic Status in US Military Recruitment of Hispanic Students," Paper presented at the American Political Science Association Annual Meeting, Washington, DC, September 2–5 describes military recruitment as a "black box," calling for more explicit analysis of recruiting methods and the experience of potential soldiers as they interact with military recruiters. See Matthew Friesen and Matthew Eddy, 2019, "Selling the Service: Veteran Reflections on Their Past Experience of the Military Recruitment Process," *Critical Military Studies* 5(3):213–37; Matthew F. Rech, 2014, "Recruitment, Counter-Recruitment, and Critical Military Studies," *Global Discourse* 4(2-3):244–62.

29. Antidepressant medications have many indications and uses for both psychiatric and nonpsychiatric conditions. Nonpsychiatric conditions can include smoking cessation, neuropathic pain syndromes, hot flashes, and migraine prophylaxis. Bupropion is a nonnicotine option used to aid in smoking cessation and is considered a first-line treatment to help quit smoking by the military and VA.

30. A quick reaction force (QRF), sometimes also known as a rapid reaction force (RRF) or immediate reaction force (IRF), is a military unit designed to respond to developing situations and emergencies. Army units postured as quick reaction forces typically have a main mission of security and information gathering.

31. See, for example, Joshua Reno, 2011, "Beyond Risk: Emplacement and the Production of Environmental Evidence," *American Ethnologist* 38(3):516–30; Nicholas Shapiro, 2015, "Attuning to the Chemosphere: Domestic Formaldehyde, Bodily Reasoning, and the Chemical Sublime," *Cultural Anthropology* 30(3):368–93. On uncertainty and environmental toxicity, see Javier Auyero and Debora Swistun, 2008, "The Social Production of Toxic Uncertainty," *American Sociological Review* 73(3):357–79.

32. Serious neuropsychiatric events have been reported in patients taking bupropion for smoking cessation. The boxed warning reports that these have included changes in mood (including depression and mania), psychosis, hallucinations, paranoia, delusions, homicidal ideation, hostility, agitation, aggression, anxiety, and panic, as well as suicidal ideation, suicide attempt, and completed suicide.

CHAPTER 6. ENCAPSULATE

1. Two months was by far the longest period of unit watch I heard of. While there is no readily available data on the average amount of time spent on unit watch, one retrospective chart review of unit watches that were recommended during 2000 in the garrison setting of the Fourth Infantry Division Mental Health Section (DMHS) at Fort Hood in Texas reported that the average amount of time spent on unit watch was 33.62 hours with 87% of soldiers placed on watch for 48 hours or less. Alisa D. Hassinger, 2003, "Mentoring and Monitoring: The Use of Unit Watch in the 4th Infantry Division," *Military Medicine* 168(3):234–8, 235.

2. While much of the literature as well as many of my interlocutors use these terms interchangeably, some distinguish buddy watch as a more flexible, short-term, and informal type of watch for lower-risk individuals during the daylight hours only, while unit watch involves constant observation during a 24-hour period. For a proposal for a set of guidelines based on this distinction, see Samuel Payne et al., 2008, "The Use of Unit Watch or Command Interest Profile in the Management of Suicide and Homicide Risk: Rationale and Guidelines for the Military Mental Health Professional," *Military Medicine* 173(1):25–35.

3. Jeffrey H. Hill et al., 2006, "Suicidal and Homicidal Soldiers in Deployment Environments," *Military Medicine* 171(3):228–32.

4. Payne et al., "The Use of Unit Watch or Command Interest Profile in the Management of Suicide and Homicide Risk," 26.

5. The notion of the Army as a family that "takes care of its own" has its roots in what Jennifer Mittelstadt calls the "masculine familialism" of the Army family model, which envisioned an economic and support relationship between the Army, soldiers, and their families and emerged in the 1970s with the rise of the all-volunteer force. Mittelstadt argues that this respectable image was meant in part to relegitimize the institution after the perceived unprofessionalism, disrepute, and chaos of the Vietnam-era Army. Jennifer Mittelstadt, 2015, *The Rise of the Military Welfare State* (Cambridge, MA: Harvard University Press), 36–43.

6. Hill et al., "Suicidal and Homicidal Soldiers in Deployment Environments," 228.

7. For comparison, one study on suicidality among 272 Iraq and Afghanistan veterans found that 34 respondents (12.5%) reported contemplating suicide in the two weeks prior. Robert Pietrzak et al., 2010, "Risk and Protective Factors Associated with Suicidal Ideation in Veterans of Operations Enduring Freedom and Iraqi Freedom," *Journal of Affective Disorders* 123(1–3):102–7.

8. Hill et al., "Suicidal and Homicidal Soldiers in Deployment Environments," 228.

9. Samuel Payne et al., 2011, "Suicide and Homicide Risk Management: Rationale and Suggestions for the Use of Unit Watch in Garrison and Deployed

Settings," in *Textbook of Combat and Operational Psychiatry*, ed. E. Ritchie, 423–39 (Washington, DC: Office of the Surgeon General of the United States Army), 416. Despite this, clinicians will often pursue hospitalization in the case of the homicidal soldier to protect the potential victim.

10. Parallel to the ways suicide is distinguished from the forms of self-sacrifice and willingness to die that some soldiers ascribed to "good" soldiering, the distinction between homicide and state-sanctioned war killing is predicated on normative moralities and legal definitions in war.

11. Payne et al., "The Use of Unit Watch or Command Interest Profile in the Management of Suicide and Homicide Risk," 26.

12. United States Department of the Army, *Army Health Promotion, Risk Reduction, Suicide Prevention Report* 2010, 11.

13. Hill et al., "Suicidal and Homicidal Soldiers in Deployment Environments," 228.

14. In proposing the utility of unit watch in reducing "secondary gain," Payne et al. introduce the terms "military-specific suicidal ideation" and "military-specific homicidal ideation," which they define as "the verbal expression of suicidal (or homicidal) thoughts with the implicit (as determined by the clinician) or explicit goal of avoiding military duty. . . . The soldiers essentially imply or state that they may or will kill themselves, or a leader in their unit, unless allowed to achieve a stated goal." Payne et al., "The Use of Unit Watch or Command Interest Profile in the Management of Suicide and Homicide Risk," 27.

15. Hill et al., "Suicidal and Homicidal Soldiers in Deployment Environments," 288.

16. Rose, "Governing Risk Individuals."

17. Rose "Governing Risky Individuals," 179.

18. Rose "Governing Risky Individuals," 179.

19. Paul Brodwin and Livia Velpry, 2014, "The Practice of Constraint in Psychiatry: Emergent Forms of Care and Control," *Culture, Medicine & Psychiatry* 38(4):524–6, 524. Ethnographic accounts have explored the diverse institutions, practices, and rationales that facilitate tactics of constraint-as-treatment, both within and beyond the walls of clinical institutions. See João Biehl, 2013, *Vita: Life in a Zone of Social Abandonment* (Berkeley: University of California Press); Paul Brodwin, 2013, *Everyday Ethics: Voices from the Front Line of Community Psychiatry* (Berkeley: University of California Press); Angela Garcia, 2024, *The Way That Leads among the Lost: Life, Death, and Hope in Mexico City's Anexos* (New York: Macmillan Press); Sarah Pinto, 2014, *Daughters of Parvati: Women and Madness in Contemporary India* (Philadelphia: University of Pennsylvania Press); Lorna Rhodes, 2004, *Total Confinement: Madness and Reason in Maximum Security Prison* (Berkeley: University of California Press); Julio Villa-Palomino, 2025, "Home Sweet Harm: Confinement and *Tranquilidad* in Post-Asylum Peru," *Medical Anthropology Quarterly*:e70032.

20. For more on the medicolegal issues surrounding the use of unit watch in the military, see Payne et al., "Suicide and Homicide Risk Management," 436–7.

21. Christopher Brown and Richard Sheridan, 2015, "Case Study Illustrating Risks of Garrison Unit Watch for Soldiers at Risk of Suicide," *Military Medicine* 180(6):e721–e722, e721.

22. See, for example, Gary Junker et al., 2005, "Using Trained Inmate Observers for Suicide Watch in a Federal Correctional Setting: A Win-Win Solution," *Psychological Services* 2(1):20–7.

23. Hassinger, "Mentoring and Monitoring," 235.

24. Elspeth Reeve, 2009, "Suicidal Soldiers," *The Daily Beast,* May 11; Brown and Sheridan, "Case Study Illustrating Risks of Garrison Unit Watch for Soldiers at Risk of Suicide," e721.

25. Payne et al., "The Use of Unit Watch or Command Interest Profile in the Management of Suicide and Homicide Risk, 25–6.

26. Hassinger, "Mentoring and Monitoring," 234.

27. Payne et al., "The Use of Unit Watch or Command Interest Profile in the Management of Suicide and Homicide Risk," 25.

28. In one case study, two NCOs were delegated with the responsibility of serving as watchers for a junior enlisted soldier. By the second night, unit watch responsibility had been delegated to junior soldiers, some of whom were themselves pending separation for drug use and some of whom were reportedly taunting the watched soldier to commit suicide. "This delegation had occurred at the NCO level and was apparently driven by operational demands for the most competent Soldiers to do other tasks, which were perceived to be a higher priority than watching a Soldier whose misconduct had already harmed the unit." Brown and Sheridan, "Case Study Illustrating Risks of Garrison Unit Watch for Soldiers at Risk of Suicide," e721.

29. Hassinger, "Mentoring and Monitoring," 234.

30. Jeffrey J. Hollingsworth and Jean Paul Hare, 2013, "Managing Acute Suicidal Ideation in a Forward Deployed Location in Afghanistan," *Military Medicine* 178(4):357–8, 358.

31. Hassinger, "Mentoring and Monitoring," 234.

32. Firearms have been the method used in the vast majority of suicide and homicide deaths in the US Army. Between 2014 and 2019, gunshot wounds accounted for 65% of suicide deaths and 79% of homicide deaths among US Army soldiers. Gabrielle Kaplansky and Maisha Toussaint, 2024, "US Army Mortality Surveillance in Active Duty Soldiers, 2014-2019," *Medical Surveillance Monthly Reporting* 31(5):2–8.

33. The retrospective chart review discussed in footnote 1, which analyzed new cases opened at the Fourth Infantry DMHS at Fort Hood during 2000, found that 78.8% of soldiers recommended for unit watch were age 25 years or below, and 90.4% had less than 3 years of service. It was also used almost

exclusively with soldiers in enlisted grades E1 to E4, though it should be noted that this study examined cases in a garrison, not deployed, environment. Hassinger, "Mentoring and Monitoring," 235.

34. On dirty work in medicine, see Charles Bosk, 1992, *All God's Mistakes: Genetic Counseling in a Pediatric Hospital* (Chicago: University of Chicago Press); Mara Buchbinder, 2022, "Dirty Work in Medicine: Understanding US Physicians' Agency in Contested Medical Practices," *Medical Anthropology Quarterly* 36(4):534–51; Ian Shaw, 2004, "Doctors, 'Dirty Work' Patients, and 'Revolving Doors,'" *Qualitative Health Research* 14(8):1032–45.

35. Brown and Sheridan, "Case Study Illustrating Risks of Garrison Unit Watch for Soldiers at Risk of Suicide," e721. See Payne et al., "Suicide and Homicide Risk Management," for an example of such guidelines.

36. Payne et al., "Suicide and Homicide Risk Management," 424.

37. Hassinger, "Mentoring and Monitoring," 234.

38. CQ or "charge of quarters" refers to the tasked duty in which designated military personnel handle the administration of the unit, typically for a 24-hour assignment. Thus, in the case of unit watch, "CQ watch" refers both to the area where CQ duty is performed and where the watched soldier is kept—but also to the pairing of the duty of CQ and unit watch.

39. While recommendations on unit-watch procedures, including template memoranda and information papers for commanders, have been published (see Payne et al., "Suicide and Homicide Risk Management"), no one I interviewed who spoke of unit watch recalled or mentioned receiving written instructions regarding procedures to follow.

40. Payne et al., "Suicide and Homicide Risk Management," 425.

41. Payne et al., "Suicide and Homicide Risk Management," 408.

42. See Katherine Hejtmanek, 2010, "Caring through Restraint: Violence, Intimacy and Identity in Mental Health Practice," *Culture, Medicine & Psychiatry* 34:668–74.

43. Rose, "Governing Risky Individuals;" Anne Lovell, 1996, "Coercion and Social Control: A Framework for Research on Aggressive Strategies in Community Mental Health," in *Coercion and Aggressive Treatment: A New Frontier in Mental Health Law*, ed. D. Dennis and J. Monahan, 147–66 (New York: Plenum Publishing).

44. The stigma attached to unit watch resembles the stigma associated with injury and with soldiers being placed on a physical or psychiatric profile, a temporary or permanent designation based on the soldier's capacity to perform their duties as defined by military standards. See chapter 5.

45. The Army banned the use of orange road guard vests to single out soldiers in response to the article. See Reeve, "Suicidal Soldiers," for General Pete Chiarelli's response and the original article published in *The Daily Beast*.

46. Robert Ursano et al., 2017, "Risk of Suicide Attempt among Soldiers in Army Units with a History of Suicide Attempts," *JAMA Psychiatry* 74(9):924–31.

47. The psychiatric asylum has been positioned as the epitome of such expulsion. See Michel Foucault, 1961, *Madness and Civilization* (New York: Vintage); Erving Goffman, 1961, *Asylums: Essays on the Social Situation of Mental Patients and Other Inmates* (New York: Anchor Books).

48. The Army PT uniform, or physical training uniform, refers to a uniform designed for comfort and performance while working out. It can include sweatpants, shorts, and long and short-sleeve shirts.

49. On the protection of life against the threat of suicide, see also Jocelyn Lim Chua, 2014, *In Pursuit of the Good Life: Aspiration and Suicide in Globalizing South India* (Berkeley: University of California Press); Lauren Sealy Krishnamurti, 2020, "The Potential of 'Watchful' Care: Preventing Suicide with Aloha in Hawaii," *Medical Anthropology Quarterly* 35(1):120–35.

50. Zöe Wool, 2019, "Afterwar Work for Life," in *War and Health: The Medical Consequences of the Wars in Iraq and Afghanistan*, ed. C. Lutz and A. Mazzarino, 210–30 (New York: New York University Press), 222.

51. Angela Garcia, 2010, *The Pastoral Clinic: Addiction and Dispossession along the Rio Grande* (Berkeley: University of California Press), 133; see also Krishnamurti, "The Potential of 'Watchful' Care."

EPILOGUE

1. This now well-known quote by Petraeus, cited in the epigraph, comes from an interview with *Washington Post* reporter Rick Atkinson when Petraeus was commanding the 101st Airborne Division. Rick Atkinson, 2003, "The Long, Blinding Road to War," *The Washington Post*, March 6.

2. Gerry Shih, Niha Masih, and Dan Lamothe, 2021, "The Story of an Afghan Man Who Fell from the Sky," *The Washington Post,* August 21.

3. Barbara Plett-Usher, 2021, "US Admits Drone Strike Killed Civilians," *The Washington Post,* September 17.

4. Daulatzai and Ghumkhor, "Afghanistan, Racial Melancholia, and Loss That Exceeds Loss," 202-203; El-Haj, *Combat Trauma*, 250, italics in original.

5. While the discourse of "allyship" presumes a mutual and symmetric relationship, the risks of allyship were not equally borne. Iraqis and Afghans who were seen to be collaborating with US occupation faced death threats, extortion, kidnapping, and murder throughout the span of the war on terror. See chapter 5 of Nadia El-Shaarawi, 2025, *Collateral Damages: Tracing the Debts and Displacements of the Iraq War* (Berkeley: University of California Press) on the dangers of collaboration for Iraqis and why "allyship" is an impoverished concept for the debts and complicities of collaborating with empire for those who bear its greatest risks and violence.

6. Kirsten Fontenrose, 2021, "PTSD Is an Endless War for Veterans. The News from Afghanistan Is Making It Worse," *New Atlanticist,* August 25, italics in original.

7. Sandy Cohen, 2021, "News, Images from Afghanistan Can Trigger PTSD in Military Veterans," *UCLA Health*, August 24.

8. Lutz and Millar, "War," 482.

9. United States Department of the Army, 2022, *Field Manual (FM) 3-0: Operations* (Washington, DC: United States Department of the Army).

10. National Institute of Mental Health, "Mental Illness," September 2024, https://www.nimh.nih.gov/health/statistics/mental-illness. After multiple years of recruitment shortfalls, all six branches of the US Armed Forces reached their respective recruiting goals for fiscal year 2025. The $900 billion National Defense Authorization Act (NDAA) for fiscal year 2026 included continued efforts to boost military recruitment. Nick Mordowanec, 2025, "Defense Bill Will 'Turbocharge' Surging Military Recruitment Numbers: Senator," *Military.com*, December 19.

11. See Cortney Weinbaum, 2023, "An Autistic Soldier Wants You to Read This." *Modern War Institute*, June 1, https://mwi.westpoint.edu/an-autistic-soldier-wants-you-to-read-this/.

12. White House, 2025, "Prioritizing Military Excellent and Readiness," January 27, https://www.whitehouse.gov/presidential-actions/2025/01/prioritizing-military-excellence-and-readiness/.

13. Quoted in Patty Neiberg, 2025, "If Common Mental Health Issues are Labeled 'Incompatible' with Service, Advocates Fear Troops Will Go 'Underground,'" *Task & Purpose*, February 19.

14. See, for example, Mason Remondelli et al., 2024, "Refocusing the Military Health System to Support Role 4 Definitive Care in Future Large-Scale Combat Operations," *Journal of Trauma and Acute Care Surgery* 97(2S Suppl 1):S145–53. On how definitions of LSCO are being updated to contemporary conditions, see John Dzwonczyk and Clayton Merkley, 2023, "Through a Glass Clearly: An Improved Definition of LSCO," *Military Review*, https://www.armyupress.army.mil/Journals/Military-Review/Online-Exclusive/2023-OLE/Through-a-Glass-Clearly/. This is hardly the first time the US military would look to historical conflicts to reimagine contemporary conflict. The Pentagon held screenings of Gillo Pontecorvo's film, *The Battle of Algiers*, circulated texts written about Iraq during World War II, and drew on T. E. Lawrence to develop counterinsurgency strategy and training programs for commanders and staff officers in the war on terror—reducing people to imperial representations and discourse in the process. See Joseph Masco, "Counterinsurgency, *The Spook*, and Blowback," in *Anthropology and Global Counterinsurgency*, ed. by J. Kelly, B. Jauregui, S. Mitchell, and J. Walton, 193–208 (Chicago: University of Chicago Press).

15. Sections of this paragraph have been paraphrased from Tim Hoyt and Christina Hein, 2021, "Combat and Operational Stress Control in the Prolonged Field Environment," *Military Review*, September–October: 55–64, 57–58.

16. Tim Hoyt and Christina Hein, "Combat and Operational Stress Control in the Prolonged Field Environment," 58.

Bibliography

Abrams, David. 2012. *Fobbit.* New York: Black Cat.

Açıksöz, Salih Can. 2019. *Sacrificial Limbs: Masculinity, Disability, and Political Violence in Turkey.* Berkeley: University of California Press.

Adler, Amy and Ian Guttierez. 2022. "Acute Stress Reaction in Combat: Emerging Evidence and Peer-Based Interventions." *Current Psychiatry Reports* 24:277–84.

Agard-Jones, Vanessa. 2013. "Bodies in the System." *Small Axe: A Caribbean Journal of Criticism* 17(3):182–92.

Aggarwal, Neil Krishnan. 2015. *Mental Health in the War on Terror: Culture, Science, and Statecraft.* New York: Columbia University Press.

Al-Mohammad, Hayder. 2012. "A Kidnapping in Basra: The Struggles and Precariousness of Life in Postinvasion Iraq." *Cultural Anthropology* 27(4):597–614.

American Anthropological Association. 2007. "American Anthropological Association Executive Board Statement on the Human Terrain System Project." https://americananthro.org/about/committees-and-task-forces/human-terrain-system-hts-project/.

American Psychiatric Association. 2013. *Diagnostic and Statistical Manual of Mental Disorders 5th ed.* Washington, DC: American Psychiatric Publishing.

Anderson, Ben. 2011a. "Facing the Future: US Counterinsurgency Doctrine and the Pre-insurgent." *Theory, Culture & Society* 28(7-8):216–40.

Anderson, Ben. 2011b. "Population and Affective Perception: Biopolitics and Anticipatory Action in US Counterinsurgency Doctrine." *Antipode* 43(2):205–36.

Andreas, Peter. 2022. *Killer High: A History of War in Six Drugs*. Oxford: Oxford University Press.

Applewhite, Larry, Nathan Keller, and Adam Borah. 2012. "Mental Health Care Used by Soldiers Conducting Counterinsurgency Operations." *Military Medicine* 177(5):501–6.

Aretxaga, Begoña. 2003. "Maddening States." *Annual Review of Anthropology* 32(1):393–410.

Asad, Talal. 2007. *On Suicide Bombing*. New York: Columbia University Press.

Associated Press. 2007. "Military Granting More Criminal Waivers," February 14.

Atkinson, Rick. 2003. "The Long, Blinding Road to War." *The Washington Post*. March 6.

Auyero, Javier and Debora Swistun. 2008. "The Social Production of Toxic Uncertainty." *American Sociological Review* 73(3):357–79.

Axinn, Sidney. 1989. *A Moral Military*. Philadelphia, PA: Temple University Press.

Baard, Erik. 2003. The Guilt-Free Soldier. *The Village Voice*, January 21.

Baiocchi, Dave. 2013. "Measuring Army Deployments to Iraq and Afghanistan." RAND Corporation.

Bajjani-Gebara, Jouhayna, Sherrie L. Wilcox, John W. Williams Jr., Andrzej S. Kosinski, Rhonda J. Allard, Candy Wilson, and Ryan Landoll. 2021. "Adjustment Disorders in US Active Duty Military Women: A Scoping Review for the Years 2000 to 2018." *Women's Health Issues* 31:S33–S42.

Baran, Madeleine. 2024. "The Haditha Massacre Photos That the Military Didn't Want the World to See." *The New Yorker*, August 27.

Barry, Andrew. 2005. "Pharmaceutical Matters: The Invention of Informed Materials." *Theory, Culture & Society* 22(1):51–69.

Basham, Victoria. 2015. "Waiting for War: Soldiering, Temporality, and the Gendered Politics of Boredom and Joy in Military Spaces." In *Emotions, Politics and War*, edited by L. Åhäll and T. Gregory, 128–49. New York: Routledge.

Beck, Ulrich. 1992. *Risk Society: Towards a New Modernity*. Thousand Oaks, CA: Sage.

Ben-Ari, Eyal. 1998. *Mastering Soldiers: Conflict, Emotions, and the Enemy in an Israeli Military Unit*. New York: Berghahn Books.

Bergen-Cico, Dessa. 2012. *War and Drugs: The Role of Military Conflict in the Development of Substance Abuse*. New York: Routledge.

Berlant, Lauren. 2007. "Slow Death (Sovereignty, Obesity, Lateral Agency)." *Critical Inquiry* 33(4):754–80.

Bey, Douglas. 2006. *Wizard 6: A Combat Psychiatrist in Vietnam*. College Station, TX: Texas A&M University Press.

Bickford, Andrew. 2020. *Chemical Heroes: Pharmacological Supersoldiers in the US Military*. Durham, NC: Duke University Press.

Biehl, João. 2007. "Pharmaceuticalization: AIDS Treatment and Global Health Politics." *Anthropological Quarterly* 80(4):1083–126.

Biehl, João. 2013. *Vita: Life in a Zone of Social Abandonment.* Berkeley: University of California Press.

Blanc, J-R Sébastien, Christopher Warner, Gary Ivey, and Deanna Messervey. 2018. "Association Between Unethical Battlefield Conduct and Mental Health: Implications for Leaders and Ethical Risk Assessment." *Psychology of Violence* 8(2):250–8.

Board on the Health of Select Populations. 2010. *Returning Home from Iraq and Afghanistan: Preliminary Assessment of Readjustment Needs of Veterans, Service Members, and Their Families.* Washington, DC: National Academies Press.

Bosk, Charles. 1992. *All God's Mistakes: Genetic Counseling in a Pediatric Hospital.* Chicago: University of Chicago Press.

Bourne, Peter G. 1970. "Military Psychiatry and the Viet Nam Experience." *American Journal of Psychiatry* 127(4):481–8.

Brænder, Morten. 2016. "Adrenalin Junkies: Why Soldiers Return from War Wanting More." *Armed Forces & Society* 42(1):3–25.

Braswell, Harold and Howard Kushner. 2012. "Suicide, Social Integration, and Masculinity in the US Military." *Social Science & Medicine* 74(4):530–6.

British Forces Broadcasting Service. 2024. "British Army Dishing Out Too Many Antidepressants to Treat PTSD, Says Former Soldier." *Forces News,* March 31.

Brodwin, Paul. 2013. *Everyday Ethics: Voices from the Front Line of Community Psychiatry.* Berkeley: University of California Press.

Brodwin, Paul and Livia Velpry. 2014. "The Practice of Constraint in Psychiatry: Emergent Forms of Care and Control." *Culture, Medicine & Psychiatry* 38(4):524–6.

Brown, Christopher and Richard Sheridan. 2015. "Case Study Illustrating Risks of Garrison Unit Watch for Soldiers at Risk of Suicide." *Military Medicine* 180(6):e721–e722.

Brown, Ethan. 2023. "The Ghost of GWOT Haunting the Military Recruiting Crisis." The Modern War Institute at West Point. https://mwi.westpoint.edu/the-ghost-of-gwot-haunting-the-military-recruiting-crisis/.

Brown, Keith and Catherine Lutz. 2007. "Grunt Lit: The Participant-Observers of Empire." *American Ethnologist* 34(2):322–8.

Brusher, Edward. 2011. "Combat and Operational Stress Control." In *Combat and Operational Behavioral Health,* edited by E. Ritchie, 59–74. Falls Church, VA: Office of the Surgeon General of the United States Army.

Buchbinder, Mara. 2022. "Dirty Work in Medicine: Understanding US Physicians' Agency in Contested Medical Practices." *Medical Anthropology Quarterly* 36(4):534–51.

Burns, Robert. 2004. "Pentagon: 40,000 US Troops Being Sent to Iraq for a Year." *Associated Press*, May 3.
Butler, Judith. 2016. *Frames of War: When is Life Grievable?* London: Verso Books.
Camp, Norman. 2011. "US Army Psychiatry Legacies of the Vietnam War." In *Combat and Operational Behavioral Health*, edited by E. Ritchie, 9–42. Falls Church, VA: Office of the Surgeon General of the United States Army.
Capaldi, Vincent F. and Hanna D. Zembrzuska. 2015. "Thrust into the Breach: Psychiatry in a Combat Zone within 1 Year of Residency Completion." *Academic Psychiatry* 39:410–5.
Castañeda, Sheila F., Jennifer N. Belding, Claire A. Kolaja, Cynthia A. Leard-Mann, Isabel G. Jacobson, Anna C. Rivera, Felicia R. Carey et al. 2023. "Cohort Profile Update: The US Millennium Cohort Study—Evaluating the Impact of Military Experiences on Service Members and Veteran Health." *International Journal of Epidemiology* 52(4):e222–31.
Chandrasekharan, Rajiv. 2007. *Imperial Life in the Emerald City: Inside Iraq's Green Zone*. New York: Vintage Books.
Chappelle, Wayne and Vicki Lumley. 2006. "Outpatient Mental Health Care at a Remote US Air Base in Southern Iraq." *Professional Psychology: Research and Practice* 37(5):523–30.
Chedekel, Lisa and Matthew Kaufman. 2006. "Mentally Unfit, Forced to Fight." *Hartford Courant*, May 14.
Chua, Jocelyn Lim. 2014. *In Pursuit of the Good Life: Aspiration and Suicide in Globalizing South India*. Berkeley: University of California Press.
Chua, Jocelyn Lim. 2018. "Fog of War: Psychopharmaceutical 'Side Effects' and the United States Military." *Medical Anthropology* 37(1):17–31.
Chua, Jocelyn Lim. 2020a. "Bloody War: Menstruation, Soldiering, and the 'Gender-Integrated' United States Military." *Critical Military Studies* 8(2):139–58.
Chua, Jocelyn Lim. 2020b. "Medication by Proxy: The Devolution of Psychiatric Power and Shared Accountability to Pharmaceutical Use among Soldiers in America's Post-9/11 Wars." *Culture, Medicine & Psychiatry* 44:565–85.
Chua, Jocelyn Lim. 2020c. "Pharmaceutical Creep: US Military Power and the Global and Transnational Mobility of Psychopharmaceuticals." *Medical Anthropology Quarterly* 34(1):41–58.
Chua, Jocelyn Lim. 2022. "Escaping the Clinic: Exposure as Care among Military Medical Professionals at War." *Medicine Anthropology Theory* 9(2):1–25.
Chua, Jocelyn Lim and Lacy Jo Evans. 2018. "Collaborative Research Between Student Veterans and Faculty in Higher Education." *Journal of Veteran Studies* 3(1):122–38.
Cohen, Sandy. 2021. "News, Images from Afghanistan Can Trigger PTSD in Military Veterans." *UCLA Health*, August 24.

Congressional Research Service. 1998. "Military Readiness, Operations Tempo (OPTEMPO) and Personnel Tempo (PERSTEMPO): Are US Forces Doing Too Much?" January 14.

Congressional Record. 2007. "Text of Amendments." Congressional Record, Vol. 153, No. 139. September 19.

Congressional Record. 2009. "The Current Status of US Ground Forces." Senate Hearing 111–66. April 22.

Cooper, Marc A., Sharon Newton, and Jeffrey Yarvis. 2011. "Provision of Mental Health Services in Operation Iraqi Freedom 05-07." In *Textbook of Combat and Operational Psychiatry*, edited by E. Ritchie, 137-49. Washington, DC: Office of the Surgeon General of the United States Army.

Cooter, Roger. 1993. "War and Modern Medicine." In *Companion Encyclopedia of the History of Medicine, Vol. 2*, edited by W. F. Bynum and R. Porter, 1536–73. London and New York: Routledge.

Crawford, Neta. 2013. *Accountability for Killing: Moral Responsibility for Collateral Damage in America's Post-9/11 Wars*. Oxford: Oxford University Press.

D'Arcy, Michael. 2019. "'It Tastes Like Order': Psychotic Evidence for Antipsychotic Efficacy and Medicated Subjectivity." *Ethos* 47(1):89–107.

Datel, William and Arnold Johnson Jr. 1978. *Psychotropic Prescription Medication in Vietnam*. Washington, DC: Walter Reed Army Institute of Research.

Daulatzai, Anila and Sahar Ghumkhor. 2023. "Afghanistan, Racial Melancholia, and Loss That Exceeds Loss." *Critical Times* 6(2):202–11.

Dauphinee, Elizabeth and Cristina Masters, eds. 2007. *The Logics of Biopower and the War on Terror*. London: Palgrave MacMillan.

Defense Health Board. 2010a. "Defense Health Board Psychotropic Medication Work Group Complementary and Alternative Medicine Work Group Meeting Minutes." November 3. Arlington, VA.

Defense Health Board. 2010b. "Defense Health Board Joint Meeting Psychological Health External Advisory Subcommittee Psychotropic Medication Work Group Complementary and Alternative Medicine Work Group." December 2–3. Rockville, MD.

Defense Health Board. 2011a. "Defense Health Board Joint Meeting Psychological Health External Advisory Subcommittee Psychotropic Medical Work Group Complementary and Alternative Medicine Work Group." February 24–5. Bethesda, MA.

Defense Health Board. 2011b. "Defense Health Board Recommendation Memorandum Pertaining to Psychotropic Medication Prescription Practices and Use and Complementary and Alternative Medicine Use 2011–09." September 23. Falls Church, VA.

Dewachi, Omar. 2020. *Ungovernable Life: Mandatory Medicine and Statecraft in Iraq*. Stanford: Stanford University Press.

Dewachi, Omar, Mac Skelton, Vinh-Kim Nguyen, et al. 2014. "Changing Therapeutic Geographies of the Iraqi and Syrian Wars." *The Lancet* 383(9915):449–57.

Donovan, Elise. 2010. "Propranolol Use in the Prevention and Treatment of Posttraumatic Stress Disorder in Military Veterans: Forgetting Therapy Revisited." *Perspectives in Biology and Medicine* 53(1):61–74.

Dzwonczyk, John and Clayton Merkley. 2023. "Through a Glass Clearly: An Improved Definition of LSCO." *Military Review*. https://www.armyupress.army.mil/Journals/Military-Review/Online-Exclusive/2023-OLE/Through-a-Glass-Clearly/.

Eide, Richard and Shauna Stahlman. 2018. "Polypharmacy Involving Opioid, Psychotropic, and Central Nervous System Depressant Medications, Period Prevalence and Association with Suicidal Ideation, Active Component, US Armed Forces, 2016." *Medical Surveillance Monthly Report* 25(6):2–9.

El-Haj, Nadia Abu. 2022. *Combat Trauma: Imaginaries of War and Citizenship in Post-9/11 America*. New York: Verso.

El-Shaarawi, Nadia. 2025. *Collateral Damages: Tracing the Debts and Displacements of the Iraq War*. Berkeley: University of California Press.

Ender, Morten G. 2012. "Boredom: *Groundhog Day* as Metaphor for Iraq." In *The Oxford Handbook of Military Psychology*, edited by J. Laurence and M. Matthews, 311–24. New York: Oxford University Press.

Fassin, Didier. 2012. *Humanitarian Reason: A Moral History of the Present*. Berkeley: University of California Press.

Fassin, Didier and Richard Rechtman. 2009. *The Empire of Trauma: An Inquiry into the Condition of Victimhood*. Princeton: Princeton University Press.

Finley, Erin. 2011. *Fields of Combat: Understanding PTSD among Veterans of Iraq and Afghanistan*. Ithaca, NY: Cornell University Press.

Floersch, Jerry. 2004. "The Subjective Experience of Youth Psychotropic Treatment." *Social Work in Mental Health* 1(4):51–69.

Flore, Jacinthe, Renata Kokanovic, Felicity Callard, Alex Broom, and Cameron Duff. 2019. "Unraveling Subjectivity, Embodied Experience and (Taking) Psychotropic Medication." *Social Science and Medicine* 230:66–73.

Fontenrose, Kirsten. 2021. "PTSD Is an Endless War for Veterans. The News from Afghanistan Is Making It Worse." *New Atlanticist*, August 25.

Forte, Maximillian. 2011. "The Human Terrain System and Anthropology: A Review of Ongoing Public Debates." *American Anthropologist* 113(1):149–53.

Fortun, Kim. 2012. "Ethnography in Late Industrialism." *Cultural Anthropology* 27(3):446–64.

Foucault, Michel. 1961. *Madness and Civilization*. New York: Vintage.

Foucault, Michel. 1977. *Discipline and Punish: The Birth of the Prison*. New York: Pantheon Books.

Foucault, Michel. 1991. "Governmentality." In *The Foucault Effects: Studies in Governmentality,* edited by G. Burchill, C. Gordon, and P. Miller, 87–104. London: Hargraves.

Friedman, Richard. 2013. "Wars on Drugs." *New York Times,* April 6.

Friedman, Thomas L. 2004. "'Groundhog Day' in Iraq." *New York Times,* November 12.

Friesen, Matthew and Matthew Eddy. 2019. "Selling the Service: Veterans' Reflections on Their Past Experience of the Military Recruitment Process." *Critical Military Studies* 5(3):213–37.

Gaines, Atwood. 2012. "From DSM-I to III-R; Voices of Self, Mastery and the Other: A Cultural Constructivist Reading of US Psychiatric Classification." *Social Science and Medicine* 35(1):3–24.

Garcia, Angela. 2010. *The Pastoral Clinic: Addiction and Dispossession along the Rio Grande.* Berkeley: University of California Press.

Garcia, Angela. 2024. *The Way That Leads Among the Lost: Life, Death, and Hope in Mexico City's Anexos.* New York: Macmillan Press.

Gilbert, Emily. 2015. "The Gift of War: Cash, Counterinsurgency, and 'Collateral Damage.'" *Security Dialogue* 46(5):403–21.

Goffman, Erving. 1961. *Asylums: Essays on the Social Situation of Mental Patients and Other Inmates.* New York: Anchor Books.

González, Roberto J. 2009. *American Counterinsurgency: Human Science and the Human Terrain.* Chicago: Prickly Paradigm Press.

González, Roberto J. 2015. "Seeing into Hearts and Minds: 'Big Data,' Algorithms, and Computational Counterinsurgency." *Anthropology Today* 31(4):13–18.

González, Roberto J. 2024. *War Virtually: The Quest to Automate Conflict, Militarize Data, and Predict the Future.* Berkeley: University of California Press.

Graham, Stephen. 2009. "Cities as Battlespace: The New Military Urbanism." *City* 13(4):383–402.

Greene, Jeremy. 2011. "Making Medicines Essential: The Emergent Centrality of Pharmaceuticals in Global Health." *BioSocieties* 6(1):10–33.

Gregory, Derek. 2008a. "The Biopolitics of Baghdad: Counterinsurgency and the Counter-City." *Human Geography* 1(1):1–21.

Gregory, Derek. 2008b. "The Rush to the Intimate." *Radical Philosophy* 150(1):8–23.

Gregory, Derek. 2010. "Seeing Red: Baghdad and the Event-ful City." *Political Geography* 29(5):266–79.

Gregory, Derek. 2011. "The Everywhere War." *The Geographic Journal* 177(3):238–50.

Gregory, Thomas. 2012. "Potential Lives, Impossible Deaths: Afghanistan, Civilian Casualties and the Politics of Intelligibility." *International Feminist Journal of Politics* 14(3):327–47.

Gregory, Thomas. 2019. "Dangerous Feelings: Checkpoints and the Perception of Hostile Intent." *Security Dialogue* 50(2):131–47.

Gregory, Thomas. 2020. "The Costs of War: Condolence Payments and the Politics of Killing Civilians." *Review of International Studies* 46(1):156–76.

Gupta, Sugandh. 2021. "A Shifting Hospital and Shifting Dependencies in Jammu and Kashmir." *Somatosphere*, January 26. https://somatosphere.com/2021/shifting-hospital-dependencies-jammu-kashmir.html/.

Gusterson, Hugh. 2017. *Drone: Remote Control Warfare*. Cambridge, MA: MIT Press.

Han, Clara. 2020. *Seeing Like a Child: Inheriting the Korean War*. New York: Fordham.

Hanson, Frederick. 1949. *Combat Psychiatry: Experiences in the North African and Mediterranean Theaters of Operation, American Ground Forces, World War II, Vol. 9*. Washington, DC: United States Government Printing Office.

Hardon, Anita, Nurul Ilmi Idrus, and Takeo David Hymans. 2013. "Chemical Sexualities: The Use of Pharmaceutical and Cosmetic Products by Youth in South Sulawesi, Indonesia." *Reproductive Health Matters* 21(41):214–24.

Hardon, Anita and Emilia Sanabria. 2017. "Fluid Drugs: Revisiting the Anthropology of Pharmaceuticals." *Annual Review of Anthropology* 46:117–32.

Hardt, Michael and Antonio Negri. 2001. *Empire*. Cambridge, MA: Harvard University Press.

Harp, Seth. 2025. *The Fort Bragg Cartel: Drug Trafficking and Murder in the Special Forces*. New York: Penguin Books.

Harvey, David. 2003. *The New Imperialism*. Oxford: Oxford University Press.

Hassinger, Alisa D. 2003. "Mentoring and Monitoring: The Use of Unit Watch in the 4th Infantry Division." *Military Medicine* 168(3):234–8.

Hautzinger, Sarah and Jean Scandlyn. 2014. *Beyond Post-Traumatic Stress: Homefront Struggles with the Wars on Terror*. New York: Routledge.

Healy, David. 2012. *Pharmageddon*. Berkeley: University of California Press.

Hecht, Gabrielle. 2012. *Being Nuclear: Africans and the Global Uranium Trade*. Cambridge, MA: MIT Press.

Hejtmanek, Katherine. 2010. "Caring through Restraint: Violence, Intimacy and Identity in Mental Health Practice." *Culture, Medicine & Psychiatry* 34:668–74.

Hervouet-Zeiber, Grégoire. 2026. *War and the Pull of Life: Ex-Combatants in Putin's Russia*. New York: Fordham University Press.

Hill, Jeffrey H., Robert C. Johnson, and Richard A. Barton. 2006. "Suicidal and Homicidal Soldiers in Deployment Environments." *Military Medicine* 171(3):228–32.

Hoge, Elizabeth, John Worthington, John Nagurney et al. 2012. "Effect of Acute Posttrauma Propranolol on PTSD Outcome and Physiological Responses During Script-Driven Imagery." *CNS Neuroscience & Therapeutics* 18:21–7.

Hollingsworth, Jeffrey J. and Jean Paul Hare. 2013. "Managing Acute Suicidal Ideation in a Forward Deployed Location in Afghanistan." *Military Medicine* 178(4):357–8.

Hoque, Romy and Andrew Chesson Jr. 2009. "Zolpidem-Induced Sleepwalking, Sleep-Related Eating Disorder, and Sleep-Driving: Fluorine-18-Flourodeoxyglucose Positron Emission Tomography Analysis, and a Literature Review of Other Unexpected Clinical Effects of Zolpidem." *Journal of Clinical Sleep Medicine* 5(5):471–6.

Howard, Jeffrey T., Russ S. Kotwal, Caryn A. Stern, Jud C. Janak, Edward L. Mazuchowski, Frank K. Butler, Zsolt T. Stockinger, Barbara R. Holcomb, Raaquel C. Bono, and David J. Smith. 2019. "Use of Combat Casualty Care Data to Assess the US Military Trauma System During the Afghanistan and Iraq Conflicts, 2001–2017." *JAMA Surgery* 154(7):600–8.

Howell, Alison. 2011. *Madness in International Relations: Psychology, Security, and the Global Governance of Mental Health.* New York: Routledge.

Hoyt, Tim. 2025. "Preparing Mental Health Support for Multi-Domain, Large-Scale Combat Operations: Current Progress and Future Directions." *Military Medicine* 190(2):50–6.

Hoyt, Tim and Christina Hein. 2021. "Combat and Operational Stress Control in the Prolonged Field Environment." *Military Review.* September–October: 55–64.

Hyman, Jeffrey, Robert Ireland, Lucinda Frost, and Linda Cottrell. 2012. "Suicide Incidence and Risk Factors in an Active Duty Military Population." *American Journal of Public Health* 102(S1):S138–46.

Jain, Sarah Lochlann. 2006. *Injury: The Politics of Product Design and Safety Law in the United States.* Princeton: Princeton University Press.

Jain, Sarah Lochlann. 2007. "Living in Prognosis: Toward an Elegiac Politics." *Representations* 98(1):77–92.

Jenkins, Janis H, ed. 2011. *Pharmaceutical Self: The Global Shaping of Experience in an Age of Psychopharmacology.* Santa Fe, NM: School for Advanced Research Press.

Joint Chiefs of Staff. 2004. *The National Military Strategy of the United States of America: A Strategy for Today; A Vision for Tomorrow.* Washington, DC: Joint Chiefs of Staff.

Jones, Edgar. 2006. "Historical Approaches to Post-Combat Disorders." *Philosophical Transactions of the Royal Society B* 361:533–42.

Jones, Edgar and Simon Wessely. 2003. "'Forward Psychiatry' in the Military: Its Origins and Effectiveness." *Journal of Traumatic Stress* 16(4):411–9.

Jones, Edgar and Simon Wessely. 2005. *Shell Shock to PTSD: Military Psychiatry from 1900 to the Gulf War.* East Sussex, UK: Psychology Press.

Junger, Sebastian. 2010. *War.* New York: Twelve Books.

Junker, Gary, Art Beeler, and Jeffrey Bates. 2005. "Using Trained Inmate Observers for Suicide Watch in a Federal Correctional Setting: A Win-Win Solution." *Psychological Services* 2(1):20–7.

Kamieński, Łukasz. 2016a. "The Drugs That Built a Super Soldier." *The Atlantic*, April 8.

Kamieński, Łukasz. 2016b. *Shooting Up: A Short History of Drugs and War.* New York: Oxford University Press.

Kan, Paul R. 2009. *Drugs and Contemporary Warfare.* Sterling, VA: Potomac Books.

Kaplansky, Gabrielle and Maisha Toussaint. 2024. "US Army Mortality Surveillance in Active Duty Soldiers, 2014-2019." *Medical Surveillance Monthly Reporting* 31(5):2–8.

Kenard, Matt. 2012. *Irregular Army: How the US Military Recruited Neo-Nazis, Gang Members, and Criminals to Fight the War on Terror.* London: Verso.

Kerry, John F. 2004. "Address Accepting the Presidential Nomination at the Democratic National Convention in Boston." https://www.presidency.ucsb.edu/documents/address-accepting-the-presidential-nomination-the-democratic-national-convention-boston.

Khayyat, Munira. 2022. *A Landscape of War: Ecologies of Resistance and Survival in South Lebanon.* Berkeley: University of California Press.

Khayyat, Munira. 2023. "War, from the South." *Public Culture* 35(1):113–34.

Kieran, David. 2019. *Signature Wounds: The Untold Story of the Military's Mental Health Crisis.* New York: New York University Press.

Kilshaw, Susie. 2009. *Impotent Warriors: Gulf War Syndrome, Vulnerability, and Masculinity.* New York: Berghahn Books.

Kim, Eleana. 2016. "Toward an Anthropology of Landmines: Rogue Infrastructure and Military Waste in the Korean DMZ." *Cultural Anthropology* 31(2):162–87.

King, Anthony. 2025. *AI, Automation, and War: The Rise of a Military-Tech Complex.* Princeton: Princeton University Press.

Kitanaka, Junko. 2014. *Depression in Japan: Psychiatric Cures for a Society in Distress.* Princeton: Princeton University Press.

Klappe, Ben. 2011. "Rules of Engagement." In *International Military Missions and International Law,* edited by M. Odello and R. Piotrowicz. Boston: Martinus Nijhoff Publishers.

Klein, Naomi. 2007. *The Shock Doctrine: The Rise of Disaster Capitalism.* New York: Metropolitan Books.

Korb, Lawrence J. and Sean E. Duggan. 2007. "Caught Off Guard: The Link Between Our National Security and Our National Guard." Center for American Progress. https://www.americanprogress.org/article/changing-to-meet-new-challenges/.

Krishnamurti, Lauren Sealy. 2020. "The Potential of 'Watchful' Care: Preventing Suicide with Aloha in Hawaii." *Medical Anthropology Quarterly* 35(1):120–35.

Kuzmarov, Jeremy. 2009. *The Myth of the Addicted Army: Vietnam and the Modern War on Drugs*. Amherst, MA: University of Massachusetts Press.
Lakoff, Andrew. 2005. *Pharmaceutical Reason: Knowledge and Value in Global Psychiatry*. Cambridge, UK: Cambridge University Press.
Latour, Bruno. 1987. *Science in Action: How to Follow Scientists and Engineers through Society*. Cambridge, MA: Harvard University Press.
Laugesen, Amanda. 2016. *"Boredom is the Enemy": The Intellectual and Imaginative Lives of Australian Soldiers in the Great War and Beyond*. Oxfordshire, UK: Routledge.
Lineberry, Timothy and Stephen O'Connor. 2012. "Suicide in the US Army." *Mayo Clinic Proceedings* 87(9):871–8.
Lipov, Eugene and Elspeth Cameron Ritchie. 2015. "A Review of the Use of Stellate Ganglion Block in the Treatment of PTSD." *Current Psychiatry Reports* 17(8):63.
Lollis, Blake, Royden Marsh, Timothy Sowin, and William Thompson. 2009. "Major Depressive Disorder in Military Aviators: A Retrospective Study of Prevalence." *Aviation, Space, and Environmental Medicine* 80(8):734–7.
Lomsky-Feder, Edna, Nir Gazit, and Eyal Ben-Ari. 2008. "Reserve Soldiers as Transmigrants: Moving Between the Civilian and Military Worlds." *Armed Forces & Society* 34(4):593–614.
Lovell, Anne. 1996. "Coercion and Social Control: A Framework for Research on Aggressive Strategies in Community Mental Health." In *Coercion and Aggressive Treatment: A New Frontier in Mental Health Law*, edited by D. Dennis and J. Monahan, 147–66. New York: Plenum Publishing.
Lovell, Anne. 2006. "Addiction Markets." In *Global Pharmaceuticals: Ethics, Markets, Practices*, edited by A. Petryna, A. Lakoff, and A. Kleinman, 136–69. Durham, NC: Duke University Press.
Lupton, Deborah. 1999. *Risk*. New York: Routledge.
Lutz, Catherine. 1996. "Engendered Emotion: Gender, Power, and the Rhetoric of Emotional Control in American Discourse." In *The Emotions: Social, Cultural, and Biological Dimension*, edited by R. Harre and W. Gerrod Parrot, 151–70. Thousand Oaks, CA: Sage.
Lutz, Catherine. 2006. "Empire is in the Details." *American Ethnologist* 33(4):593–611.
Lutz, Catherine. 2019. "Bureaucratic Weaponry and the Production of Ignorance in Military Operations on Guam." *Current Anthropology* 60(S19):S108-21.
Lutz, Catherine and Andrea Mazzarino, eds. 2019. *War and Health: The Medical Consequences of the Wars in Iraq and Afghanistan*. New York: New York University Press.
Lutz, Catherine and Kathleen Millar. 2012. "War." In *A Companion to Moral Anthropology*, edited by D. Fassin, 482–99. Hoboken, NJ: John and Wiley Sons.
Mac Ginty, Roger. 2012. "Against Stabilization." *Stability: International Journal of Security and Development* 1(1):20–30.

MacLeish, Kenneth. 2009. "Wounds of War and the Dilemmas of Stereotypes." *Savage Minds*, September 27. https://savageminds.org/2009/09/27/wounds-of-war-and-the-dilemmas-of-stereotype/.
MacLeish, Kenneth. 2012. "Armor and Anesthesia: Exposure, Feeling, and the Soldier's Body." *Medical Anthropology Quarterly* 26(1):49–68.
MacLeish, Kenneth. 2013. "'Our Job is Not to Decide': War-Making and the Limits of Moral Injury." Meeting of the American Ethnological Society, Chicago, IL.
MacLeish, Kenneth. 2020. "Churn: Mobilization-Demobilization and the Fungibility of American Military Life." *Security Dialogue* 51(2-3):194–210.
MacLeish, Kenneth. 2022. "Moral Injury and the Psyche of Counterinsurgency." *Theory, Culture & Society* 39(6):63–86.
MacLeish, Kenneth and Zoë Wool. 2022. "Burn Pits: US Military Waste as War Violence." Society for Cultural Anthropology, January 25. https://www.culanth.org/fieldsights/burn-pits-us-military-waster-as-war-violence.
Maddow, Rachel. 2013. *Drift: The Unmooring of American Military Power.* New York: Crown.
Madsen, Cathaleen, Ronald Poropatich, and Tracey Perez Koehlmoos. 2023. "Telehealth in the Military Health System: Impact, Obstacles, and Opportunities." *Military Medicine* 188(1):15–23.
Mæland, Bård and Paul Brunstad. 2009. *Enduring Military Boredom: From 1750 to the Present.* New York: Springer.
Maguen, Shira and Brett Litz. 2012. "Moral Injury in Veterans of War." *PTSD Research* 23(1):1–6.
Malone, Lauren and Neil Carey. 2011. "Waivered Recruits: An Evaluation of Their Performance and Attrition Risk." *CNA Analysis and Solutions.* https://apps.dtic.mil/sti/tr/pdf/ADA541209.pdf.
Mareth, Thomas and Alan Brooker. 1985. "Combat Stress Reaction: A Concept in Evolution." *Military Medicine* 150(4):186–90.
Masco, Joseph. 2010. "Counterinsurgency, *The Spook,* and Blowback." In *Anthropology and Global Counterinsurgency,* edited by J. Kelly, B. Jauregui, S. Mitchell, and J. Walton, 193–208. Chicago: University of Chicago Press.
Matson, Liana, Amy Adler, Phillip Quartana, Connie Thomas, and Emily Lowery-Gionta. 2022. "Management of Acute Stress Reactions in the Military: A Stepped Care Approach." *Current Psychiatry Reports* 24:799–808.
Mayhew, Emily. 2017. *A Heavy Reckoning: War, Medicine and Survival in Afghanistan and Beyond.* London: Profile Books.
McCarroll, James E., David T. Orman, and Allan C. Lundy. 1993. "Clients, Problems, and Diagnoses in a Military Community Mental Health Clinic." *Military Medicine* 158(11):701–5.
McCarthy, Rory and Peter Beaumont. 2004. "Civilian Cost of Battle for Falluja Emerges." *The Guardian*, November 13.

McChrystal, Stanley. 2009. "Tactical Directive." Kabul, Afghanistan: International Security Assistance Force.

McCormick, David. 1998. *The Downsized Warrior: America's Army in Transition*. New York: New York University Press.

McFate, Montgomery. 2005. "Anthropology and Counterinsurgency: The Strange Story of Their Curious Relationship." *Military Review* 85(2):24–37.

McGranahan, Carole and John F. Collins, ed. 2018. *Ethnographies of US Empire*. Durham, NC: Duke University Press.

McKenzie, Amber, Howard Burdett, Bethany Croak, Laura Rafferty, Neil Greenberg, and Sharon A. M. Stevelink. 2023. "Adjustment Disorder in the Armed Forces: A Systematic Review." *Journal of Mental Health* 32(5):962–84.

McKeon, Joseph, James Persson, James McGhee, and Martin Quattlebaum. 2009. *A Review of the US Army Experience Using Selective Serotonin Reuptake Inhibitors in Aircrew*. Rucker, AL: United States Army Aeromedical Research Laboratory.

McSorley, Kevin. 2013. *War and the Body*. Oxfordshire, UK: Routledge.

Messinger, Seth. 2003. "Incorporating the Prosthetic: Traumatic Limb Loss, Rehabilitation and Refigured Military Bodies." *Disability and Rehabilitation* 31(25):2130–4.

Middleton, Townsend. 2024. *Quinine's Remains: Empire's Medicine and the Life Thereafter*. Berkeley: University of California Press.

Miles, Donna. 2006. "Concept Perfected in Iraq, Afghanistan Used along US Border." American Forces Press Service, December 4.

Millar, Katharine and Joanna Tidy. 2017. "Combat as a Moving Target: Masculinities, the Heroic Soldier Myth, and Normative Martial Violence." *Critical Military Studies* 3(2):142–60.

Miller, T. Christian. 2007. "Contractors Outnumber Troops in Iraq." *Los Angeles Times*, July 4.

Mitchell, Timothy. 2011. *Carbon Democracy: Political Power in the Age of Oil*. London: Verso.

Mittelstadt, Jennifer. 2015. *The Rise of the Military Welfare State*. Cambridge, MA: Harvard University Press.

Monforti, Jessica Lavariega and Adam McGlynn. 2010. "The Poverty Draft? Exploring the Role of Socioeconomic Status in US Military Recruitment of Hispanic Students." Paper presented at the American Political Science Association Annual Meeting, Washington, DC, September 2–5.

Moniz, Dave. 2004. "Rate of Guard Deaths Is Higher." *The Spokesman-Review*, December 13.

Moore, Bret and Gregory Reger. 2007. "Historical and Contemporary Perspectives of Combat Stress and the Army Combat Stress Control Team." In *Combat Stress Injury: Theory, Research, and Management*, edited by C. Figley and W. Nash, 161–81. Oxfordshire, UK: Routledge.

Moore, Bret A., Shawn T. Mason, and Bruce E. Crow. 2012. "Assessment and Management of Acute Combat Stress on the Battlefield." In *Military Psychology: Clinical and Operational Applications*, edited by C. Kennedy and E. Zillmer, 73–92. New York: Guilford Press.

Mordowanec, Nick. 2025. "Defense Bill Will 'Turbocharge' Surging Military Recruitment Numbers: Senator." *Military.com*, December 19.

Moreno, Jonathan D. 2006. *Mind Wars: Brain Science and the Military in the 21st Century*. New York: Bellevue Literary Press.

Morgan, Maria, Kevin O'Gallagher, Marija Spanovic Kelber, et al. 2023. "Adjustment Disorder in US Service Members: Factors Associated with Early Separation." *Military Medicine* 188(7-8):e1501–07.

National Center for PTSD. 2004. *Iraq War Clinician Guide*, 2nd ed. White River Junction, VT: National Center for PTSD.

Neiberg, Patty. 2025. "If Common Mental Health Issues are Labeled 'Incompatible' with Service, Advocates Fear Troops Will Go 'Underground." *Task & Purpose*, February 19.

Nevin, Remington Lee. 2017. "To Squander the Fighting Strength? Personal Experience with Preventive Psychiatry and the Dilemma of Wartime Public Mental Health." In *Psychiatrists in Combat: Mental Health Clinicians' Experiences in the War Zone*, edited by E. Ritchie, C. Warner, and R. McLay, 145–56. New York: Springer.

O'Brien, Tim. 1990. *The Things They Carried*. Boston: Mariner Books.

Oldani, Michael. 2014. "Deep Pharma: Psychiatry, Anthropology, and Pharmaceutical Detox." *Culture, Medicine and Psychiatry* 38(2):255–78.

Osman, Wazhmah and Robert D. Crews, ed. 2025. *Decolonizing Afghanistan: Countering Imperial Knowledge and Power*. Durham, NC: Duke University Press.

Owens, Patricia. 2015. *Economy of Force: Counterinsurgency and the Historical Rise of the Social*. Cambridge, UK: Cambridge University Press.

Pagonis, William. 1994. *Moving Mountains: Lessons in Leadership and Logistics from the Gulf War*. Cambridge, MA: Harvard Business School Press.

Palka, Eugene J. 2016. "Operation Iraqi Freedom (OIF) and the Use of Forwarding Operating Bases (FOBs)." In *Military Geosciences and Desert Warfare: Past Lessons and Modern Challenges*, edited by E. McDonald and T. Bullard, 205–19. New York: Springer.

Payne, Samuel, Jeffrey Hill, and David Johnson. 2008. "The Use of Unit Watch or Command Interest Profile in the Management of Suicide and Homicide Risk: Rationale and Guidelines for the Military Mental Health Professional." *Military Medicine* 173(1):25–35.

Payne, Samuel, Jeffrey Hill, and David Johnson. 2011. "Suicide and Homicide Risk Management: Rationale and Suggestions for the Use of Unit Watch in Garrison and Deployed Settings." In *Textbook of Combat and Operational*

Psychiatry, edited by E. Ritchie, 423–39. Washington, DC: Office of the Surgeon General of the United States Army.

Pedersen, Thomas Randrup. 2017. "Get Real: Chasing Danish Warrior Dreams in the Afghan 'Sandbox.'" *Critical Military Studies* 3(1):7-26.

Pedersen, Thomas Randrup. 2019. "Ambivalent Anticipations: On Soldierly Becomings in the Desert of the Real." *Cambridge Journal of Anthropology* 37(1):77–92.

Perlman, Michael. 1975. "Basic Problems of Military Psychiatry: Delayed Reaction in Vietnam Veterans." *International Journal of Offender Therapy and Comparative Criminology* 19(2):129–38.

Petersen, Melody. 2009. "US Military: Heavily Armed and Medicated." *NBCNews*, May 19.

Petryna, Adriana, Arthur Kleinman, and Andrew Lakoff, eds. 2006. *Global Pharmaceuticals: Ethics, Markets, Practices*. Durham, NC: Duke University Press.

Pietrzak, Robert, Marc Goldstein, James Malley, Alison Riverts, Douglas Johnson, and Steven Southwick. 2010. "Risk and Protective Factors Associated with Suicidal Ideation in Veterans of Operations Enduring Freedom and Iraqi Freedom." *Journal of Affective Disorders* 123(1–3):102–7.

Pincus, Simon H. and David M. Benedek. 1998. "Operational Stress Control in the Former Yugoslavia: A Joint Endeavor." *Military Medicine* 163(6):358–62.

Pinto, Sarah. 2014. *Daughters of Parvati: Women and Madness in Contemporary India*. Philadelphia: University of Pennsylvania Press.

Pitman, Roger, Kathy Sanders, Randall Zusman, Anna R. Healy, Farah Cheema, Natasha B. Lasko, Larry Cahill, and Scott P. Orr. 2002. "Pilot Study of Secondary Prevention of Posttraumatic Stress Disorder with Propranolol." *Biological Psychiatry* 51(20):189–92.

Plett-Usher, Barbara. 2021. "US Admits Drone Strike Killed Civilians." *The Washington Post*, September 17.

Pols, Hans and Stephanie Oak. 2006. "War and Military Mental Health: The US Psychiatric Response in the 20th Century." *American Journal of Public Health* 97(12):2132–42.

Price, David. 2016. *Cold War Anthropology: The CIA, the Pentagon, and the Growth of Dual Use Anthropology*. Durham, NC: Duke University Press.

Pupavac, Vanessa. 2001. "Therapeutic Governance: Psycho-Social Intervention and Trauma Risk Management." *Disasters* 25(4):358–72.

Purnell, Kandida. 2018. "Grieving, Valuing, and Viewing Differently: The Global War on Terror's American Toll." *International Political Sociology* 12(2):156–71.

Ranson, Stephen W. 1949. "The Normal Battle Reaction: Its Relation to the Pathologic Battle Reaction." *Bulletin of the US Army Medical Department* 9, Supplement:3–11.

Rasmussen, Nicolas. 2009. *On Speed: From Benzedrine to Adderall.* New York: New York University Press.
Rech, Matthew F. 2014. "Recruitment, Counter-Recruitment, and Critical Military Studies." *Global Discourse* 4(2-3):244–62.
Redfield, Peter. 2008. "Vital Mobility and the Humanitarian Kit." In *Biosecurity Interventions: Global Health and Security in Question*, edited by A. Lakoff and S. Collier, 147–72. New York: Columbia University Press.
Redfield, Peter. 2013. *Life In Crisis: The Ethical Journey of Doctors without Borders.* Berkeley: University of California Press.
Reeve, Elspeth. 2009. "Suicidal Soldiers." *The Daily Beast,* May 11.
Reid, Julian. 2013. *The Biopolitics of the War on Terror: Life Struggles, Liberal Modernity, and the Defence of Logistical Societies.* Manchester, UK: Manchester University Press.
Remondelli, Mason, Matthew McDonough, Kyle Remick, Eric Elster, Benjamin Potter, and Danielle Holt. 2024. "Refocusing the Military Health System to Support Role 4 Definitive Care in Future Large-Scale Combat Operations." *Journal of Trauma and Acute Care Surgery* 97(2S Suppl 1):S145–53.
Reno, Joshua. 2011. "Beyond Risk: Emplacement and the Production of Environmental Evidence." *American Ethnologist* 38(3):516–30.
Rhee, Taeho Greg and Robert A. Rosenheck. 2019. "Initiation of New Psychotropic Prescriptions without a Psychiatric Diagnosis among US Adults: Rates, Correlates, and National Trends from 2006 to 2015." *Health Services Research* 54(1):139–48.
Rhodes, Lorna. 2004. *Total Confinement: Madness and Reason in Maximum Security Prison.* Berkeley: University of California Press.
Ritchie, Elspeth Cameron. 1994. "Psychiatric Medications for Deployment." *Military Medicine* 159:647–8.
Ritchie, Elspeth Cameron. 2011. "A Mixed Message about Stigma in Military Mental Health Care." *Time,* July 5.
Rivers, W. H. R. 1919. "Psychiatry and War." *Science* 49(1268):367–9.
Roberts, Elizabeth. 2017. "What Gets Inside: Violent Entanglements and Toxic Boundaries in Mexico City." *Cultural Anthropology* 32(4):592–619.
Rose, Nikolas. 1998. "Governing Risky Individuals: The Role of Psychiatry in New Regimes of Control." *Psychiatry, Psychology and Law* 5(2):177–95.
Rose, Nikolas. 2003. "The Neurochemical Self and its Anomalies." In *Risk and Morality,* edited by R. Ericson and A. Doyle, 407–37. Toronto: University of Toronto Press.
Ruamcharoen, Boyd. 2024. "Tropicalizing the Portable Radio: Electronics and the US Military's Battle against Fungi in the Pacific War." *Technology and Culture* 65(2):497–529.
Rubaii, Kali. 2019. "Tripartheid: How Sectarianism Became Internal to Being in Anbar, Iraq." *PoLAR* 42(1):125–41.

Rubaii, Kali. 2020. "Birth Defects and the Toxic Legacy of War in Iraq." *Middle East Research and Information Project*. https://www.merip.org/2020/09/birth-defects-and-the-toxic-legacy-of-war-in-iraq/.

Rubaii, Kali. 2023. "Decentering Death: The War on Terror and the Less-Than-Lethal Paradigm." *American Anthropologist* 126(3):497–508.

Rundell, James. 2006. "Demographics of and Diagnoses in Operation Enduring Freedom and Operation Iraqi Freedom Personnel Who Were Psychiatrically Evacuated from the Theater of Operations." *General Hospital Psychiatry* 28(4):352–6.

Ryan, Maria. 2019. *Full Spectrum Dominance: Irregular Warfare and the War on Terror*. Stanford: Stanford University Press.

Said, Edward W. 1979. *Orientalism*. New York: Vintage Books.

Saleh, Zainab. 2020. *Return to Ruin: Iraqi Narratives of Exile and Nostalgia*. Stanford: Stanford University Press.

Sasson-Levy, Oma. 2003. "Feminism and Military Gender Practices: Israeli Women Soldiers in 'Masculine' Roles." *Sociological Inquiry* 73(3):440–65.

Savitala, Murty and George Dydek. 2004. "US Army Reserve (Medical) Soldier Prescription Challenges during Operation Iraqi Freedom." *Military Medicine* 169(12):937–41.

Scahill, Jeremy. 2007. *Blackwater: The Rise of the World's Most Powerful Mercenary Army*. New York: Nation Books.

Schaefer, Hillary, Dave Cotting, Eliot Proctor, Diane Ryan, and Richard Lerner. 2021. "The Military Hypermasculine Mystique: Sex, Status, and Emotional Control at the United States Military Academy." *Psychology of Men & Masculinities* 22(4):611–26.

Schlosser, Allison and Kristi Ninnemann. 2012. "The Anthropology of Psychopharmaceuticals: Cultural and Pharmacological Efficacies in Context." *Culture, Medicine, and Psychiatry* 36(1):2–9.

Schmitt, Eric. 2004. "US Army Lowers Recruit Standards." *Deseret News*, October 1.

Schmitz, Kimberly, Emily Schmied, Jennifer Webb-Murphy, Paul S. Hammer, Gerald E. Larson, Terry L. Conway, Michael R. Galarneau, Wayne C. Boucher, Nathan Edwards, and Douglas C. Johnson. 2012. "Psychiatric Diagnoses and Treatment of US Military Personnel While Deployed to Iraq." *Military Medicine* 177(4):380–9.

Schneider, Brett, John Bradley, and David Benedek. 2007. "Psychiatric Medications for Deployment: An Update." *Military Medicine* 172(7):681–5.

Schneider, Brett, John Bradley, Christopher Warner, and David Benedek. 2011. "Psychiatric Medications in Military Operations." In *Textbook of Combat and Operational Psychiatry*, edited by E. Ritchie, 151–62. Washington, DC: Office of the Surgeon General of the United States Army.

Schor, Elana. 2008. "US Army Increases Use of Moral Waivers to Meet Demand for Troops." *The Guardian*, April 21.

Schüll, Natasha Dow. 2014. *Addiction by Design: Machine Gambling in Las Vegas*. Princeton: Princeton University Press.

Scurfield, Raymond. 1993. "Posttraumatic Stress Disorder in Vietnam Veterans." In *International Handbook of Traumatic Stress Syndromes*, edited by J. P. Wilson and B. Raphael, 285–96. New York: Plenum Publication.

Senior, Jennifer. 2011. "The Prozac, Paxil, Zoloft, Wellbutrin, Celexa, Effexor, Valium, Klonopin, Ativan, Restoril, Xanax, Adderall, Ritalin, Haldol, Risperdal, Seroquel, Ambien, Lunesta, Elavil, Trazodone War." *New York Magazine*, February 6.

Shapiro, Nicholas. 2015. "Attuning to the Chemosphere: Domestic Formaldehyde, Bodily Reasoning, and the Chemical Sublime." *Cultural Anthropology* 30(3):368–93.

Shapiro, Nicholas and Eben Kirksey. 2017. "Chemo-Ethnography: An Introduction." *Cultural Anthropology* 32(4):481–93.

Shaw, Ian. 2004. "Doctors, 'Dirty Work' Patients, and 'Revolving Doors.'" *Qualitative Health Research* 14(8):1032–45.

Shephard, Ben. 2003. *A War of Nerves: Soldiers and Psychiatrists in the Twentieth Century*. Cambridge, MA: Harvard University Press.

Shih, Gerry, Niha Masih, and Dan Lamothe. 2021. "The Story of an Afghan Man Who Fell from the Sky." *The Washington Post*, August 21.

Singer, P. W. 2003. *Corporate Warriors: The Rise of the Privatized Military Industry*. Ithaca, NY: Cornell University Press.

Spencer, Jack. 2000. "The Facts about Military Readiness." The Heritage Foundation, September 15.

Stone, Nomi. 2022. *Pinelandia: An Anthropology and Field Poetics of War and Empire*. Berkeley: University of California Press.

Suitt, Thomas Howard, III,. 2021. "High Suicide Rates among United States Service Members and Veterans of the Post-9/11 Wars." Costs of War Research Series. June 21. https://costsofwar.watson.brown.edu/sites/default/files/papers/Suitt-Suicides.pdf.

Terry, Jennifer. 2017. *Attachments to War: Biomedical Logics and Violence in Twenty-First-Century America*. Durham, NC: Duke University Press.

Thompson, Mark. 2008. "America's Medicated Army." *Time*, June 5.

Tidy, Joanna. 2016. "The Gender Politics of 'Ground Truth' in the Military Dissent Movement: The Power and Limits of Authenticity Claims Regarding War." *International Political Sociology* 10(2):99–114.

Tilghman, Andrew and Brendan McGarry. 2010. "Medicating the Military." *Military Times*, March 17.

United States Army Surgeon General. 2003. *Operation Iraqi Freedom* (OIF) *Mental Health Advisory Team (MHAT) Report (MHAT-I)*. Washington, DC: Army Medical Command.

United States Army Surgeon General. 2006. *Mental Health Advisory Team (MHAT) IV Operation Iraqi Freedom 05-07 Final Report.* Washington, DC: Army Medical Command.

United States Army Surgeon General. 2008. *Mental Health Advisory Team (MHAT) V Operation Iraqi Freedom 06-08.* Washington, DC: Army Medical Command.

United States Central Command. 2019. *MOD 14 to USCENTCOM Individual Protection and Individual/Unit Deployment Policy (3 Oct), Tab A: Amplification of the Minimal Standards of Fitness for Deployment to the CENTCOM AOR.* (Washington, DC: USCENTCOM).

United States Department of the Army. 1998. *Combat Stress Control in a Theater of Operations: Field Manual 8–51.* Washington, DC: United States Department of the Army.

United States Department of the Army. 2006a. *Combat and Operational Stress Control: Field Manual 4-02.51.* Washington, DC: United States Department of the Army.

United States Department of the Army. 2006b. *Counterinsurgency Field Manual* 3-24. Washington, DC: United States Department of the Army.

United States Department of the Army. 2008. *Stability Operations Field Manual 3-07.* Washington, DC: United States Department of the Army.

United States Department of the Army. 2010. *Army Health Promotion, Risk Reduction, Suicide Prevention Report.* Washington, DC: United States Department of the Army.

United States Department of the Army. 2022. *Field Manual (FM) 3-0: Operations.* Washington, DC: United States Department of the Army.

United States Department of Defense. 2006. *Policy Guidance for Deployment-Limiting Psychiatric Conditions and Medications.* Washington, DC: Assistant Secretary of Defense.

United States Department of Defense. 2010. *DoD Instruction 6490.07 Deployment Limiting Medical Conditions for Service Members and DoD Civilian Employees.* https://www.esd.whs.mil/Portals/54/Documents/DD/issuances/dodi/649007p.pdf.

United States Department of Defense. 2011. *Department of Defense Suicide Event Report: Calendar Year 2010.* https://www.dspo.mil/Portals/113/Documents/2010-DoDSER-Annual-Report.pdf.

United States Department of Defense. 2018. "DoDI 6130.03, Vol. 1: Medical Standards for Military Service: Appointment, Enlistment or Deduction." Washington, DC: Department of Defense. https://www.esd.whs.mil/Portals/54/Documents/FOID/Reading%20Room/Personnel_Related/15-F-1724_DoDI_6130.3_V1.pdf.

United States Department of Defense. 2023. "Profile of the Military Community." https://download.militaryonesource.mil/12038/MOS/Reports/2023-demographics-report.pdf.

United States Government Accountability Office. 2009. "Military Personnel: Army Needs to Focus on Cost-Effective Use of Financial Incentives and Quality Standards in Managing Force Growth." GAO Report Number GAO-09-256.

Ursano, Robert, Ronald Kessler, and James Naifeh. 2017. "Risk of Suicide Attempt among Soldiers in Army Units with a History of Suicide Attempts." *JAMA Psychiatry* 74(9):924–31.

Van Wijk, Charles H. 2024. "Prevalence Estimate for Adjustment Disorders in the South African Navy." *Clinical Practice and Epidemiology in Mental Health* (20):e17450179301661.

Varley, Emma and Saiba Varma. 2019. "Medicine's Shadowside: Revisiting Clinical Iatrogenesis." *Anthropology & Medicine* 28(2):141–55.

Varma, Saiba. 2020. *The Occupied Clinic: Militarism and Care in Kashmir.* Durham, NC: Duke University Press.

Villa-Palomino, Julio. 2025. "Home Sweet Harm: Confinement and *Tranquilidad* in Post-Asylum Peru." *Medical Anthropology Quarterly*:e70032.

Vine, David. 2015. *Base Nation: How US Military Bases Abroad Harm America and the World.* New York: Metropolitan Books.

von Hippel, Frank. 2020. *The Chemical Age: How Chemists Fought Famine and Disease, Killed Millions, and Changed Our Relationship with the Earth.* Chicago: University of Chicago Press.

Von Schnitzler, Antina. 2013. "Traveling Technologies: Infrastructure, Ethical Regimes, and the Materiality of Politics in South Africa." *Cultural Anthropology* 28(4):670–93.

Wallerstein, Immanuel. 2005. *The Decline of American Power: The US in a Chaotic World.* New York: New Press.

Warner, Christopher H., Jill E. Brietbach, George N. Appenzeller, Virginia Yates, Thomas Grieger, and William G. Webster. 2007. "Division Mental Health in the New Brigade Combat Team Structure: Part I Predeployment and Deployment." *Military Medicine* 172(9):907–11.

Warner, Christopher H., George N. Appenzeller, Matthew J. Barry, Anthony Morton, and Thomas Grieger. 2007. "The Evolving Role of the Division Psychiatrist." *Military Medicine* 172(9):918–24.

Weinbaum, Cortney. 2023. "An Autistic Soldier Wants You to Read This." *Modern War Institute*, June 1. https://mwi.westpoint.edu/an-autistic-soldier-wants-you-to-read-this/.

Wessely, Simon. 2006. "Twentieth-Century Theories on Combat Motivation and Breakdown." *Journal of Contemporary History* 41(2):268–86.

West, James C. 2016. "Guest Perspective: Deployment, Mental Health Conditions and Psychotropic Medications—Good to Go?" Center for Deployment Psychology, April 19. https://deploymentpsych.org/blog/guest-perspective-deployment-mental-health-conditions-and-psychotropic-medictions-good-to-go.

Whaley, Dave, John Spain, Teresa Overman, and Vincent Valinotti. 2018. "Considerations for Retrograding Deployed Army Pharmacy Operations: What about Department of Defense Civilian Contractors? Lessons from Kosovo." *Military Medicine* 183(1–2):e19–23.

White House. 2023. "US Withdrawal from Afghanistan." April 6. https://bidenwhitehouse.archives.gov/wp-content/uploads/2023/04/US-Withdrawal-from-Afghanistan.pdf.

White House. 2025. "Prioritizing Military Excellent and Readiness." January 27. https://www.whitehouse.gov/presidential-actions/2025/01/prioritizing-military-excellence-and-readiness/.

Wojcik, Barbara E., Fatema Z. Akhtar, and Harrison Hassell. 2009. "Hospital Admissions Related to Mental Disorders in US Army Soldiers in Iraq and Afghanistan." *Military Medicine* 174(10):1010–18.

Wolfendale, Jessica. 2008. "Performance-Enhancing Technologies and Moral Responsibility in the Military." *American Journal of Bioethics* 8(2):28–38.

Wong, Leonard. 2006. *CU @ the FOB: How the Forward Operating Base is Changing the Life of Combat Soldiers*. Carlisle Barracks, PA: Strategic Studies Institute.

Wool, Zöe. 2015. *After War: The Weight of Life at Walter Reed*. Durham, NC: Duke University Press.

Wool, Zöe. 2019. "Afterwar Work for Life." In *War and Health: The Medical Consequences of the Wars in Iraq and Afghanistan*, edited by C. Lutz and A. Mazzarino, 210–30. New York: New York University Press.

Wool, Zöe. 2023. "All That is Solid Burns into Smoke: US Military Burn Pits, Petrochemical Toxicity, and the Racial Geopolitics of Displacement." *Catalyst* 9(1):1–22.

Yates-Doerr, Emily. 2015. *The Weight of Obesity: Hunger and Global Health in Postwar Guatemala*. Berkeley: University of California Press.

Young, Allan. 1995. *The Harmony of Illusions: Inventing Post-Traumatic Stress Disorder*. Princeton: Princeton University Press.

Zulaika, Joseba. 2014. "Drones and Fantasy in US Counterterrorism." *Journal for Cultural Research* 18(2):171–87.

Zulaika, Joseba and William Douglas. 2016. *Terror and Taboo: The Follies, Fables, and Faces of Terrorism*. Oxfordshire, UK: Routledge.

Index

NOTE: Locators ending with *fig.* indicate figures and/or illustrations.

Founded in 1893,
UNIVERSITY OF CALIFORNIA PRESS
publishes bold, progressive books and journals on topics in the arts, humanities, social sciences, and natural sciences—with a focus on social justice issues—that inspire thought and action among readers worldwide.

The UC PRESS FOUNDATION
raises funds to uphold the press's vital role as an independent, nonprofit publisher, and receives philanthropic support from a wide range of individuals and institutions—and from committed readers like you. To learn more, visit ucpress.edu/supportus.

www.ingramcontent.com/pod-product-compliance
Ingram Content Group UK Ltd.
Pitfield, Milton Keynes, MK11 3LW, UK
UKHW042355130926
475321UK00002B/17

9 780520 428638